Handbook of Neurochemistry

Handbook of Neurochemistry

Editor: Winston Coleman

AMERICAN
MEDICAL PUBLISHERS
www.americanmedicalpublishers.com

AMERICAN
MEDICAL PUBLISHERS
www.americanmedicalpublishers.com

Cataloging-in-publication Data

Handbook of neurochemistry / edited by Winston Coleman.
p. cm.
Includes bibliographical references and index.
ISBN 979-8-88740-150-8
1. Neurochemistry. 2. Neurosciences. 3. Biochemistry.
4. Brain chemistry. I. Coleman, Winston.
QP356.3 .H36 2023
612.804 2--dc23

American Medical Publishers,
41 Flatbush Avenue,
1st Floor, New York,
NY 11217, USA

ISBN 979-8-88740-150-8 (Hardback)

Contents

Preface

Neurochemistry is the branch of neuroscience concerned with the study of neurochemicals, which are organic molecules that participate in neural activity. Oxytocin, serotonin, dopamine, glutamate, neurotransmitters and neurotransmitter-regulating substances are some examples of neurochemicals. Oxytocin plays an important role in controlling the maternal behavior. Hypothalamus is the reservoir of oxytocin from where it is transported to the posterior lobe of the pituitary. Finally, it is released into the blood stream, which transports it to the target tissues such as the mammary glands. Dopamine is a common neurotransmitter that is involved in the functioning of the limbic system, which is responsible for emotional function and control. Serotonin is a neurochemical that plays a regulatory role in several areas, such as mood and sleep. This book unravels the recent studies in the field of neurochemistry. It aims to serve as a resource guide for students and experts alike and contribute to the growth of the discipline.

This book has been the outcome of endless efforts put in by authors and researchers on various issues and topics within the field. The book is a comprehensive collection of significant researches that are addressed in a variety of chapters. It will surely enhance the knowledge of the field among readers across the globe.

It gives us an immense pleasure to thank our researchers and authors for their efforts to submit their piece of writing before the deadlines. Finally in the end, I would like to thank my family and colleagues who have been a great source of inspiration and support.

Editor

1

Cytosolic Calcium Homeostasis in Neurons — Control Systems, Modulation by Reactive Oxygen and Nitrogen Species and Space and Time Fluctuations

Carlos Gutierrez-Merino, Dorinda Marques-da-Silva,
Sofia Fortalezas and Alejandro K. Samhan-Arias

1. Introduction

Cytosolic calcium plays a major and central role in neuronal activity and functions both in brain and in peripheral nervous systems, and its sustained alteration is a critical event that leads to neuronal death. On these grounds, it is not surprising that a sustained alteration of intracellular calcium homeostasis in neurons is a point of convergence of the cellular mechanisms underlying many neurodegenerative processes in the brain. Indeed, this has been shown to be the case for the brain's neurodegenerative diseases of higher incidence to humans, like Alzheimer's and Parkinson's, or in the acute neurodegeneration observed in amyotrophic lateral sclerosis, and also for major brain insults, such as excitotoxicity in trauma and ischemia-reperfusion, inflammation and neurotoxicity by drugs and environmental chemicals.

Sustained deregulation of cytosolic calcium concentration have been reported in neuronal apoptosis and necrosis, the two major cellular death pathways involved in brain neurodegeneration. It has been experimentally demonstrated and confirmed by many investigations using cell cultures that a sustained rise of cytosolic calcium concentration in the neuronal soma within the range 0.5-1 μM elicits a rapid necrotic neuronal death, mediated by calcium-dependent proteases activation, like calpains. On the other hand, long-term sustained cytosolic calcium concentrations below 60-70 nM in the neuronal soma promote the slow development of apoptotic neuronal death of neurons in culture [1,2]. Since the central role of calcium in neurotransmitter secretion and neuronal plasticity is also well known, the basal steady state cytosolic calcium concentration in the neuronal soma can be considered as a bioenergetics marker of neuronal activity and survival. We shall then present the major calcium transport systems that control the cytosolic calcium homeostasis in the wider space within neurons, i.e. in the neuronal soma. Owing to the large subcellular regionalization of neuronal processes essential for the normal activity of neurons and especially in neuronal signal transduction pathways, we shall also place a particular emphasis in the subcellular compartmentation of these calcium transport systems.

Noteworthy, neurodegenerative processes in the brain also share another common metabolic deviation, namely, that neurons are also exposed to an enhanced oxidative stress in the brain. Using different types of neuronal cultures, many investigators have shown during the last 15 years that the cellular oxidative stress produced by reactive oxygen species (ROS) and reactive nitrogen species (RNS) and a sustained alteration of the intracellular calcium homeostasis are metabolic deregulations usually observed during the early stages of the development of the process of neuronal death and before the cell viability loss induced entry in the irreversible steps characterized by the activation of proteases. In addition, it has been proposed that alterations of the intracellular calcium homeostasis of glial cells can also contribute to inflammation and damage in the brain in neurodegenerative processes [3]. Therefore, a better knowledge of the major molecular pathways contributing to induce the oxidative stress in the brain and the deregulation of intracellular calcium homeostasis in neurons should be expected to lead to the development of novel and more efficient therapies against brain neurodegeneration.

The fact that the most relevant calcium transport systems for the fine tuning of cytosolic calcium homeostasis in neurons have been shown to be molecular targets for ROS/RNS generated in neurodegenerative insults and diseases will be analyzed next in this context. As most of neurotoxic ROS/RNS species react with many intracellular molecules and these species are short-lived within the cells, the extent of chemical modification of each calcium transport system by ROS/RNS is strongly dependent on its relative proximity to the ROS/RNS source. In functional terms, it has been shown by many studies that ROS/RNS can elicit estimulation or inhibition of key proteins of calcium signalling pathways in neurons, and that these effects are strongly dependent on the specific protein, on the ROS/RNS concentration in the micro-environment and on the accummulated dose of ROS/RNS (time of exposure). Therefore, clustering of these systems within subcellular microdomains plays a major role in cross-modulation between calcium and ROS/RNS intracellular signalling, and this point will be specifically addressed thereafter in this chapter.

Furthermore, the accummulated experimental evidences pointing out that there is an intimate cross-talk between calcium and ROS/RNS intracellular signalling pathways are now ovel-whelming, including the modulation of ROS/RNS sources by calcium in neurons and the redox modulation of calcium transport systems. Both, calcium and ROS/RNS intracellular signalling show a clear pattern of local and focalized transients of intracellular concentration (peaks). Therefore, clustering of calcium transport systems responsible of the rise of cytosolic calcium and ROS/RNS sources within the same subcellular microcompartments will generate over-lapping focalized points of high concentration of calcium and ROS/RNS. In addition, this clustering will produce transient and highly focalized cytosolic calcium concentration peaks near the calcium entry points and associated calcium concentration waves owing to the rapid diffusion coefficient of calcium ions. Thus, we shall discuss the space and time fluctuations of cytosolic calcium concentrations that are known to be produced by the activity of calcium transport systems more relevant for the control of cytosolic calcium homeostasis in the neuronal soma. Finally, the last section of this chapter is focussed in the most relevant calcium buffering systems expressed in neurons and their modulation by oxidative stress, since calcium buffering systems of the neuronal cytosol play a major role to attenuate the local gradients of calcium concentration.

2. Neuronal cytosolic calcium homeostasis is attained by functional coupling between different types of calcium transport systems

A highly efficient spatial and temporal coupling between the activity of transport systems producing calcium entry to the cytosol and those extruding calcium out of the cytosol is a basic bioenergetics need for brain neurons, as they establish many functional synapses and have to maintain and rapidly restore cytosolic calcium in the neuronal soma within the narrow concentration window that allows for neuron survival. Extensive experimental studies carried out during last thirty years have settled the major molecular actors that allow neurons to achieve this goal, see for example the reviews [4-7], and these are schematically presented in the diagram of the Figure 1. Thus, the control of cytosolic calcium homeostasis in neurons is primarily the result of the activity of transport systems at the plasma membrane acting in concert, with the help of calcium transport systems located in intracellular stores, mainly in the endoplasmic reticulum and mitochondria. The concentration gradient of calcium ions across the neuronal plasma membrane in the brain is by far larger than the concentration gradients of other ions involved in the control of neuronal excitability, like potassium, sodium and chloride. In addition, cytosolic calcium binding proteins provide the neurons with buffering capacity to attenuate the peak height of free cytosolic calcium concentration spikes after focal neuronal stimulation by some neurotransmitters or after high frequency repetitive neuronal stimulation [8].

In primary cultures of cerebellar granule neurons, calcium entry through L-type voltage-operated calcium channel (L-VOCC) accounts for more than 75% of the increase of the steady-state cytosolic calcium in the neuronal soma after partial depolarization of the plasma membrane upon raising the extracellular potassium concentration from 5 to 25 mM [9]. The particular relevance of this observation for neuronal survival is highlighted by the fact that the apoptosis of these neurons induced by low potassium (5 mM) in the extracellular medium can be blocked simply by raising the extracellular potassium concentration up to 25 mM [1,10].

Many other experimental data accumulated along the last two decades point out that the transport systems more potent to elicit a fast and sustained increase of cytosolic calcium in neurons are located at the plasma membrane, i.e. ionotropic receptors and VOCC. These calcium transport systems are activated by extracellular stimuli, neurotransmitters or neuro-modulators, either directly or indirectly through plasma membrane depolarization. Let us recall here, for example, that high frequency stimulation of neurons by application of electrical

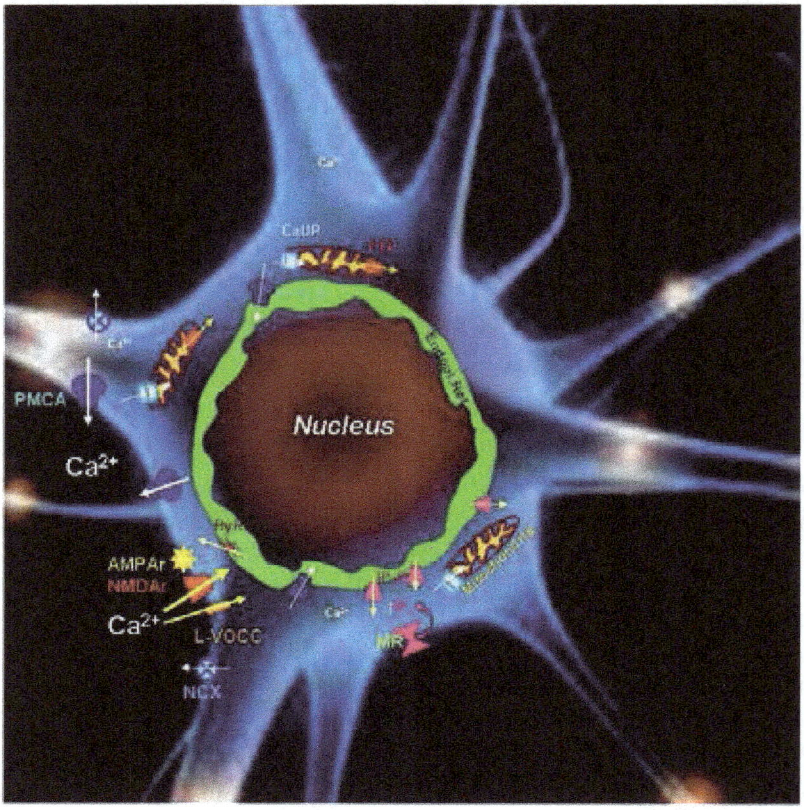

Figure 1. Diagrammatic image illustrating the major calcium transport systems controlling the concentration of cytosolic calcium in the neuronal soma. Yellow and white arrows indicate cytosolic calcium entry and extrusion transport systems, respectively. The thickness of the arrow indicates the relative relevance. Abbreviations: Endopl.Ret., endoplasmic reticulum (green space); NMDAr, NMDA receptor; AMPAr, AMPA receptor; L-VOCC, L-type voltage- operated calcium channel; PMCA, plasma membrane calcium pump; NCX, sodium-calcium exchanger; MR, metabotropic receptor; RyR, ryanodine receptor; IP_3R, IP_3 receptor; SERCA, endoplasmic reticulum calcium pump; PTP, mitochondrial permeability transition pore; CaUP, mitochondrial calcium uniporter.

depolarizing pulses or of the appropriate neurotransmitter (chemical stimulation) can lead to neuronal tetanic activity. Because of their focalized distribution pattern in the neurons and also because of the large differences in the intensity of calcium currents across activated ionotropic receptors and VOCC, significant calcium concentration gradients between different cytosolic regions of the neuron during normal neuronal activity are expected to develop at least transiently. In contrast, the rise of IP_3 following activation of phospholipase C after stimulation of members of the large family of G-coupled neurotransmitter receptors [5], also located at the plasma membrane, promoted calcium release from intracellular stores displaying calcium spikes of smaller intensity and a more widespread increase of calcium concentration within the cytosol.

Taking into consideration the large number of different chemical molecules that promote neuronal stimulation within the brain and the high frequency of the stimulation events, it is wonderful for its simplicity that the concerted action of only a few calcium transport systems can maintain neurons functional and alive for so many years during human lifetime. Why such a simple design? As the evolution selects the living structures and organisms that optimize the use of metabolic energy [11] and the bioenergetics costs for building a complex structural design is always higher than the costs for building simpler structures, probably the answer is: to optimize the use of the metabolic energy in neurons. Let us recall here that the large needs of metabolic energy to continuously restore the electric potential of the plasma membrane of active brain neurons, which is essential for their proper biological functions, would not allow them to develop a safe system for the control of cytosolic calcium homeostasis of a high-bioenergetics cost of maintenance and repair. Noteworthy, maximal energy optimization within the cells can be attained when the coupling between molecules involved in energy transduction makes use of the information or entropic energy stored in subcellular structures, i.e. minimizing stochastic collisional events that dissipate a large amount of energy, and this seems to be the case. For example, the subcellular distribution of the calcium transport systems in neurons enables them to use cytosolic calcium for highly polarized, rapid and specific synaptic responses, and also for more slowly developing adaptative responses, like long term post-synaptic potentiation or depression [4,5]. Furthermore, the different levels of expression of ionotropic and metabotropic receptors in distinct types of neurons allows for differential selectivity and sensitivity in calcium modulation of neuronal threshold excitability, thereby linking regionalization of neuronal responses within the brain structures with the major neurotransmitter pathways.

2.1. The calcium entry systems of the neuronal plasma membrane

All neurons express different types of functional VOCC. On the basis of their unitary conductance, on their rate of inactivation and their subcellular location the most relevant for neuronal calcium homeostasis are the L-VOCC. The L-VOCC unitary conductance has been reported to be in the range of 20-25 pS, while reported unitary conductances for N-, P/Q- and R-type range between 10 and 20 pS, and L-VOCC inactivation kinetics is slower than that of the other VOCC types [12-17]. In addition, L-VOCC are polarised in the neuronal soma and at the conical neck leading to neurite extensions [18], whereas N-, P/Q and R-types of VOCC are largely enriched in the presynaptic plasma membranes and its activation serves largely to elicit neurotransmitter release at the synapses [14,19-21]. On these grounds, taking also into consideration the rate of kinetics inactivation of the P/Q-VOCC, these channels should afford a contribution to the cytosolic calcium homeostasis of the neuronal soma much lower than that of L-VOCC but higher than that of N-, R- and T-types of VOCC. Indeed, using specific channels blockers we have experimentally assessed that the sum of the contributions of non-L-VOCC calcium channels to the cytosolic calcium homeostasis of the neuronal soma of primary cultures of cerebellar granule neurons in a standard Locke's medium with 25 mM K^+ is lower than 20%, while the L-VOCC contribution is 80% or higher (*unpublished results*).

L-VOCC, which are expressed in all neurons, are by far the most relevant calcium channels not only for the tuning of steady-state cytosolic calcium homeostasis in neurons (see above), but also for the overall threshold neuronal excitability, see [22-24]. The L-VOCC family, also known as Ca_V1, has four subtypes: $Ca_V1.1$, $Ca_V1.2$, $Ca_V1.3$ and $Ca_V1.4$ [25]. $Ca_V1.2$ and $Ca_V1.3$ are expressed in neurons, cardiac and endocrine cells, while $Ca_V1.1$ and $Ca_V1.4$ are specific of skeletal muscle and retina, respectively [26]. In brain, near 80% of L-VOCC belongs to the $Ca_V1.2$ subtype and 10-25% to the subtype $Ca_V1.3$ [27]. It has been reported that inactivation of the gene encoding for $Ca_V1.2$ in the hippocampus and neocortex of mouse ($Ca_V1.2$HKO) leads to a selective loss of N-methyl-D-aspartate (NMDA) receptors-independent long-term potentiation [28]. The activity of these calcium channels is modulated not only by the plasma membrane potential but it is also dependent upon their phosphorylation by protein kinases. Meanwhile the activation of different isoforms of protein kinase C (PKC) has been reported to produce stimulation or inhibition of L-VOCC activity in different cellular types [29], the activation of protein kinase A (PKA) and of calcium/calmodulin-dependent protein kinase II (CaMKII) have been shown to increase the activity of L-VOCC. Moreover, both PKA and CaMKII have been shown to form complexes with L-VOCC subunits. In brain, PKA associates with L-VOCC subunit α1c [30]. L-VOCC subunits α1c and β2 are phosphorylated by PKA [31-34], and this produces an increase of L-VOCC activity. It has been demonstrated that this increase of L-VOCC activity is mediated by phosphorylation of Ser478 and Ser479 of the β-subunit and also by phosphorylation of Ser1928 of the α1c-subunit, as their mutations led to complete elimination of the PKA-induced increase of calcium currents catalyzed by L-VOCC [29,35]. Regarding CaMKII, the amino acids sequence near Thr498 of the L-VOCC subunit β2a shows a high homology with the self-inhibitory domain of the CaMKII and with the binding domain of this kinase in the NR2B subunit of NMDA receptors [36]. Indeed, it has been shown the co-localization within neurons of the L-VOCC ($Ca_V1.2$ type) and CaMKII [37] and also of the L-VOCC subunit β2a with CaMKII, and this has led to the suggestion that the L-VOCC subunit β2a can act as an associated protein of CaMKII *in vivo* [36]. Phosphorylation of L-VOCC by CaMKII takes place not only in Thr498 of the β2a subunit but also in Ser1512 and Ser1570 of the α1 subunit and leads to an increase of the intensity of calcium currents through these channels [36, 38-40]. It has been proposed that the modulation of L-VOCC by CaMKII can be relevant to potentiate the raise of cytosolic calcium concentration in response to hormones and growth factors [41,42]. In contrast, the excessive activation of the L-VOCC ($Ca_V1.3$ type) by CaMKII over-stimulation has been correlated with the loss of dendritic spines in the striatum observed after dopamine depletion in animal models of parkinsonism [43].

The most potent calcium ionotropic receptors present in the neurons of the mammalian brain are L-glutamate receptors of the NMDA and α-amino-3-hydroxy-5-methylisoxazole-4-propionic acid (AMPA) subtypes, except those AMPA receptors formed only with GluR2 subunits [44,45], and P_{2X}-purinergic receptors [46]. NMDA and AMPA receptors are present in most fast excitatory synapses in the brain, allowing for neuronal responses in the milliseconds time scale range, and P_{2X}-purinergic receptors display also a widespread distribution in the brain. The more limited distribution in brain of L-glutamate receptors of the kainate subtype, its low ionic selectivity for calcium and the slight calcium currents generated upon its activation compared to those observed upon activation of AMPA and NMDA receptors [47], suggest that they can play at most a secondary role in the tuning of cytosolic calcium homeostasis of a very limited number of brain neurons.

The L-glutamate receptors are expressed in the vast majority of glutamatergic neurons, and they are present in the major structures of mammalian brain (neocortex, striatum, hippocampus and cerebellum). NMDA, AMPA and kainate receptors are oligomeric integral membrane proteins, being their calcium channel structure predominantly formed by a combination of different, though highly homologous, subunits [48]. Among these receptors, NMDA receptors play an outstanding role in neurosciences, as supported by many experimental evidences in studies of brain development [49], long term post-synaptic potentiation [4] or brain damage after ischemia-reperfusion [44,45]. Three major reasons allows to explain the dominant role of NMDA receptors over AMPA and kainate receptors in the brain: (1) the NMDA single channel conductance is higher than AMPA single channel conductance, 40-50 pS versus ~20 pS [16,50]; (2) their higher affinity for the endogenous agonist L-glutamate, e.g. the EC_{50} for L-glutamate is ~10 μM for NMDA receptors and ~200 μM for AMPA receptors, and (3) the slower desensitization rate of NMDA receptors, e.g. several hundreds of milliseconds for NMDA receptors while it is ~10 milliseconds for AMPA receptors [48]. Nevertheless, the maximal activation of NMDA receptors not only requires the presence of L-glutamate but also co-stimulation by glycine or D-serine in the brain and relief of Mg^{2+} inhibition [48,51]. Both, AMPA and P_{2x} receptors can potentiate NMDA receptor activation in the brain. AMPA receptors co-localization with NMDA receptors allows that plasma membrane depolarization induced by activation of AMPA receptors elicits the relief of Mg^{2+} inhibition of NMDA receptors. Phosphorylation by PKC and CaMKII promotes synaptic incorporation of AMPA receptors during long-term post-synaptic potentiation (LTP), and the latter kinase also enhances the channel conductance of this receptor [52-54]. On the other hand, it has been shown that facilitation of L-glutamate release by P_{2x} activation can lead to a stronger NMDA receptor activation. The calcium channel in the NMDA-receptor structure can be formed by different combinations of subunit 1 (NR1) and one of the isoforms of subunit 2 (NR2A, NR2B, NR2C and NR2D) [55]. The expression of functional NMDA receptors is a relatively slow process during the maturation of neurons [56]. Therefore, in molecular terms there are different isoforms of functional NMDA receptors whose level of expression varies from one type of neurons to another, and also during neuronal maturation. In addition, NMDA receptors are found in synaptic and in extra-synaptic locations [56-58]. As activation of extra-synaptic NMDA receptors can lead to a less focalized increase of cytosolic calcium, the extra-synaptic NMDA receptors are likely to play a role more relevant than synaptic NMDA receptors in the control of cytosolic calcium homeostasis in the neuronal soma. Phosphorylation of NMDA receptors *in vitro* by PKA and by some PKC isoforms increases their activity [59]. The co-stimulation of PKA and PKC elicits the phosphorylation of Ser896 and Ser897 leading to activation of NMDA receptors, while phosphorylation of Ser890 by only PKC leads to a subcellular re-localization of the NR1 subunit of NMDA receptors, which is reverted upon dephosphorylation [60].

2.2. Transport systems that release calcium from intracellular stores

The long-term control of neuronal calcium homeostasis also involves several major calcium transport systems of the subcellular organelles that behave as relevant neuronal intracellular stores, namely, endoplasmic reticulum and mitochondria.

The endoplasmic reticulum Ca^{2+}-ATPase (SERCA) helps to pump calcium out from the cytosol to the endoplasmic reticulum internal space [5], while calcium release from the endoplasmic reticulum involves the activation of IP_3 receptors and/or ryanodine receptors in different neuronal responses and in synaptic plasticity [5,61-63]. Although the neuronal endoplasmic reticulum can accumulate much lower amounts of calcium than the sarcoplasmic reticulum of muscle cells, it is still significant for hippocampal neurons as shown in several studies, see e.g. [4,64]. In these cases, calcium release from the endoplasmic reticulum can sustain a moderate increase of cytosolic calcium, which has been shown to play a significant role in the process of LTP in hippocampal neurons [4,64]. By itself, calcium filling of the endoplasmic reticulum is relevant for neuronal survival to ensure the correct protein folding of many proteins, particularly proteins of the plasma membrane or to be secreted to the extracellular space, as the activity of several endoplasmic reticulum protein-chaperones is dependent on the calcium concentration in the internal space of the endoplasmic reticulum [65]. Depletion of calcium in the endoplasmic reticulum has been shown to elicit the opening of specific calcium channels of the plasma membrane, the store-operated calcium entry (SOCE) [5,66-67]. The presence of SOCE in neurons has been documented during last years [4,68], and its opening elicits a transient increase of cytosolic calcium under neuronal stress conditions to restore the calcium levels of intracellular stores. The inhibition of SERCA by selective inhibitors, thapsigargin or cyclopiazonic acid, is needed to induce the large calcium depletion in the endoplasmic reticulum required for SOCE in experiments with cells in culture. Thus, this process can be seen as a 'rescue call' at the cellular level and operates under conditions of severe energetic depletion of the neurons. Indeed, it is to be recalled here that these channels and in particular the isoforms TRPC-3 and -6 have been also involved in neuronal survival of CGN [69]. More recently, Selvaraj *et al.* [70] have demonstrated that in a mouse neurotoxin-based model of Parkinson's disease, reduced Ca^{2+} influx through transient receptor potential C1 (TRPC1) channels in the plasma membrane of dopaminergic neurons triggers a cell death-inducing endoplasmic reticulum-stress response. These latter results highlighted for the first time the relevance of calcium homeostasis in Parkinson's disease.

In contrast, the large population of neuronal mitochondria can store relatively large amounts of calcium, high enough to elicit a large increase of cytosolic calcium as shown by several studies, see e.g. [71,72]. Nevertheless, the rate of calcium fluxes across the mitochondrial membrane transporters in normal cells is much slower than that measured for the major endoplasmic reticulum calcium transport systems listed above. However, calcium release from mitochondria high enough to promote a large and sustained rise of cytosolic calcium in neurons has been observed only during the development of neuronal cell death, as a consequence of the steady opening of the high permeability mitochondrial transition pore [73]. On these grounds, large calcium release from mitochondria has been proposed to be part of the molecular mechanism that triggers irreversible events in neuronal cell death through calpains activation. On the other hand, the uptake of calcium by mitochondria takes place through a calcium uniporter [71,73], with a rate of uptake in the submicromolar calcium range much lower than the major cytosolic calcium extrusion pathways, namely, PMCA and SERCA in neurons [4,6].

2.3. The transport systems involved in calcium extrusion from the cytosol

The major plasma membrane calcium extrusion systems, PMCA and Na^{+}/Ca^{2+}-exchanger (NCX) are expressed in all neuronal types. PMCA provides the major extrusion pathway operating in neurons for the maintenance of cytosolic calcium concentrations below the neurotoxic calcium range, i.e. <0.4 μM cytosolic calcium [6,74,75]. As PMCA is active at cytosolic calcium concentrations below 0.4 μM [6,74], neurons must spend a significant amount of metabolic energy (ATP) to maintain cytosolic calcium within the short concentration range which is required for neuronal survival. Therefore, the cytosolic calcium concentration can be considered a key bioenergetics marker of neuronal activity and survival. In contrast, NCX is more potent than the PMCA at cytosolic calcium concentrations ≥0.5 μM [6,76]. On these grounds, NCX can be seen as a safety system to minimise neuronal damage associated with cytosolic calcium ≥0.4 μM, as its activation when cytosolic calcium reaches this range allows neurons to rapidly reset cytosolic calcium to the concentration window that allows neuronal survival, see above. The expression levels of different neuronal isoforms of PMCA undergo significant changes during neuronal maturation [77], and a similar observation has been reported for NCX isoforms [78]. This has been seen as a neuronal adaptative response to the fine set of free cytosolic calcium concentration and control of cytosolic calcium homeostasis, since it has been demonstrated that different PMCA isoforms show different affinity for calcium [79]. On the other hand, although both PMCA and NCX are found in the plasma membrane of the neuronal soma and neuronal dendrites, recent data cast doubt on the current assumption that both PMCA and NCX are homogeneously distributed in the plasma membrane. For example, regulatory effects of actin cytoskeleton have been recently reported on the NCX activity [80], and actin filaments are components of caveolin-rich structures associated with 'lipid rafts' [81].

SERCA, which catalyzes the ATP-dependent calcium uptake by this subcellular organelle, plays only a secondary role as a system for calcium extrusion from the cytosol because in neurons PMCA is a calcium pump more potent than SERCA [4]. The calcium uptake by mitochondria is performed mainly via the Ca^{2+} uniporter driven by the large mitochondrial inner membrane potential [73], although the contribution of an alternate transport system yet ill-defined in molecular terms cannot be excluded under conditions of high frequency of cytosolic calcium peaks [82]. Nevertheless, in neurons the rate of calcium uptake by mitochondria is much slower than the rate of calcium extrusion from the cytosol via the plasma membrane systems, i.e. the PMCA and NCX, and via the SERCA.

3. Compartmentation of calcium transport systems relevant for the control of cytosolic calcium homeostasis in nanodomains of the neuronal plasma membrane and functional implications

Many recent experimental evidences have demonstrated that the calcium transport systems of the neuronal plasma membrane more relevant for the control of cytosolic calcium homeostasis are clustered within focalized nanodomains of a diameter size lower or equal to few hundreds of nanometers. Lipid rafts of the plasma membrane are dynamic nanodomains of a dimension between 10 and 200 nm [83], which define cellular sub-microdomains of the plasma membrane anchoring caveolins, see e.g. [81], and it has been suggested that caveolin-rich nanodomains associated with neuronal plasma membrane lacking the morphological appearance of "caveola invaginations" can serve to focalize signal transduction in neurons [84]. Indeed, the putative implication of lipid rafts in the regulation of intracellular calcium homeostasis and calcium signalling pathways was already suggested in the 1970's [85,86], but only during the last decade this hypothesis has been experimentally demonstrated, see [87,88].

Lipid rafts are enriched in cholesterol and sphingolipids [83], including a lipid family particularly enriched in the plasma membrane of neurons: the gangliosides [89], and define nanodomains of the plasma membrane for the anchoring of caveolins, flotillin, actin microfilaments and also an increasingly higher number of palmitoylated or farnesylated proteins, see [81]. The isoform caveolin-1 binds to cholesterol and sphingolipids [90-92], and also promotes the transport of cholesterol from the endoplasmic reticulum to the plasma membrane [93]. These nanodomains are merging as unique platforms for intracellular signalling in neurons, as pointed out in [84,94,95], and their stability is currently rationalized in terms of specific protein/protein or protein/lipid interactions. Noteworthy, as caveolins can act as scaffolding proteins in protein/protein interactions within these nanodomains [96,97], these interactions also bear functional relevance for the protein partners and, therefore, these nanodomains cannot be solely seen as structural elements of the plasma membrane. In this regard, it has been reported that cholesterol depletion with methyl-β-cyclodextrin, a chemical widely used to solubilise lipid rafts, alters the basal current of L-VOCC in foetal mouse skeletal muscle cells and cardiomyocytes [98,99]. Also the calcium-dependent exocytosis in synaptosomes is sensible to the cholesterol content of the plasma membrane [100], and probably one of the best documented functions of caveolins is their implication in the maintenance of intracellular cholesterol homeostasis [101].

Noteworthy, using hippocampal neurons in culture it has been demonstrated the regulation of caveolins expression by L-glutamate [102], and an increased level of caveolins expression has been reported in Alzheimer's disease which has been correlated with the increased level of cellular cholesterol observed in these patients [103]. On the other hand, knockout mice in caveolin-1 have impaired nitric oxide and calcium signalling pathways, displaying severe vascular and pulmonary anomalies and uncontrolled cellular proliferation [104], and caveolins mutations has been associated with muscle disorders and cancer [96]. Moreover, lipid rafts alterations have been reported in a significant number of pathologies [105,106].

The association of the muscle type of L-VOCC with lipid rafts sub-microdomains in cardiomyocytes was established nearly 10 years ago [81,107]. Later, we have demonstrated L-VOCC association with lipid rafts nanodomains in mature primary cultures of cerebellar granule neurons using FRET microscopy imaging [108]. This association of L-VOCC with lipid rafts nanodomains has a major functional relevance for the regulation by protein kinases of the calcium influx through these channels in neurons. First, as noted previously in this chapter within the brain the α1c subunit of L-VOCC forms a complex with PKA [30] and Razani *et al.* [109] have demonstrated the co-localization and direct interaction between the scaffolding domain of caveolin-1 and the catalytic subunit of PKA *in vivo* and *in vitro*, respectively. Second, some experimental data have suggested the possibility of direct association of CaMKII with lipid rafts [110], which is consistent with the reported co-localization of $Ca_V1.2$, the predominant L-VOCC subtype in the brain, and CaMKII [37]. Functional regulation of L-VOCC by lipid rafts is also supported by the modulation of the level of phosphorylation of L-VOCC by cholesterol depletion in cardiomyocytes [99].

Since the two major subtypes of L-VOCC present in the brain, namely $Ca_V1.2$ and $Ca_V1.3$, directly interact with many proteins having the PDZ binding domain [111,112], proteins that also bind to the NMDA receptor [113], the association of these receptors with lipid rafts nanodomains is not an unexpected finding. The presence of NMDA receptors in isolated lipid rafts has been shown by different investigators [114-117], and using fluorescence resonance energy transfer (FRET) microscopy imaging their association with lipid rafts nanodomains in mature primary cultures of cerebellar granule neurons has been demonstrated in a recent work of our laboratory [117]. The critical role of proteins with PDZ domains in the association of NMDA receptors with neuronal lipid rafts has been experimentally demonstrated using genetically modified mice, as mutations in the NR2A and NR2B subunits which impair their interaction with PDZ domains led to a reduction of NMDA receptors association with lipid rafts [118]. It has been suggested that the clustering of NMDA receptors in lipid rafts-associated sub-microdomains can potentiate the activation of these receptors, thereby serving as a molecular mechanism for potentiation of the synaptic efficiency in neuronal connections [116,117]. Because AMPA receptor clustering near NMDA receptors plays a key role for NMDA receptor activation and LTP induction, it is of special neurophysiological relevance to note here that the association of AMPA receptors with molecular components of the lipid rafts of neuronal plasma membranes has also been experimentally demonstrated [114,119,120].

The association with lipid rafts of the major systems of the neuronal plasma membrane for extrusion of calcium from the cytosol, PMCA and NCX, has also been experimentally assessed, although to the best of our knowledge only in the case of PMCA this has been reported with neuronal plasma membranes at the time this chapter was written. PMCA association with lipid rafts has been shown using preparations of synaptic plasma membranes [121] and also in primary cultures of rat cortical and hippocampal neurons [122]. Earlier, it was shown that the C-terminal domain of the PMCA interacts with proteins with PDZ domains [123]. Moreover, Jiang *et al.* [122] showed that disruption of lipid rafts domains by chronic depletion of cholesterol elicited a marked decrease of PMCA activity, suggesting that PMCA associated with lipid rafts is more active than PMCA bound to non-raft domains. NCX has been shown to be associated with lipid rafts in the smooth muscle of coronary arteries [124], it has also been shown to be present in membrane fractions of vascular endothelial cells enriched in the lipid rafts markers caveolin-1 and e-NOS [125] and the direct interaction of cardiac NCX with caveolin-3 has been demonstrated by co-precipitation [126].

On these grounds, lipid rafts nanodomains of the neuronal plasma membrane can be seen as microchip-like structures for the fine coupling and control of systems playing a major role in the maintenance of a cytosolic calcium homeostasis within the range that allows for survival and normal functionality of neurons. Because of the relevance of oxidative stress in neurodegeneration it is of utmost importance to note that two enzymatic sources of ROS/RNS have been shown to be also associated with these lipid rafts nanodomains in the neuronal plasma membrane, namely, neuronal nitric oxide synthase (nNOS) and cytochrome b_5 reductase (Cb_5R). Sato *et al.* [127] showed that two domains of the nNOS, the oxygenase and the reductase domains, interact with the scaffolding domain of caveolin-1. More recently, using FRET microscopy imaging our group has shown that nNOS is associated with lipid rafts nanodomains enriched in NMDA receptors and L-VOCC in mature cultures of primary cerebellar granule neurons [117]. Since nitric oxide play a very important role in neuromodulation, this association bears a special relevance as protein/protein interactions regulate the enzyme activity of nNOS as well as define anchoring points for the subcellular location of this protein [127,128]. Indeed, it has been shown that the interaction of nNOS with caveolin-3 in skeletal muscle modulates the catalytic activity of NOS [128]. In addition, previous works of our laboratory have shown that the Cb_5R, whose deregulation at the onset of neuronal apoptosis generates a burst of superoxide anion that stimulates the entry in the irreversible phase characterized by caspases activation [10,129-131], is also associated with lipid rafts nanodomains enriched in L-VOCC and NMDA receptors in mature cultures of primary cerebellar granule neurons [108,130,131]. Moreover, the association with these lipid rafts nanodomains of a source of nitric oxide (nNOS) and of a source of superoxide anion (Cb_5R) point out that these nanodomains may play also a major role in the focalized generation of the harmful oxidant peroxynitrite in the plasma membrane when the neurons are exposed to sustained cellular stress conditions. Let us recall here also that some mitochondria, a widely accepted major ROS-producing subcellular compartment, are also close to the plasma membrane in many neuronal types, because the cell nucleus occupies a large volume of the neuronal soma.

This protein clustering associated with lipid rafts nanodomains of the neuronal plasma membrane is summarized in the Table 1, where proteins of the cytoskeleton typically associated with lipid rafts are also included. Noteworthy, ROS significantly alter the actin polymerisation/depolymerisation dynamics, reviewed in [132]. Because actin microfilaments are part of the structural protein network of proteins associated with lipid rafts nanodomains, ROS are expected to produce a significant distortion of this protein network, like nNOS which has been shown to associate with the neuronal cytoskeleton in synaptic terminals [133]. Indeed, regulatory effects of actin cytoskeleton have been reported on NMDA receptors activation [134], on the distribution of L-type calcium channels in myocytes [135], and on the activity of NCX [80].

Structural elements	Calcium transport systems	ROS/RNS sources	Regulatory kinases
Cholesterol, Caveolins,	L-VOCC,	nNOS and Cb_5R	PKA and CaMKII
Sphingolipids, Flotillin,	NMDA and AMPA receptors,		
Actin microfilaments,	PMCA and NCX		
PDZ-binding proteins			

Table 1 Molecules associated with lipid rafts in the neuronal plasma membrane of special relevance for cytosolic calcium homeostasis and ROS/RNS-calcium signalling cross-modulation.

In spite of the well known relevance of L-glutamate AMPA and NMDA receptors clustering in LTP, the regulation of incorporation and dissociation of proteins in nanodomains or sub-microdomains associated with lipid rafts is still poorly understood and, thus, it is a pending issue. It is to be noted also that knowledge of the time scale range of the clustering dynamics of proteins within these nanodomains is a basic need to properly understand their formation and plasticity, and this is particularly relevant to reach firm conclusions regarding their role as structural or adaptive elements in rapid and slow neuronal responses.

In conclusion, a close spatial location of these calcium transport proteins in the neuronal plasma membrane can also afford a fast and fine tuning of cytosolic calcium concentrations. Moreover, as major redox centers producing ROS are also tighly associated with lipid rafts nanodomains, this compartmentation allows also to rationalize on simple grounds the intimate cross-talk between ROS and calcium signalling in neurons, as well as between oxidative stress and sustained cytosolic calcium deregulation, reviewed in [136,137].

4. Sustained alteration of cytosolic calcium homeostasis in neuronal death

Neuronal survival is extremely dependent of the fine tuning of cytosolic calcium homeostasis, because cytosolic calcium concentration has to be maintained within a relatively narrow window for neuronal survival [1], for example, between 70 and 200 nM for cerebellar granule neurons in culture [9,138]. An overwhelming amount of experimental data reported by many investigators from different countries show that sustained deviations of cytosolic calcium concentration out of this narrow window lead to neuronal cell death. Besides rapid necrotic neuronal death induced by sustained cytosolic calcium concentration higher than 0.4 μM for periods in the minutes time scale range [1,9,44,45,138,139], it has also been shown that apoptotic neuronal death can be induced when cytosolic calcium concentration remains very low for longer periods of time, in the hours time scale range [1,2]. As the extracellular free calcium concentration is approximately 1 mM, this implies that neurons need to sustain a large calcium gradient across their plasma membranes. Owing to the large number of synaptic connections established by neurons in the brain, these cells need to spend a large amount of metabolic energy to maintain their cytosolic calcium homeostasis, because during synaptic activity calcium entry is activated through VOCC and some ionotropic receptors, mainly NMDA receptors. In addition, many neuronal processes are extremely dependent upon cytosolic calcium concentration, such as neurotransmitter secretion and synaptic plasticity [140], neurite growth and sprouting [141] and signalling pathways which mediate the metabolic neuronal responses to a large number of relevant extracellular stimuli [4,5]. Therefore, the cytosolic calcium concentration should be considered a major bioenergetic marker for neuronal activity and survival.

The increase of oxidative stress in brain is a biochemical marker associated with neurodegenerative insults, like ischemia-reperfusion or inflammation, or neurodegenerative diseases of high prevalence and relevance to humans, for example, Alzheimer's, Parkinson's, amyotrophic lateral sclerosis and Huntington's diseases. Many studies have shown that cellular oxidative stress is caused by an imbalance between endogenous antioxidant defences and ROS production in favour of the latter, which results in an excessive exposure of cells to harmful ROS/RNS. On the other hand, it is well established now that the calcium transport systems most relevant for the cytosolic calcium homeostasis in neurons are molecular targets for ROS/RNS and that their chemical modification by these reactive species lead to their functional impairment. Indeed, oxidative chemical modifications of these calcium transport systems have been reported to take place *in vivo*. Moreover, many experimental studies reported during last 10 years led to the conclusion that ROS produce a sustained deregulation of cytosolic calcium homeostasis in neurons. For example, neuronal death mediated by calpains activation can be taken as a biological marker of a sustained rise of cytosolic calcium concentration [142-144]. Another examples are provided by the central role of L-VOCC and ROS in the apoptosis induced by low extracellular potassium concentration [2,9,10,129,131,145], and also by L-glutamate excitoxicity-induced neuronal death [44,45,146]. Thus, sustained alterations of neuronal cytosolic calcium are expected to be a convergent cellular mechanism in brain neurodegeneration. Consistent with this hypothesis, alterations of neuronal calcium homeostasis and brain oxidative stress have been reported in the case for the brain neurodegenerative diseases of higher incidence to humans, like Alzheimer's [147,148] and Parkinson's [149,150], or in the acute neurodegeneration observed in amyotrophic lateral sclerosis [146,151], and also for major brain insults, such as excitotoxicity in trauma and ischemia-reperfusion [44,45], inflammation [152,153] and neurotoxicity by drugs and environmental chemicals [139,154].

Most ROS/RNS that are produced in cellular oxidative stress in mammalian tissues have been demonstrated to be strongly neurotoxic to neurons *in vitro*. This is a relatively large list of ROS/RNS, and we shall concentrate in this chapter in those most studied as agents in brain neurodegeneration, namely, superoxide anion, H_2O_2, hydroxyl radicals, lipid hydroperoxides, and nitric oxide-derived ROS, mainly peroxynitrite and nitrogen dioxide. Because of the calcium dependence of the activity of nNOS, the main enzymatic system responsible for the production of nitric oxide in neurons [133], RNS should be expected to play a particularly relevant role as intracellular biomarkers of the level of coordination or deregulation of calcium and ROS signalling pathways in neurons. However, it is still a matter of debate whether *in vivo* all of these ROS/RNS can reach concentrations high enough to act as causal agents or merely as agents that potentiate or accelerate the rate of an ongoing neuronal death process in the brain. Moreover, the analysis and dissection of the chemical reaction pathways of each one of this ROS/RNS is further complicated by the fact that *in vivo* they generate radicalic chain chemical reactions. Therefore, it is critical to identify the major subcellular primary sources of these ROS/RNS in different neurons and in different degenerative processes in the brain, and this is an issue yet to be settled in many cases, as during lasts years the experimental evidences have pointed out that the relative relevance of different ROS/RNS seems to be largely dependent on the neurodegenerative disease or brain insult.

5. Modulation by ROS/RNS of calcium transport systems relevant for the control of neuronal cytosolic calcium homeostasis

ROS and RNS producing oxidative stress to neurons can be generated by neuronal and also by non-neuronal cells, like microglia or endothelial cells of the brain blood vessels. It is to be noted that oxidative stress-induced brain degeneration is a relatively slow process, in most neurodegenerative diseases developing in periods of time of years and in acute brain ischemia-reperfusion in a time range from minutes to several days, depending upon the intensity of the oxidative stress insult. Thus, in a brain suffering oxidative stress neurons are exposed for relatively large time periods to either extracellularly and/or intracellularly generated ROS/RNS. Because the extracellular liquid bathing the brain and stem neurons is poorer in antioxidants than the blood, due to the low permeability and high selectivity of the blood-brain barrier, the extracellular antioxidant protection in the brain is notably lower than that of other organs and tissues in mammals. Under these environmental conditions the plasma membrane of neurons, where major calcium transport systems controlling the cytosolic calcium homeostais are located, is particularly sensitive to the oxidative stress generated in the brain by vicinal neuronal and non-neuronal cells. The major ROS/RNS reported to play a significant role in the enhanced brain oxidative stress associated with neurodegenerative diseases and insults like ischemia-reperfusion and inflammation can be split into three major groups: (i) primary biochemical ROS/RNS, i.e. chemical species directly generated by some enzymes or proteins during brain activity in normal or pathophysiological conditions, (ii) secondary biochemical ROS/RNS, chemical species derived by rapid reaction between the primary biochemical ROS/RNS or by systems involved in their detoxification, and (iii) radicalic chain ROS/RNS, chemical radicals involved in the initiation of radical reaction chains or that are largely generated within radical reaction chains.

Superoxide anion is a primary biochemical ROS that plays a key role in the generation of many of the more harmful ROS and RNS detected in the oxidative stress-induced degeneration of the brain. Superoxide anion can be produced by neuronal and non-neuronal cells within the brain. Because of the relatively low permeability to superoxide anion of lipid bilayers [155], extracellular superoxide anion must be largely generated by redox centres of the plasma membrane of neuronal and non-neuronal cells. In glial, macrophages and endothelial cells there are NADPH oxidases of the NOX family, which are under the control of transcriptional antioxidant-responsive elements (ARE), reviewed in [156]. In contrast, we found that in the plasma membrane of neurons the NADH-dependent production of superoxide anion associated with their NADH oxidase activity was nearly ten-fold higher than their NADPH activity [157,158]. Indeed, an overshot of superoxide anion production at the plasma membrane is an early event in the apoptosis of cerebellar granule neurons induced by extracellular K^+ deprivation [10,131], an overshot that we have found to be largely catalyzed by deregulation of cytochrome b_5 reductase associated with plasma membrane lipid rafts sub-microdomains [130,131]. Mitochondria is now widely accepted as the major source of intracellular superoxide anion in oxidative stress-induced neuronal death in cultures *in vitro*, particularly by complexes I and III of the mitochondrial respiratory chain [159]. In addition, non-mitochondrial enzymes that use oxygen as substrate can also become a source of intracellular superoxide anion in neurons, such as the conversion of xanthine dehydrogenase into xanthine oxidase either by direct oxidation and/or by proteolytic activation during oxidative stress-induced neuronal death [160].

Nitric oxide is the major primary biochemical RNS produced in oxidative stress-induced brain degeneration, and although not harmful by itself, its reaction with superoxide anion yields peroxynitrite (a secondary biochemical ROS/RNS), probably the most neurotoxic ROS/RNS generated during oxidative stress-mediated brain neurodegeneration, see e.g. [161,162]. The reaction between nitric oxide and superoxide anion is very fast, such that it is considered a diffusion-controlled chemical reaction due to the very high value of the bimolecular rate constant, (4-7) 10^9 M^{-1} s^{-1} [163]. Peroxynitrite, in spite of its short lifetime within the cells [162], has been shown to be a very harmful ROS/RNS involved in the brain damage produced by ischemia-reperfusion [161], by inflammation and spinal cord injury [164,165] and also in neurodegenerative diseases and aging [166,167]. Peroxynitrite can elicit functional damage of biomolecules and subcellular structures acting either as a potent oxidant ($E^{0'}$ = 1.2-1.4 V) or through the generation of harmful radicals such as hydroxyl and nitrogen dioxide free radicals, reviewed in [162,168]. Due to this, peroxynitrite can produce oxidation of protein cysteines to disulfide bonds, sulfenic and sulfinic acids eventually leading to sulfonic acids, oxidation of protein methionines, nitration of protein tyrosines and lipids, lipid peroxidation, coenzyme Q oxidation, and DNA and RNA oxidation. Because the activation of neuronal nitric oxide synthase requires an increase of cytosolic calcium, peroxynitrite is one of the more harmful ROS/RNS produced in the oxidative stress accompanied by sustained alterations of the neuronal cytosolic calcium homeostasis. Indeed, this has been shown to be the case for the excitotoxic neuronal death elicited by L-glutamate through activation of NMDA receptors [166,169].

ROS/RNS initiating lipid oxidation and peroxidation, i.e. self-accelerating chemical radical chains, are the other group of ROS/RNS playing a major role in brain damage by oxidative stress. Among them, H_2O_2 has required a large attention because is one of the major products generated under conditions that elicit over-production of superoxide anion, as it is a product of superoxide dismutase activity. In addition, intracellular traces of metal ions such as Fe^{3+} or Cu^{2+} can catalyse Fenton-like reactions in neurons, generating hydroxyl radical from superoxide and H_2O_2 [170]. Hydroxyl radical is one of the most potent cytotoxic oxygen radicals, which can attack a large variety of important biomolecules, from small biomolecules such as coenzyme Q or α-tocopherol [171] up to large biomolecules like proteins, RNA and DNA [170,172]. Since hydroxyl radical can be also generated from peroxynitrite decomposition (see above), it turns out that it is a converging point between the oxidative stress pathways involving ROS and RNS derived from nitric oxide. The involvement of hydroxyl radical in oxidative stress-induced neuronal damage has been suggested, for example, in the pathophysiological case of spinal cord trauma [173], amyotrophic lateral sclerosis [174] and Parkinson's disease [170,175].

Lipid ROS are a family of harmful ROS detected in oxidative stress-mediated brain degeneration that also catalyze chemical radical reaction chains. They can be produced as primary biochemical ROS by cyclooxygenases (COX) and lipoxygenases in some brain oxidative stress insults, such as ischemia-reperfusion [176], or Parkinson's disease [177]. Indeed, inhibitors of the neuronal COX-2 isoform have been reported to attenuate brain damage after ischemia-reperfusion [176]. Moreover, the oxidation of dopamine by the microglial COX-1 isoform and also by COX-2 isoform in the dopaminergic neurons of the substantia nigra has been involved in the pathogenesis of Parkinson's disease [177]. It is to be noted though that lipid ROS are also generated during hydroxyl radical- and hydrogen peroxide-induced lipid oxidation and peroxidation, respectively [170]. In addition, lipid oxidation and peroxidation also release the aldehydes malondialdehyde and 4-hydroxynonenal, which have been shown to be highly neurotoxic compounds [178,179]. Because of the self-propagating properties of lipid radical chains once they are initiated, and also due to the high toxicity for neurons of lipid breakdown compounds released, the possibility of cell rescue after the threshold antioxidant barrier against lipid oxidation/peroxidation is surpassed can be considered negligible. The extent of lipid oxidation marking the 'point of no return' for neurons survival has not been firmly established yet, but it is likely to be at most only a few per cent of the total lipids [180]. On these grounds, an enhanced lipid oxidation should be expected to be a late and largely irreversible step in neuronal death. This view is consistent with the many reports showing that largely damaged brain areas after an ischemia-reperfusion insult display a marked increase of lipid peroxidation.

5.1. Modulation by ROS/RNS of the major calcium entry systems of the neuronal plasma membrane

5.1.1. Voltage-operated calcium channels

As indicated above in the section 2 of this chapter, the L-type are the most relevant VOCC in the fine tuning of the steady state level of cytosolic calcium concentration in the neuronal soma and, thus, in the fine tuning of threshold neuronal excitability [22-24]. L-type VOCC as a primary target for ROS in brain is also supported by the hypoxic up-regulation of these channels, which is mediated by Alzheimer's amyloid peptides [181]. L-VOCC contain two vicinal cysteines at positions 271 and 272 which are involved in their interaction with syntaxin 1A, thereby playing a major role in their regional localization in plasma membrane microdomains [182]. In addition, three cysteines are located in the calcium-pore region (Cys^{330}, Cys^{1383} and Cys^{1396}) [183]. Therefore, L-VOCC contains redox centres that have been shown to react with ROS/RNS in other proteins, for example, in NMDA-receptors (see below).

Studies with neurons in culture have provided ample experimental evidences of direct modulation of L-VOCC by the major ROS/RNS involved in brain ischemia-reperfusion, inflammation and/or neurodegeneration. The L-VOCC antagonist nifedipine has been reported to protect CNS neurons against hydrogen peroxide-induced death, which is mediated by a sustained increase of cytosolic calcium, pointing out activation of L-type VOCC by H_2O_2 [184]. H_2O_2 was shown later to activate recombinant calcium channel α_{1C} subunit stably expressed in HEK 293 cells [185]. In addition, nitric oxide has been reported to induce activation of L-VOCC in hippocampal neurons by plasma membrane depolarization [186] or to inhibit calcium channel gating via activation of cGMP-dependent protein kinases [187]. In contrast, exposure to peroxynitrite has been reported to produce decrease of calcium influx through L-VOCC at low submicromolar doses in rat cerebellar granule neurons in culture and increase of calcium influx through L-VOCC at higher micromolar doses in rat cerebellar granule neurons in culture [9] and in mouse cerebral cortical neurons [188]. Hydroxyl radicals, a radical produced during the decomposition of peroxynitrite, have been reported to suppress the calcium influx through L-VOCC in mouse cortical neurons [189]. Consistent with these results, dihydropyridine L-VOCC blockers afford protection against neuronal death induced by exposure of neurons *in vitro* to the peroxynitrite-releasing agent SIN-1 [9,190]. Because of the short lifetime and high reactivity of these radicals this is likely to be due to direct chemical modification of L-VOCC, although it is to be noted that this chemical modification is yet unknown. In addition, it has been reported that eicosanoids and ROS generated during arachidonic acid oxidative metabolism also activate L-VOCC [191], and that the lipid peroxidation product 4-hydroxynonenal causes opening of the L-VOCC, resulting in an increase of cytosolic calcium and neuronal death which is prevented by the L-VOCC blocker nimodipine [192]. Direct redox modulation of L-VOCC is further supported by its activation by hydrogen sulphide [138]. Further studies are needed to reach firm conclusions regarding the molecular mechanisms of modulation of different neuronal L-VOCC subtypes by ROS.

Only very scarce experimental studies have been done on the putative modulation of N-, P/Q- and R-type VOCC by ROS/RNS, despite the fact that N- and R-type of calcium channels are blocked by heavy metals such as Pb^{2+} and Hg^{2+} that are likely to interact with thiols [193]. $Ca_V2.2$ (N-type) channel gating is inhibited by nitric oxide via cGMP-dependent protein kinase, as it is also the Ca_V1 (L-type) channel [187]. Also, the lipid peroxidation product 4-hydroxynonenal increased the calcium influx through L-type and other ill-defined types of VOCC [178].

5.1.2. NMDA and other ionotropic receptors with calcium channel activity

It is well known the relevant role of NMDA-receptor mediated excitotoxic neuronal death in ischemia-reperfusion brain injury, see [44,45], in multiple chemical sensitivity in brain [194], in neuronal glutathione depletion [195] and in hydrogen sulfide-induced neuronal death [138,196]. Therefore, it is not surprising that the redox modulation of the NMDA-receptor is by far the most studied within the group of ionotropic receptors. The redox modulatory site of the NMDA-receptor consists of thiols groups that are vicinal in the three-dimensional structure and may form disulfide bonds under the cellular oxidative stress conditions induced by ROS [197], and it acts as a gain control for current flux through the NMDA-receptor [197,198]. Moreover, a significant number of NMDA-receptor cysteines are in the domains of this receptor facing the extracellular space, including at least one pair of vicinal thiols [199]. Thus, this receptor can also play a major role in the rapid neuronal adaptation to changes of the redox potential in the extracellular fluids within the brain, and the different types of NMDA-receptors display a redox response that is dependent on the type of NR2 forming the channels [55]. The differential redox-sensitivity of NMDA receptors isoforms led to the discovery of two redox modulatory centres within the NMDA-receptor structure, one formed by Cys744 and Cys798 on the subunit NR1 and a second one on the subunit NR2A [200,201]. Whereas the redox centre of the subunit NR1 plays a major role in the redox modulation of NR1/NR2C- and NR1/NR2B-containing receptors, the redox centre of subunit NR2A is sufficient for the expression of redox sensitivity in NR1/NR2A-containing receptors [201]. Redox active compounds modulate NMDA-receptors such that reduction of NMDA-receptor increases NMDA-receptor activity and their oxidation leads to a decrease of NMDA-receptor activity [202].

Because of the high physiological relevance of nitric oxide and of NMDA receptors in the brain, the modulation of NMDA receptors by nitric oxide is of particular relevance. Nitric oxide inhibition of NMDA-receptor response in cortical neurons in culture has been rationalized in terms of NO-induced disulfide bonds between vicinal thiols of the NMDA-receptor, and was proposed to afford neuronal protection against L-glutamate excitotoxicity [203]. Indeed, it has also been reported that thiol-reducing agents such as dithiothreitol increase the open dwell-time and opening frequency of NR1/NR2A channels [55,201]. Consistent with these findings, it has been reported that the novel neuromodulator hydrogen sulphide potentiates NMDA-receptor response in hippocampal neurons [204] and in cerebellar granule neurons [138], and that over-stimulation of NMDA-receptors by hydrogen sulphide can lead to excitotoxic neuronal death [138,196]. Glutamate-induced excitotoxic neuronal death has been shown to mediate brain injury after a transient focal cerebral ischemia episode [44,45]. Inhibitors of the H_2S-producing enzymes cystathionine β-synthase and cystathionine γ-lyase reduced the infarct volume in a dose-dependent manner, while administration of sodium hydrosulfide significantly increased the infarct volume after a transient focal cerebral ischemia insult [205]. Exposure of neurons to peroxynitrite also leads to activation of calcium entry through NMDA-receptors [166,169]. This effect of peroxynitrite has been rationalized in terms of the rise of L-glutamate concentration within the synaptic cleft, either due to potentiation by nitric oxide and/or peroxynitrite of L-glutamate secretion in synaptic terminals [194,206] or of inhibition of L-glutamate transporters catalyzing its re-uptake [207].

Besides the major role of NMDA-receptors on the neuronal damage elicited by ROS and/or oxidative stress, AMPA receptors have been also involved in the neurotoxicity of ROS. It has been reported that the increase of cytosolic calcium associated with the influx of Ca^{2+} through the ionotropic AMPA-receptors can stimulate nNOS leading to an enhanced production of nitric oxide within L-glutamatergic neurons [208]. Moreover, antagonists of AMPA/kainate-receptors have been reported to prevent the loss of cell viability induced by the peroxynitrite-releasing agent SIN-1 in mixed cortical cell cultures containing both neurons and astrocytes [209]. AMPA-receptors contain a disulfide bond between cysteines 260 and 315 in the ligand binding domain of receptor subunit GluRD, which has been proposed to act as a redox centre implicated in direct redox modulation of these receptors [210]. Nevertheless, the redox modulation of AMPA-receptors is a topic that will require further studies to develop an integrative view of its modulation by the different ROS that has been implicated in brain damage.

Finally, the response of the purinergic ionotropic P2X-receptors has been shown to be altered by acute hypoxia, an effect that has been proposed to be mediated by ROS because H_2O_2 attenuated the effect of hypoxia on homomeric P2X2 whole-cell currents, which are reversibly reduced to 38% of control by H_2O_2 [211]. Yet, studies regarding the putative modulation of P2X-receptors by other ROS are a pending issue.

5.2. Modulation by ROS/RNS of the transport systems that release calcium from intracellular stores

5.2.1. Endoplasmic reticulum

ROS/RNS have been shown to elicit a potent stimulation of calcium release from the endoplasmic reticulum, through activation of IP_3 and ryanodine receptors.

Superoxide anion and H_2O_2 have been reported to induce calcium release from the endoplasmic reticulum of neurons through activation of IP_3 receptors [212,213]. Oxidized glutathione and the alkyl mercury compound thimerosal, a thiol specific agent, increase the affinity of IP_3 receptors for IP_3, thereby sensitizing this receptor to basal IP_3 level in the cell and promoting calcium release from the endoplasmic reticulum to the cytosol [214,215]. Cysteine clusters highly reactive against ROS have been recently identified in the IP_3 receptors [216]. IP_3 receptors are inhibited by interaction with luminal endoplasmic reticulum proteins through luminal-facing domains of the receptor containing reduced cysteines, and oxidation of these cysteines weakens these interactions leading to IP_3 receptor activation [63,217]. Moreover, nitric oxide-induced increase of IP_3 binding to the IP_3 receptor in hypoxic brain has been proposed to mediate IP_3 receptors activation in calcium-dependent neuronal apoptotic death induced by hypoxia [218].

Although all ryanodine receptor isoforms are expressed in the brain, the isoform 2 is the most heavily expressed [219, 220]. Many studies have addressed the redox modulation of the ryanodine receptors in myocytes and in neurons, reviewed in [62,64,221]. Nitric oxide activates the skeletal and cardiac ryanodine receptors [222,223]. The activation of the ryanodine receptor by nitric oxide has been shown to be due to the presence of highly reactive cysteines of the receptor, which are S-nitrosylated upon exposure to nitric oxide [222-224]. The cysteines that are S-nitrosylated upon *in vitro* exposure to nitric oxide have been identified [225]. However, *in vivo* the extent of S-nitrosylation of ryanodine receptor cysteines is highly modulated by the physiological oxygen tension, leading to the concept that ryanodine receptors can operate as a coupled redox sensor for oxygen and nitric oxide [226,227]. *In vitro* studies have shown that these cysteines of the ryanodine receptor are highly sensitive to oxidative stress and are likely to mediate the redox ryanodine receptor response to another ROS, as they are also prone to reversible S-glutathionylation or oxidation to disulfide bonds [225]. The ryanodine receptors are also activated by hydroxyl radical, H_2O_2, the disulfide bond-forming agent diamide and also by oxidized glutathione [221,224,228]. Overall, oxidizing conditions favor the opening of the ryanodine receptor calcium channel, and on these grounds it has been proposed that activation of these calcium channels are also involved in the pathology of brain ischemia-reperfusion [229] and Alzheimer's disease [230]. Noteworthy, a moderate and sustained stimulation of the ryanodine receptors in the hippocampus has been involved in the sustained increase of cytosolic calcium needed for the induction of the long-term postsynaptic potentiation associated with memory formation [231,232].

Calcium accumulation within the luminal space of the endoplasmic reticulum is performed by Ca^{2+}-ATPases (SERCA), whose activity is inhibited by exposure to H_2O_2, superoxide anion and peroxynitrite [233-236], the major ROS produced in brain insults such as ischemia-reperfusion or inflammation and in neurodegeneration. Despite that the isoforms of SERCA most sensitive to ROS, i.e. SERCA2 isoforms, are expressed in brain, the relevance of the impairment of their activity to alterations of neuronal cytosolic calcium homeostasis has yet to be conclusively demonstrated, probably because in neurons the PMCA is a calcium pump more potent than SERCA for calcium extrusion from the cytosol.

The apparently higher susceptibility to ROS/RNS of the calcium release systems of the endoplasmic reticulum, ryanodine and IP_3 receptors, should lead under oxidative stress conditions to at least a partial depletion of the calcium concentration within the luminal space of this subcellular compartment, see for example [237]. It should be noted, though, that in neurons the amount of calcium stored in the endoplasmic reticulum is small compared with the amount of calcium entering through plasma membrane calcium channels and ionotropic receptors. However, in most severe cases the depletion of calcium can elicit the opening of plasma membrane SOCE, see section 2.2 of this chapter. Thus, the relevance of calcium release from the endoplasmic reticulum or of inhibition of the SERCA to the observed alterations by ROS/RNS of cytosolic calcium homeostasis will strongly depend on the differential expression of SOCE isoforms in different type of neurons. On the other hand, the depletion of calcium of the endoplasmic reticulum may lead to a dysfunctional endoplasmic reticulum by itself, because of the relevance of the endoplasmic calcium concentration for the correct folding and processing of membrane and secretory proteins [65, 238]. On these grounds, these authors have proposed that ROS/RNS-induced endoplasmic reticulum dysfunction can be a mechanism underlying slow-developing cell injury in ischemia-reperfusion, epileptic seizures and degenerative diseases of the brain like Alzheimer's and Parkinson's diseases. In addition, it has been recently shown that mutations in presenilin-1 and -2 observed in nearly 40% of familial Alzheimer's disease lead to calcium release from the endoplasmic reticulum [239]. Moreover, presenilins by themselves can form calcium leak channels in the endoplasmic reticulum whose properties are altered in mutant presenilins linked to Alzheimer's disease [240].

5.2.2. Mitochondria

A key role has been proposed for mitochondrial dysfunctions in the onset or development of neuronal death in the brain mediated by the enhanced oxidative stress observed in relevant neurodegenerative disorders, such as Alzheimer's and Parkinson's diseases, amyotrophic lateral sclerosis and Friedreich's ataxia, and in harmful brain insults like ischemia-reperfusion and glutamate excitotoxicity, reviewed in [166,241,242]. Mitochondrial calcium overload is observed in excitotoxic conditions that produce a sustained increase of neuronal cytosolic calcium or high frequency repetitive cytosolic calcium peaks [73]. ROS/RNS have been shown to promote opening of the permeability transition pore of mitochondria and this effect of ROS/RNS is enhanced by mitochondrial calcium overload [71,73,166]. Opening of the permeability transition pore leads to a significant calcium release from mitochondria which contributes to foster excitotoxic neuronal death [71, 243], and also is an important factor in necrotic cell death following ischemia-reperfusion [73] or in neurons exposed to transient hypoglycemia [244]. Consistently, calcium-dependent mitochondrial dysfunction by peroxynitrite has been demonstrated to elicit necrotic cell death via activation of calpains [245]. In addition, opening of this pore has also been shown to mediate the neuronal apoptosis elicited by 3-nitropropionic acid, an agent which has been used to mimic in model rodents the brain neurodegeneration observed in Huntington's disease [246]. Despite that most of studies concerning ROS-stimulated release of calcium from mitochondria point out a major role of the permeability transition pore, it should be recalled that the inner membrane Na^+/Ca^{2+}-exchanger, i.e. the other major mitochondrial calcium release system [71], is also sensitive to oxidative stress. It has been reported that oxidative stress mediated by H_2O_2 modulates this exchanger and can lead to activation of caspase 3-dependent apoptosis due to mitochondrial Na^+ overload [247].

The permeability transition pore opening induced by ROS/RNS is mediated by oxidation of critical thiols of proteins forming the pore, as it can be elicited by a relatively large number of oxidizing agents such as diamide, dithiopyridine, singlet oxygen, diazoxide, nitric oxide, S-nitrosothiols and selenium [221]. The adenine nucleotide transporter of the inner mitochondrial membrane and the voltage-dependent anion channel of the outer mitochondrial membrane have been proposed to be part of the molecular structure of the permeability transition pore, and both proteins have shown to be modulated by oxidative stress and exposure of mitochondria to chemically defined ROS, such that oxidation of thiols of the adenine nucleotide transporter facing to the mitochondrial matrix have been shown to elicit the opening of the permeability transition pore, reviewed in [73].

5.3. Modulation by ROS/RNS of the transport systems involved in calcium extrusion from the cytosol

Much of the interest on modulation of PMCA and Na^+/Ca^{2+}-exchanger of neurons by ROS is based on the reported decrease of these activities in synaptic plasma membranes in aging, and the possibility that this could lead to a sustained increase of the steady state cytosolic calcium in aged animals with respect to young animals [248,249].

5.3.1. PMCA

It has been shown that incubation of brain synaptic plasma membranes with Fe^{2+}/EDTA, H_2O_2, peroxyl radicals generated by azo-initiators and peroxynitrite resulted in a significant loss of PMCA activity [250-253]. Inhibition of purified PMCA by H_2O_2 has been proposed to be due to oxidation of two cysteines of this protein [253]. Also, lipid peroxidation and the lipid peroxidation product 4-hydroxynonenal have been shown to inhibit the PMCA actvity [254]. In the case of incubation with peroxynitrite, the loss of Ca^{2+}-ATPase activity was paralleled by decrease of ATP-dependent calcium uptake activity and by a significant increase of tyrosine nitration of the PMCA [252]. However, it is to be noted that all these studies were carried out *in vitro* with purified plasma membranes in an altered environment with respect to the normal redox cytosolic environment in living neurons, and this has to be taken into account since endogenous antioxidant levels of reduced glutathione has been shown to largely attenuate the inhibition of PMCA by peroxynitrite [252]. In addition, the concentrations of H_2O_2 and peroxynitrite producing approximately 50% inhibition of the PMCA in these studies, higher than 100 μM in both cases, were much higher than those reported to be attained in brain after transient focal ischemia or inflammation. For the case of neuronal exposure to peroxynitrite fluxes mimicking those attained in inflammation or ischemia-reperfusion, in a previous work of our laboratory it was shown that in cerebellar granule neurons in culture the PMCA is significantly inhibited in less than 2 hours exposure to micromolar concentrations of peroxynitrite, although it was also noted that the PMCA has nearly ten-fold lower sensitivity to peroxynitrite than L-VOCC [9].

Na^{+}/Ca^{2+}*–exchanger (NCX)*

The NCX has been reported to be less sensitive to inhibition by the peroxyl radical azo initiator 2,2'- azobis (2-amidinopropane) dihydrochloride (AAPH) and peroxynitrite than the PMCA [251], and also to be insensitive to inhibition by up to 700 μM of H_2O_2 [255]. The Na^{+}/Ca^{2+}-exchanger activity of synaptic brain plasma membranes and in transfected CHO-K1 cells has been reported to be inhibited by exposure to AAPH and also to peroxynitrite [255], although it must be noted that peroxynitrite only afforded a partial inhibition of the exchanger caused by decrease of its affinity for calcium without a significant change of the V_{max}. The inhibition induced by both oxidants correlated with the formation of higher molecular weight aggregates of the Na^{+}/Ca^{2+}-exchanger, and in addition AAPH also caused fragmentation of the exchanger protein.

In contrast, in cardiac muscle myocytes, hypoxia inhibits the Na^{+}/Ca^{2+}-exchanger and ROS are required for its rapid reactivation upon reoxygenation [256]. This is consistent with the earlier demonstration in ventricular myocytes of stimulation of the Na^{+}/Ca^{2+}-exchanger by H_2O_2 and superoxide anion [257]. Owing to the different pattern of Na^{+}/Ca^{2+}-exchanger isoforms expression in brain cells and cardiac myocytes, more experimental studies are needed to reach solid conclusions regarding the effects of oxidative stress on the activity of this exchanger in different neuronal types and also in the glial cells of the brain.

6. Space and time fluctuations of cytosolic calcium in the neuronal soma

As indicated previously in this chapter, protein compartmentation within microdomains allows for a more efficient and rapid functional coupling between influx and efflux calcium transport systems, and this is particularly relevant for neuronal activity, as neurons have to deliver fast responses to many repetitive and simultaneous extracellular stimuli coming from different neighbour cells. Studies on calcium signalling in neurons have played a pioneer role to demonstrate the outstanding role of subcellular compartmentation in the control of neuronal activity, see for example [5]. As analyzed in more detail in the section 3 of this chapter more recently reported experimental data point out that the calcium transport systems of the plasma membrane more relevant for the control of cytosolic calcium homeostasis in neurons are associated with lipid rafts sub-microdomains or nanodomains. This is an emerging scenario that opens new perspectives for the rationalization of the modulation of cytosolic calcium peaks amplitude and also of the rate of attenuation of calcium local gradients in neurons, as both parameters are strongly dependent on the spatial proximity between systems controlling calcium entry and extrusion from the cytosol. For example, the rationalization of the transient calcium gradients observed between different regions of the neuronal cytosol can be done on simple grounds taking into account a polarised or focalized distribution of the major calcium transport systems of the neuronal plasma membrane. Note that, as indicated before in this chapter, sustained cytosolic calcium concentrations higher than 0.4 μM are strongly cytotoxic to neurons, but it is a need for neurons to reach these concentrations in the environment of cytosolic proteins and enzymes having EC_{50} values for calcium between 0.4 and 1 μM. Indeed, some of these proteins play a key role in neuronal plasticity and functional responses critical for proper brain development and function, like calmodulin, nNOS, GAP-43 and CaMK, to cite only a few of well-established examples.

The calcium concentration reaches values in the micromolar range upon activation of L-VOCC and NMDA receptors in small volume elements close to the cytosolic side of their calcium channel structures [258], see also the Figure 2a. This generates a calcium concentration wave that diffuses within the cytosolic space, because the protein cytosolic buffering systems are not fast enough to trap all incoming calcium ions through these calcium channels [259, 260]. Due to the rapid diffusion of calcium ions in the aqueous space of the cytoplasm, ~300 $\mu m^2\ s^{-1}$, the calcium entry through the high conductance L-VOCC and NMDA receptors channels will rapidly raise the calcium concentration to the micromolar range within the associated lipid rafts nanodomains. As these nanodomains have sizes lower than 200 nm, it can be derived that in less than 1 microsecond the incoming calcium ions will diffuse within the whole space of the nanodomain, i.e. in the time scale range characteristic for fast conformational relaxation in proteins. Thus, this clustering serves to built up a very efficient molecular switch for signal transduction in calcium signalling pathways within neurons, with a time response as fast as the rapid conformational relaxations elicited by regulatory direct protein/protein interactions. However, nanodomains can be seen as multi-port exit molecular devices that can serve to many uni-port exit molecular devices, through regulatory direct protein/protein interactions. Therefore, the localized calcium rise within these nanodomains not only serves to guarantee the maximal possible activation of proteins or enzymes with EC_{50} values ≥0.4 micromolar, such as those listed above, but also to elicit rapid integrative cellular responses. We shall next briefly analyze several integrative responses of relevance for the rapid and fine control of cytosolic calcium homeostasis in neurons elicited by the localized calcium rise within the nanodomains associated with lipid rafts.

The association of CaMKII with L-VOCC subunit β2a and with NMDA receptors subunit NR2B, mentioned in the section 2.1 of this chapter, implies that this protein is present in neuronal nanodomains associated with lipid rafts. A direct consequence of the steep calcium concentration gradient generated by calcium entry through L-VOCC and NMDA receptors is the stronger selective activation of the pool of CaMKII that lies in their vicinity over other CaMKII pools present in neurons. Thus, this will selectively potentiate phosphorylation of CaMKII substrates present in lipid rafts associated nanodomains. Regarding the cytosolic calcium homeostasis in neurons, the more relevant effect is the activation of L-VOCC upon phosphorylation by CaMKII, as this potentiates the increase of the local gradient of calcium concentration within these nanodomains, leading to a longer lasting increase of the concentration of cytosolic calcium with the concomitant increase in neuronal secretory activity and excitability (Figure 2b). Indeed, it has been shown that L-VOCC plays a relevant physiological role in NMDA receptors-independent long-term potentiation [28]. The activation and synaptic clustering of AMPA receptors upon phosphorylation by CaMKII has been shown to potentiate NMDA receptors activation in the induction of LTP [53]. Noteworthy, L-VOCC blockers like nifedipine and nimodipine and AMPA antagonists/inhibitors have been shown to have anti-epileptic therapeutic effects, pointing out that overstimulation of L-VOCC and/or AMPA underlies, at least, some types of epileptic seizures.

The high concentration of calcium attained within the nanodomains associated with lipid rafts allows for a stronger and faster selective stimulation of the pool of nNOS localized therein. Because of the rapid diffusion coefficient of nitric oxide, these nanodomains can be seen as the most relevant plasma membrane points for focalized nitric oxide generation in neurons and, therefore, define the sub-microcompartments of neurons where higher transient concentrations of nitric oxide are attained upon nNOS stimulation. This fact and the vicinal location of nNOS and NMDA receptors within these nanodomains, i.e. separated by a distance lower than 40 nm [117], makes of NMDA receptors a major cellular target for the chemical reactivity of released nitric oxide. As the calcium currents through NMDA receptors are inhibited by exposure of these receptors to nitric oxide, see the section 5.1 of this chapter, the co-localization of nNOS and NMDA receptors within these nanodomains serves to potentiate a feedback retroinhibition mechanism for the attenuation of excessive NMDA receptors activity which would lead to neuronal excitotoxicity [117], i.e. these nanodomains can be also seen as a molecular microchip-like structure designed for neuronal protection against the harmful consequences of overstimulation by L-glutamate (Figure 2c). On these grounds, the reported stimulation of L-VOCC by nitric oxide, see the section 5.1 of this chapter, can be rationalized as a molecular compensatory mechanism for the fine tuning of NMDA receptor activity, as it will lead to an increase of L-glutamate secretion near these nanodomains and this should avoid excessive depression of NMDA receptor activity in the neuron.

The latter point already highlights a major role of the nanodomains associated with lipid rafts in the intimate cross-talk between calcium and nitric oxide signalling for the normal physiological activity of neurons, but also points out that excessive calcium entry through L-VOCC or NMDA receptors should rapidly lead to unusually large peaks of nitric oxide generation in these nanodomains. As indicated above in this chapter, it is well established now that the sustained rise of intracellular calcium and/or nitric oxide can induce neuronal death and are common features in brain degeneration. Many experimental evidences accumulated up to date reveal that in some cases the induction of oxidative stress in brain neurodegeneration takes place before a sustained cytosolic calcium homeostasis deregulation can be observed. For example, in the case of inflammation of a brain area induced either by a traumatic shock injury or cerebral stroke the neurons are exposed to a ROS/RNS overshot largely generated by vicinal glial and vascular endothelial cells. The major sources for the overshot of ROS/RNS observed in this inflammation episode are the increase of iNOS expression, which produces a nitric oxide overshot, and activation of plasma membrane NADPH oxidases, which produces a superoxide anion overshot. Therefore, within the brain area affected by inflammation neurons suffer a long-lasting exposure to an extracellular microenvironment where the simultaneous presence

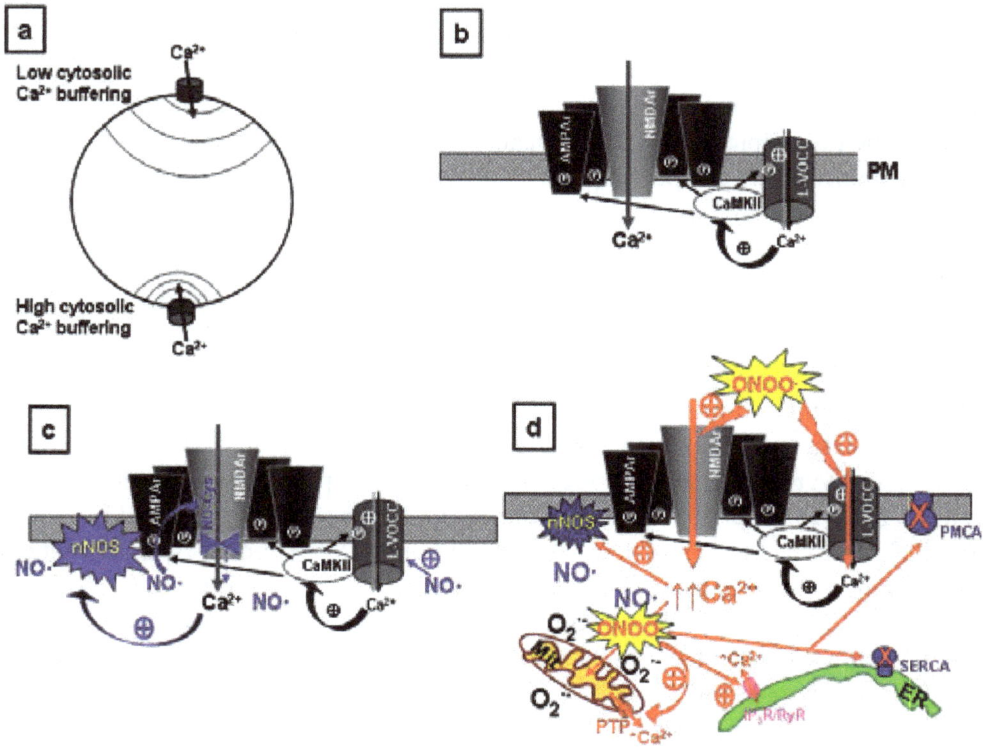

Figure 2. Functional implications of the association of calcium transport systems and ROS/RNS-sources in the neuronal plasma membrane. (a) Generation of transients of micromolar calcium concentrations within nano- or sub-micro-volume elements. The size attained by these volume elements is strongly dependent on the intensity of the total calcium inward current through the calcium transport systems clusters within lipid rafts-associated nanodomains and on the cytosolic calcium buffering capacity (see the text). (b) Faster and long-lasting potentiation of NMDA receptors (NMDAr). Calcium entry through L-VOCC triggers the activation of associated CaMKII, which elicits (i) a feedback activation of L-VOCC potentiating calcium entry and (ii) a recruitment of activated AMPA receptors (AMPAr). (c) Potentiation of NO -mediated protection against L-glutamate excitotoxicity. The co-localization of nNOS allows to reach higher NO concentrations near NMDA receptors and L-VOCC potentiating its effects on these calcium transport systems. (d) Peroxynitrite-induced sustained cytosolic calcium deregulation. A dramatic consequence of an unbalanced overstimulation of calcium transport systems that raise the cytosolic calcium concentration. Other abbreviations used in this figure: PM, plasma membrane; Mit, mitochondria; ER, endoplasmic reticulum; $ONOO^-$, peroxynitrite;, protein phosphorylation; ⊕, stimulation; ⋈ and X, inhibition or blockade.

of high nitric oxide and superoxide anion concentrations generate significant amounts of peroxynitrite, see e.g. [162,169]. In this oxidative scenario, the calcium-entry transport systems more relevant for the control of neuronal cytosolic calcium homeostasis associated with lipid rafts nanodomains, NMDA and AMPA receptors and L-VOCC, are strongly activated by peroxynitrite, see the section 5.1 of this chapter. This produces a large peak of calcium concentration within these nanodomains, large enough to elicit a large increase of cytosolic calcium and a strong stimulation of nNOS, leading to an intracellular burst of nitric oxide, and stimulation of the neuronal metabolic activity and associated intracellular superoxide anion generation, oxidative conditions that generate intracellular peroxynitrite. In turn, these intracellular oxidative conditions produce the release of calcium from endoplasmic reticulum and mitochondria (see the section 5.2 of this chapter), contributing to a further and more widespread rise of cytosolic calcium concentration, and partial inactivation of the extrusion systems of the neuronal plasma membrane, PMCA and NCX (see the section 5.3 of this chapter). These latter effects lead to impairment of the ability of neurons to restore the low cytosolic calcium concentration needed for their normal function, and as a result lead to a long-lasting rise of cytosolic calcium concentration which can eventually reach the level that elicits a rapid necrotic death. Thus, impairment of the calcium transport systems of nanodomains associated with lipid rafts results in generation of an intracellular ROS/RNS oxidative stress that amplifies the oxidative stress suffered by exposure of neurons to a combined ROS/RNS extracellular oxidative stress (Figure 2d). Indeed, many experimental studies have shown that pharmacological compounds that inhibit the calcium currents through NMDA and AMPA receptors and L-VOCC behave as protection agents against neuronal death in inflammatory brain insults.

Experimental evidences have pointed out that there is a large mesh/network of lipid rafts-associated nanodomains in the plasma membrane of the soma of primary cultures of cerebellar granule neurons, where they are particularly enriched in neuron/neuron contact areas [130], and microscopy images have also shown a distribution map that closely overlap with the distribution map of flavoproteins bound to the plasma membrane [130,261], consistent with the association of the flavoproteins nNOS and cytochrome b_5 reductase with these nanodomains. Because of the strong impairment of the activity of calcium transport systems present in these nanodomains by many ROS/RNS that can be generated in the neuronal cytoplasm under a variety of cellular stress conditions, it should be expected that even exposure of neurons to a relatively mild oxidative stress should elicit a partial failure of the control of calcium homeostasis within these neurons. Owing to the large intracellular space occupied by nuclei in these neurons, partial failure in the control of cytosolic calcium homeostasis should elicit significant fluctuations of the cytosolic calcium concentration even in the absence of neuronal stimulation. The occurrence of basal endogenous oscillations of the cytosolic calcium concentration have been reported in *in vitro* cultures of different types of neurons, see for example [186,262-264]. We have recorded synchronized fluctuations of the cytosolic calcium concentration in primary cultures of rat cerebellar granule neurons, of an average amplitude of ±0.15 units of the ratio 340/380 in cells loaded with fura-2, by simply increasing the intensity of UV-irradiation in the epifluorescence microscope [Marques-da-Silva D and Gutierrez-Merino C, *unpublished results*], conditions that promote an increase of H_2O_2 production by cellular flavoproteins. The implication of nanodomains associated with lipid rafts in the generation of these cytosolic calcium fluctuations is unravelled by their attenuation by specific inhibitors or blockers of the calcium transport systems associated with these nanodomains. In this particular case the calcium entry through L-VOCC plays a major role in the modulation of the amplitude of the UV-induced fluctuations of cytosolic calcium concentrations. However, it is to be noted that other calcium transport systems associated with lipid rafts can also play a major role under different experimental conditions, as it has been shown that NCX interactions with another proteins bound to lipid rafts can elicit cytosolic calcium oscillations in oocytes [265].

6.1. The role and relevance of cytosolic calcium buffering systems

The activation of a channel with a typical conductance of 2.6 pS, like that of some calcium channels, can generate a calcium diffusion sub-microcompartment where the calcium concentration is higher than 1 μM, but the effective dimensions of this volume element is largely dependent upon the calcium buffering capacity of the microenvironment, increasing from only several nanometers with a millimolar calcium buffering capacity up to 82 nm in presence of a calcium buffering capacity equal to that afforded by 0.1 mM fura-2 [258]. The higher the conductance of the calcium channel, the higher the effective dimension of this sub-microcompartment. Using the equations derived in [260], for channels with unitary calcium conductances in the range of 20 to 40 pS, i.e. that of L-VOCC and NMDA receptors (section 2.1 of this chapter), effective dimensions of a sub-microcompartment with calcium concentrations higher than 1 μM can extend to several hundreds of nanometers taking into account that only micromolar concentrations of calcium buffering systems are present in the neuronal cytosol (Figure 2a). Because of the high neurotoxicity of cytosolic calcium concentrations in the micromolar range, a decrease of the calcium buffering capacity of the cytosol shall increase the propensity for rapid degeneration of neurons.

On these grounds, it can be easily understood that the role of the cytosolic calcium buffering in neurons has attracted considerable interest, not only because of the abundance of calcium-binding proteins in the nervous system but also because of the specificity of their regional distribution in the brain. It is also relevant herein to note that an altered expression of the major calcium-binding proteins has been noticed in damaged brain regions of patients suffering from acute insults, such as stroke or epileptic seizures, and from chronic human neurodegenerative disorders which develop with an enhanced oxidative stress in the brain, such as Alzheimer's, Huntington's, Parkinson's and Pick's diseases [266]. Several of the major calcium-buffering proteins present in the brain have been reported to show altered expression levels in degenerating brain regions, namely, parvalbumin, calbindin-D28K and S100, all of them members of the EF-hand calcium binding proteins like the calcium-binding protein calmodulin ubiquitously expressed in all mammalian cells. Furthermore, it has been proposed that the lack of calcium buffering proteins parvalbumin and calbindin-D28K may be considered one of the factors that render human motor neurons particularly vulnerable to calcium toxicity following glutamate receptor activation in amyotrophic lateral sclerosis [267]. Consistently, it has been reported that parvalbumin overexpression delays disease onset in a transgenic model of familial amyotrophic lateral sclerosis [268], a devastating and oxidative stress-mediated neurodegenerative disease of the brain.

Because of the high relevance of calmodulin as a multifunctional modulator of cellular calcium homeostasis and also of cellular calcium signalling pathways [4-6], this is the calcium binding protein of the EF-hand family whose functional and structural alterations by ROS have been more extensively studied [269]. In this regard, calmodulin-dependent proteins particularly relevant for the control of calcium homeostasis in neurons are the calcium transport systems

PMCA and IP_3-receptors, see above. In addition, calmodulin modulates signalling pathways controlling neuronal activity and synaptic plasticity like the protein phosphatase calcineurin, CaMK and IQ motif-containing proteins, such as myosins, Ras exchange proteins and GAP-43 among others [141,270,271]. Noteworthy, the activity of calcineurin has been reported to be decreased in sporadic and familial amyotrophic lateral sclerosis [272]. Calmodulin has been shown to become more oxidized in aged animals [269], pointing out that the physiological oxidative stress developed in the tissues is enough to lead to a sustained chemical modification of this protein. *In vitro* calmodulin suffers chemical oxidative modifications upon exposure to either H_2O_2 or peroxynitrite, for a review on this topic see [269]. Two vicinal methionine residues close to the carboxyl-terminus of calmodulin, Met-144 and Met145, are oxidized to methionine sulfoxide in aged tissues and also by H_2O_2 and more efficiently by peroxynitrite. Calmodulin oxidation leads to inhibition of the target proteins by non-productive association and stabilization of their inactive state. This has been experimentally demonstrated for the PMCA [273-275]. The oxidation of these methionines is reversible *in vivo*, as methionine sulfoxide reductases can efficiently reduce them back to methionine, restoring normal calmodulin function [269]. The fact that in aged tissues this oxidation is not fully reverted indicates a functional loss of this recycling process during aging. Thus, oxidation of calmodulin leads to a transient inactivation of neuronal PMCA. On these grounds, the fact that high levels of expression of calcium binding proteins are observed in neurons expressing nNOS [276-279] can be seen as a protective mechanism to attenuate long-lasting calcium transients in these neurons, which could eventually elicit cell death through calpains activation.

The widespread expression of calmodulin in the brain, its high level of expression in neurons relative to other cell types and its pleiotropic cellular functions confer a high relevance to the oxidative modifications of this protein by ROS/RNS. Regarding specifically the calcium transport systems associated with lipid rafts nanodomains, a loss of functional calmodulin leads to a marked decrease of the CaMK activity and this, in turn, leads to a decrease of the activity of the calcium entry systems L-VOCC and AMPA and NMDA receptors. As a result, the calcium concentration within these sub-microcompartments will be lowered up to levels closer to those found in the overall cytosol. Although the PMCA will also be inhibited, this inhibition by itself cannot compensate a large decrease of the inward calcium currents for two major reasons: (i) in neurons PMCA is also stimulated by phosphatidylserine and in these cells calmodulin stimulation is weak relative to other cell types [280], and (ii) the higher potency for transport across the open calcium channels of L-VOCC and NMDA receptors with respect to that of PMCA. Therefore, these nanodomains can eventually enter in a latent state regarding calcium and nitric oxide signalling in neurons. A simple and rational hypothesis merges from this conclusion, namely, that this could be a molecular mechanism underlying the observed loss of neuronal threshold excitability in aging and brain neurodegeneration. Owing to its putative relevance for the search of new therapeutic drugs and treatments for slow-developing neurodegenerative processes, this hypothesis deserve to be experimentally assessed in future studies.

7. Concluding remarks

The organization of the major calcium transport systems controlling the cytosolic calcium homeostasis within nanodomains of the neuronal plasma membrane associated with lipid rafts is opening new perspectives for regulation and deregulation of calcium signalling in neurons. In addition to the relevance of this fact for the efficient neuronal function in brain associative structures, like the concerted activity in neuronal circuits and LTP, the co-localization of ROS/RNS enzyme sources within these nanodomains is of particular relevance for neurodegenerative insults and diseases. The basic reason for this conclusion is that the calcium transport systems playing a major role in cytosolic calcium homeostasis and calcium-mediated neuronal activity are highly sensitive to modulation by ROS/RNS, and that oxidative stress is a common feature observed during the development of brain damage elicited in the most frequent brain insults and neurodegenerative diseases of high prevalence in humans. Yet, the actual knowledge of the molecular structure and plasticity of these nanodomains is still very limited, both in terms of their molecular composition in different types of neurons and of the factors controlling its formation and structural organization. Moreover, the molecular mechanisms leading to deregulation of the ROS/RNS enzyme sources associated with these nanodomains remain to be established, as well as the structural changes induced in these nanodomains by exposure to the different ROS/RNS that are generated in neurodegenerative insults and diseases. Because of the central role of cytosolic calcium in the control of neuronal activity, plasticity and survival it can be foreseen that these nanodomains will become a relevant pharmacological target in the search for alternate and novel therapies aiming to prevent or slowdown neurodegenerative processes in the brain.

Abbreviations used in the text

AAPH, 2,2'- azobis (2-amidinopropane) dihydrochloride; AMPA, α-amino-3-hydroxy-5-methylisoxazole-4-propionic acid; CaMKII, calcium/calmodulin-dependent protein kinase, isoform II; Cb_5R, cytochrome b_5 reductase; cGMP, 3′,5′-cyclic guanosine monophosphate; CNS, central nervous system; COX, cyclooxygenase; EDTA, ethylenediamine-tetraacetic acid; FRET, fluorescence resonance energy transfer; LTP, long-term post-synaptic potentiation; NCX, sodium-calcium exchanger; NMDA, N-methyl-D-aspartate; nNOS, neuronal nitric oxide synthase; NOX, ROS-generating NADPH oxidases; PKA, protein kinase A; PKC, protein kinase C; PMCA, plasma membrane calcium pump; ROS, reactive oxygen species; RNS, reactive nitrogen species; SIN-1, 3-morpholinosydnonimine; SOCE, store-operated calcium entry; UV, ultraviolet; VOCC, voltage-operated caclium channels (L-VOCC, L-type VOCC; N-VOCC, N-type VOCC; etc).

Acknowledgements

This work has been supported by Grant BFU2011-30178 of the Spanish Plan Nacional de I+D +I and by Grant GR10092 of the Gobierno de Extremadura to the Research Group "Estrés oxidativo y bioenergética en neuronas y cerebro", both with co-financing by the European Funds for Structural Development (FEDER). DMS and SF have been supported by predoctoral fellowships of the Spanish Ministerio de Ciencia y Tecnología and of the Portuguese Fundação para a Ciência e a Tecnologia (FCT), respectively, and AKSA by a post-doctoral fellowship of the Gobierno de Extremadura with FEDER co-financing (reference number RE000008).

Author details

Carlos Gutierrez-Merino, Dorinda Marques-da-Silva, Sofia Fortalezas and Alejandro K. Samhan-Arias

*Address all correspondence to: carlosgm@unex.es

Dept. Biochemistry and Molecular Biology, School of Sciences, University of Extremadura, Badajoz, Spain

References

[1] Franklin JL, Johnson EMJr. Suppression of programmed neuronal death by sustained elevation of cytoplasmic calcium. Trends Neurosci 1992;15: 501-508.

[2] Franklin JL, Johnson EMJr. Block of neuronal apoptosis by a sustained increase of steady-state free Ca2+ concentration. Philos Trans R Soc Lond B Biol Sci 1994;345: 251-256.

[3] Mattson MP, Chan SL. Neuronal and glial calcium signaling in Alzheimer's disease. Cell Calcium 2003;34: 385-397.

[4] Berridge MJ. Neuronal calcium signaling. Neuron 1998;21: 13-26.

[5] Berridge MJ, Lipp P, Bootman MD. The versatility and universality of calcium signalling. Nat Rev Mol Cell Biol 2000; 1: 11-21.

[6] Carafoli E, Santella L, Branca D, Brini M. Generation, control, and processing of cellular calcium signals. Crit Rev Biochem Mol Biol 2001;36: 107-260.

[7] Carafoli E. Calcium signaling: a tale for all seasons. Proc Natl Acad Sci USA 2002;99: 1115-1122.

[8] Baimbridge KG, Celio MR, Rogers JH. Calcium-binding proteins in the nervous system. Trends Neurosci 1992;15: 303-308.

[9] Gutierrez-Martin Y, Martin-Romero FJ, Henao F, Gutierrez-Merino C. Alteration of cytosolic free calcium homeostasis by SIN-1: high sensitivity of L-type Ca2+ channels

to extracellular oxidative/nitrosative stress in cerebellar granule cells. J Neurochem 2005;92: 973-989.

[10] Martin-Romero FJ, Garcia-Martin E, Gutierrez-Merino C. Inhibition of the oxidative stress produced by plasma membrane NADH oxidase delays low-potassium induced apoptosis of cerebellar granule cells. J Neurochem 2002;82: 705–715.

[11] Harold FM. The Vital Force: A Study of Bioenergetics. New York: WH Freeman and Co; 1986.

[12] Tsien RW, Lipscombe D, Madison DV, Bley KR, Fox AP. Multiple types of neuronal calcium channels and their selective modulation. Trends Neurosci 1988;11: 431-438.

[13] Forti L, Tottene A, Moretti A, Pietrobon D. Three novel types of voltage-dependent calcium channels in rat cerebellar neurons. J Neurosci 1994;14: 5243-5256.

[14] Olivera BM, Miljanich GP, Ramachandran J, Adams ME. Calcium channel diversity and neurotransmitter release: the omega-conotoxins and omega-agatoxins. Annu Rev Biochem 1994;63: 823-867.

[15] Catterall WA. Structure and function of voltage-gated ion channels. Annu Rev Biochem 1995;64: 493-531.

[16] Hammond C., editor. Cellular and Molecular Neurobiology. San Diego: Academic Press; 1996.

[17] Tottene A, Moretti A, Pietrobon D. Functional diversity of P-type and R-type calcium channels in rat cerebellar neurons. J Neurosci 1996;16: 6353-6363.

[18] Schild D, Geiling H, Bischofberger J. Imaging of L-type Ca2+ channels in olfactory bulb neurones using fluorescent dihydropyridine and a styryl dye. J Neurosci Methods 1995;59: 183-190.

[19] Cohen R, Atlas D. R-type voltage-gated Ca(2+) channel interacts with synaptic proteins and recruits synaptotagmin to the plasma membrane of Xenopus oocytes. Neuroscience 2004;128: 831-841.

[20] Khanna R, Sun L, Li Q, Guo L, Stanley EF. Long splice variant N type calcium channels are clustered at presynaptic transmitter release sites without modular adaptor proteins. Neuroscience 2006;138: 1115-1125.

[21] Tai C, Kuzmiski JB, MacVicar BA. Muscarinic enhancement of R-type calcium currents in hippocampal CA1 pyramidal neurons. J Neurosci 2006;26: 6249-6258.

[22] Marchetti C, Usai C. High affinity block by nimodipine of the internal calcium elevation in chronically depolarized rat cerebellar granule neurons. Neurosci Lett 1996;207: 77-80.

[23] Maric D, Maric I, Barker JL. Developmental changes in cell calcium homeostasis during neurogenesis of the embryonic rat cerebral cortex. Cereb Cortex 2000;10: 561-573.

[24] Arakawa Y, Nishijima C, Shimizu N, Urushidani T. Survival-promoting activity of nimodipine and nifedipine in rat motoneurons: implications of an intrinsic calcium toxicity in motoneurons. J Neurochem 2002;83: 150-156.

[25] Ertel EA, Campbell KP, Harpold MM, Hofmann F, Mori Y, Perez-Reyes E, Schwartz A, Snutch TP, Tanabe T, Birnbaumer L, Tsien RW, Catterall WA. Nomenclature of voltage-gated calcium channels. Neuron 2000;25: 533–535.

[26] Catterall WA. Structure and regulation of voltage-gated Ca2+ Channels. Annu Rev Cell Dev Biol 2000;16: 521–555.

[27] Clark NC, Nagano N, Kuenzi FM, Jarolimek W, Huber I, Walter D, Wietzorrek G, Boyce S, Kullmann DM, Striessnig J, Seabrook GR. Neurological phenotypeand synaptic function in mice lacking the CaV1.3 alpha subunit of neuronal L-type voltage-dependent Ca2+ channels. Neuroscience 2003;120: 435 – 442.

[28] Moosmang S, Haider N, Klugbauer N, Adelsberger H, Langwieser N, Müller J, Stiess M, Marais E, Schulla V, Lacinova L, Goebbels S, Nave KA, Storm DR, Hofmann F, Kleppisch T. Role of hippocampal Cav1.2 Ca2+ channels in NMDA receptor-independent synaptic plasticity and spatial memory. J Neurosci 2005;25: 9883 – 9892.

[29] Kamp TJ, Hell JW. Regulation of Cardiac L-Type Calcium Channels by Protein Kinase A and Protein Kinase C. Circ Res 2000;87: 1095-1102.

[30] Davare MA, Dong F, Rubin CS, Hell JW. The A-kinase anchor protein MAP2B and cAMP-dependent protein kinase are associated with class C L-type calcium channels in neurons. J Biol Chem 1999;274: 30280–30287.

[31] De Jongh KS, Murphy BJ, Colvin AA, Hell JW, Takahashi M, Catterall WA. Specific phosphorylation of a site in the full-length form of the alpha 1 subunit of the cardiac L-type calcium channel by adenosine 3',5'-cyclic monophosphate-dependent protein kinase. Biochemistry 1996;35: 10392–10340.

[32] Mitterdorfer J, Froschmayr M, Grabner M, Moebius FF, Glossmann H, Striessnig J. Identification of PK-A phosphorylation sites in the carboxyl terminus of L-type calcium channel alpha 1 subunits. Biochemistry 1996;35: 9400–9406.

[33] Gao T, Yatani A, Dell'Acqua ML, Sako H, Green SA, Dascal N, Scott JD, Hosey MM. cAMP-dependent regulation of cardiac L-type Ca2+ channels requires membrane targeting of PKA and phosphorylation of channel subunits. Neuron 1997;19: 185–196.

[34] Puri TS, Gerhardstein BL, Zhao XL, Ladner MB, Hosey MM. Differential effects of subunit interactions on protein kinase A- and C-mediated phosphorylation of L-type calcium channels. Biochemistry 1997;36: 9605–9615.

[35] Bünemann M, Gerhardstein BL, Gao T, Hosey MM. Functional Regulation of L-type Calcium Channels via Protein Kinase A-mediated Phosphorylation of the β2 Subunit. J Biol Chem 1999;274: 33851–33854.

[36] Grueter CE, Abiria SA, Dzhura I, Wu Y, Ham AJL, Mohler PJ, Anderson ME, Colbran RJ. L-Type Ca2+ Channel Facilitation Mediated by Phosphorylation of the β Subunit by CaMKII. Mol Cell 2006;23: 641–650.

[37] Pinard CR, Mascagni F, McDonald AJ. Neuronal localization of Cav1.2 L-type calcium channels in the rat basolateral amygdala. Brain Res 2005;1064: 52 – 55.

[38] Hudmon A, Schulman H, Kim J, Maltez JM, Tsien RW, Pitt GS. CaMKII tethers to L-type Ca2+ channels, establishing a local and dedicated integrator of Ca2+ signals for facilitation. J Cell Biol 2005;171: 537–547.

[39] Lee TS, Karl R, Moosmang S, Lenhardt P, Klugbauer N, Hofmann F, Kleppisch T, Welling A. Calmodulin kinase II is involved in voltage-dependent facilitation of the L-type Cav1.2 calcium channel: Identification of the phosphorylation sites. J Biol Chem 2006;281: 25560–25567.

[40] Grueter CE, Abiria SA, Wu Y, Anderson ME, Colbran RJ. Differential regulated interactions of calcium/calmodulin-dependent protein kinase II with isoforms of voltage-gated calcium channel beta subunits. Biochemistry 2008;47: 1760-1767.

[41] O-Uchi J, Komukai K, Kusakari Y, Obata T, Hongo K, Sasaki H, Kurihara S. Alpha1-adrenoceptor stimulation potentiates L-type Ca2+ current through Ca2+/calmodulin-dependent PK II (CaMKII) activation in rat ventricular myocytes. Proc Natl Acad Sci USA 2005;102: 9400–9405.

[42] Gao L, Blair LA, Salinas GD, Needleman LA, Marshall J. Insulin-like growth factor-1 modulation of CaV1.3 calcium channels depends on Ca2+ release from IP3-sensitive stores and calcium/calmodulin kinase II phosphorylation of the alpha1 subunit EF hand. J Neurosci 2006;26: 6259–6268.

[43] Brown AM, Deutch AY, Colbran RJ. Dopamine depletion alters phosphorylation of striatal proteins in a model of Parkinsonism. Eur J Neurosci 2005;22: 247–256.

[44] Choi DW, Rothman SM. The role of glutamate neurotoxicity in hypoxic-ischemic neuronal death. Annu Rev Neurosci 1990;13: 171-182.

[45] Choi DW. Glutamate neurotoxicity and diseases of the nervous system. Neuron 1998;1: 623–634.

[46] Robertson SJ, Ennion SJ, Evans RJ, Edwards FA. Synaptic P2X receptors. Curr Opin Neurobiol 2001;11: 378-386.

[47] Huettner JE. Kainate receptors and synaptic transmission. Prog Neurobiol 2003;70: 387-407.

[48] Dingledine R., McBain C.J. Glutamate and aspartate. In: Siegel G.J., Agranoff B.W., Albers R.W., Fisher S.K., Uhler M.D. (eds.). Basic Neurochemistry. Molecular, Cellular and Medical Aspects (6th ed.). Philadelphia: Lippincott Williams & Wilkins; 1998. p. 315-333.

[49] Contestabile A. Roles of NMDA receptor activity and nitric oxide production in brain development. Brain Res Brain Res Rev 2000;32: 476-509.

[50] Smith TC, Wang L-Y, Howe JR. Heterogeneous conductance levels of native AMPA receptors. J Neurosci 2000;20: 2073-2085.

[51] Mothet JP, Parent AT, Wolosker H, Brady ROJr, Linden DJ, Ferris CD, Rogawski MA, Snyder SH. D-serine is an endogenous ligand for the glycine site of the N-methyl-D-aspartate receptor. Proc Natl Acad Sci USA 2000;97: 4926-4931.

[52] Derkach V, Barria A, Soderling TR. Ca2+/calmodulin-kinase II enhances channel conductance of alpha-amino-3-hydroxy-5-methyl-4-isoxazolepropionate type glutamate receptors. Proc Natl Acad Sci USA 1999;96: 3269–3274.

[53] Hayashi Y, Shi SH, Esteban JA, Piccini A, Poncer JC, Malinow R. Driving AMPA receptors into synapses by LTP and CaMKII: requirement for GluR1 and PDZ domain interaction.Science 2000;287: 2262–2267.

[54] Boehm J, Kang MG, Johnson RC, Esteban J, Huganir RL, Malinow R. Synaptic incorporation of AMPA receptors during LTP is controlled by a PKC phosphorylation site on GluR1. Neuron 2006;51: 213–225.

[55] Kohr G, Eckardt S, Luddens H, Monyer H, Seeburg PH. NMDA receptor channels: subunit-specific potentiation by reducing agents. Neuron 1994;12: 1031-1040.

[56] Rumbaugh G, Vicini S. Distinct synaptic and extrasynaptic NMDA receptors in developing cerebellar granule neurons. J Neurosci 1999;19: 10603-10610.

[57] Petralia RS, Wang YX, Hua F, Yi Z, Zhou A, Ge L, Stephenson FA, Wenthold RJ. Organization of NMDA receptors at extrasynaptic locations. Neuroscience 2010;167:68-87.

[58] Li ST, Ju JG. Functional roles of synaptic and extrasynaptic NMDA receptors in physiological and pathological neuronal activities. Curr Drug Targets 2012;13: 207-221.

[59] Leonard AS, Hell JW. Cyclic AMP-dependent Protein Kinase and Protein Kinase C Phosphorylate N-Methyl-D-aspartate Receptors at Different Sites. J Biol Chem 1997;272: 12107–12115.

[60] Tingley WG, Ehlers MD, Kameyama K, Doherty C, Ptak JB, Riley CT, Huganir RL. Characterization of Protein Kinase A and Protein Kinase C Phosphorylation of the N-Methyl-D-aspartate Receptor NR1 Subunit Using Phosphorylation Site-specific Antibodies. J Biol Chem 1997;272: 5157–5166.

[61] Fill M, Copello JA. Ryanodine receptor calcium release channels. Physiol Rev 2002;82: 893-922.

[62] Hamilton SL. Ryanodine receptors. Cell Calcium 2005;38: 253-260.

[63] Mikoshiba K. Inositol 1,4,5-trisphosphate IP(3) receptors and their role in neuronal cell function. J Neurochem 2006;97: 1627-1633.

[64] Hidalgo C. Cross talk between Ca2+ and redox signalling cascades in muscle and neurons through the combined activation of ryanodine receptors/Ca2+ release channels. Philos Trans R Soc Lond B Biol Sci 2005;360: 2237-2246.

[65] Paschen W, Frandsen A. Endoplasmic reticulum dysfunction-a common denominator for cell injury in acute and degenerative diseases of the brain? J Neurochem 2001;79: 719-725.

[66] Montero M, Alvarez J, Garcia-Sancho J. Agonist-induced Ca2+ influx in human neutrophils is secondary to the emptying of intracellular calcium stores. Biochem J 1991;277: 73-79.

[67] Parekh AB, Putney JWJr. Store-operated calcium channels. Physiol Rev 2005;85: 757-810.

[68] Arakawa N, Sakaue M, Yokoyama I, Hashimoto H, Koyama Y, Baba A, Matsuda T. KB-R7943 inhibits store-operated Ca(2+) entry in cultured neurons and astrocytes. Biochem Biophys Res Commun 2000;279: 354-357.

[69] Jia Y, Zhou J, Tai Y, Wang Y. TRPC channels promote cerebellar granule neuron survival. Nat Neurosci 2007 ;10 : 559-567.

[70] Selvaraj S, Sun Y, Watt JA, Wang S, Lei S, Birnbaumer L, Singh BB. Neurotoxin-induced ER stress in mouse dopaminergic neurons involves downregulation of TRPC1 and inhibition of AKT/mTOR signaling. J Clin Invest 2012;122: 1354-1367.

[71] Smaili SS, Hsu YT, Youle RJ, Russell JT. Mitochondria in Ca2+ signaling and apoptosis. J Bioenerg Biomembr 2000;32: 35-46.

[72] Simpson PB. The local control of cytosolic Ca2+ as a propagator of CNS communication-integration of mitochondrial transport mechanisms and cellular responses. J Bioenerg Biomembr 2000;32: 5-13.

[73] Crompton M. The mitochondrial permeability transition pore and its role in cell death. Biochem J. 1999;341: 233-249.

[74] Garcia-Martin E, Gutierrez-Merino C. Rate of Na+/Ca2+ exchange across the plasma membrane of synaptosomes measured using the fluorescence of chlorotetracycline. Implications to calcium homeostasis in synaptic terminals. Biochim Biophys Acta 1996;1280: 257-264.

[75] Garcia ML, Strehler EE. Plasma membrane calcium ATPases as critical regulators of calcium homeostasis during neuronal cell function. Front Biosci 1999;4: D869–D882.

[76] Gill DL, Chueh SH, Whitlow LC. Functional importance of the synaptic plasma membrane calcium pump and sodium-calcium exchanger. J Biol Chem 1984;259: 10807-10813.

[77] Guerini D, García-Martín E, Gerber A, Volbracht C, Leist M, Gutierrez-Merino C, Carafoli E. The expression of plasma membrane Ca2+ pump isoforms in cerebellar granule neurons is modulated by cytosolic free Ca2+. J Biol Chem 1999;274: 1667-1676.

[78] Kip SN, Gray NW, Burette A, Canbay A, Weinberg RJ, Strehler EE. Changes in the expression of plasma membrane calcium extrusion systems during the maturation of hippocampal neurons. Hippocampus 2006;16: 20-34.

[79] Hilfiker H, Guerini D, Carafoli E. Cloning and expression of isoform 2 of the human plasma membrane Ca2+ ATPase. Functional properties of the enzyme and its splicing products. J Biol Chem 1994;269: 26178-26183.

[80] Condrescu M, Reeves JP. Actin-dependent regulation of the cardiac Na+/Ca2+ exchanger. Am J Physiol Cell Physiol 2006;290: C691-C701.

[81] O′ Connell KMM, Martens JR, Tamkun MM. Localization of ion channels to lipid raft domains within the cardiovascular system. Trends Cardiovasc Med 2004;14: 37–42.

[82] Gunter TE, Yule DI, Gunter KK, Eliseev RA, Salter JD. Calcium and mitochondria. FEBS Lett 2004;567: 96-102.

[83] Pike LJ. Rafts defined: a report on the keystone symposium on lipid rafts and cell function. J Lipid Res 2006;47: 1597–1598.

[84] Head BP, Insel PA. Do caveolins regulate cells by actions outside of caveolae? Trends Cell Biol 2007;17: 51–57.

[85] Gabella G. Caveolae intracellulares and sarcoplasmic reticulum in smooth muscle. J Cell Sci 1971;8: 601–609.

[86] Popescu LM, Diculescu I, Zelck U, Ionescu N. Ultrastructural distribution of calcium in smooth muscle cells of guinea-pig taenia coli. A correlated electron microscopic and quantitative study. Cell Tissue Res 1974;154: 357–378.

[87] Brazer SC, Singh BB, Liu X, Swaim W, Ambudkar IS. Caveolin-1 contributes to assembly of store-operated Ca2+ influx channels by regulating plasma membrane localization of TRPC1. J Biol Chem 2003;278: 27208–27215.

[88] Murata T, Lin MI, Stan RV, Bauer PM, Yu J, Sessa WC. Genetic evidence supporting caveolae microdomain regulation of calcium entry in endothelial cells. J Biol Chem 2007;282: 16631–16643.

[89] Anderson RG. The caveolae membrane system. Annu Rev Biochem 1998;67: 199–225.

[90] Fra AM, Masserini M, Palestini P, Sonnino S, Simons K. A photo-reactive derivative of ganglioside GM1 specifically cross-links VIP21-caveolin on the cell surface. FEBS Lett 1995;375: 11-14.

[91] Murata M, Peranen J, Schreiner R, Weiland F, Kurzchalia T, Simons K. VIP21/caveolin is a cholesterol-binding protein. Proc Natl Acad Sci USA 1995;92: 10339–10343.

[92] Thiele C, Hannah MJ, Fahrenholz F, Huttner WB. Cholesterol binds to synaptophysin and is required for biogenesis of synaptic vesicles. Nat Cell Biol 2000;2: 42-49.

[93] Smart EJ, Ying Y-S, Donzell WC, Anderson RGW. A Role for Caveolin in Transport of Cholesterol from Endoplasmic Reticulum to Plasma Membrane. J Biol Chem 1996;271: 29427–29435.

[94] Toselli M, Biella G, Taglietti V, Cazzaniga E, Parenti M. Caveolin-1 expression and membrane cholesterol content modulate N-type calcium channel activity in NG108-15 cells. Biophys J 2005;89: 2443–2457.

[95] Head BP, Patel HH, Tsutsumi YM, Hu Y, Mejia T, Mora RC, Insel PA, Roth DM, Drummond JC, Patel PM. Caveolin-1 expression is essential for N-methyl-D-aspartate receptor-mediated Src and extracellular signal-regulated kinase 1/2 activation and protection of primary neurons from ischemic cell death. FASEB J 2008;22: 828–840.

[96] Razani B, Woodman SE, Lisanti MP. Caveolae: From Cell Biology to Animal Physiology. Pharmacol Rev 2002;54: 431–467.

[97] van Deurs B, Roepstorff K, Hommelgaard AM, Sandvig K. Caveolae: anchored, multifunctional platforms in the lipid ocean. Trends Cell Biol 2003;13: 92-100.

[98] Pouvreau S, Berthier C, Blaineau S, Amsellem J, Coronado R, Strube C. Membrane cholesterol modulates dihydropyridine receptor function in mice fetal skeletal muscle cells. J Physiol 2004;555: 365-381.

[99] Tsujikawa H, Song Y, Watanabe M, Masumiya H, Gupte SA, Ochi R, Okada T. Cholesterol depletion modulates basal L-type Ca2+ current and abolishes its β-adrenergic enhancement in ventricular myocytes. Am J Physiol Heart Circ Physiol 2008;294: H285–H292.

[100] Waseem TV, Kolos VA, Lapatsina LP, Fedorovich SV. Influence of cholesterol depletion in plasma membrane of rat brain synaptosomes on calcium-dependent and calcium-independent exocytosis. Neurosci Lett 2006;405: 106–110.

[101] Fielding CJ, Fielding PE. Intracellular cholesterol transport. J Lipid Res 1997;38: 1503–1521.

[102] Bu J, Bruckner SR, Sengoku T, Geddes JW, Estus S. Glutamate regulates caveolin expression in rat hippocampal neurons. J Neurosci Res 2003;72: 185-190.

[103] Gaudreault SB, Dea D, Poirier J. Increased caveolin-1 expression in Alzheimer's disease brain. Neurobiol Aging 2004;25: 753-759.

[104] Drab M, Verkade P, Elger M, Kasper M, Lohn M, Lauterbach B, Menne J, Lindschau C, Mende F, Luft FC, Schedl A, Haller H, Kurzxhalia TV. Loss of caveolae, vascular

dysfunction, and pulmonary defects in caveolin-1 gene disrupted mice. Science 2001;293: 2449-2452.

[105] Simons K, Ehehalt R. Cholesterol lipid rafts, and disease. J Clin Invest 2002;110: 597-603.

[106] Cohen AW, Hnasko R, Schubert W, Lisanti P. Role of caveolae and caveolins in health and disease. Physiol Rev 2004;84: 1341-1379.

[107] Balijepalli RC, Foell JD, Hall DD, Hell JW, Kamp TJ. Localization of cardiac L-type Ca2+ channels to a caveolar macromolecular signaling complex is required for b2-adrenergic regulation. Proc Natl Acad Sci USA 2006;103: 7500–7505.

[108] Marques-da-Silva D, Samhan-Arias AK, Tiago T, Gutierrez-Merino C. L-type calcium channels and cytochrome b5 reductase are components of protein complexes tightly associated with lipid rafts microdomains of the neuronal plasma membrane. J Proteomics 2010;73: 1502-1510.

[109] Razani B, Rubin CS, Lisanti MP. Regulation of cAMP-mediated Signal Transduction via Interaction of Caveolins with the Catalytic Subunit of Protein Kinase A. J Biol Chem 1999;274: 26353–26360.

[110] Suzuki T, Du F, Tian Q-B, Zhang J, Endo S. Ca2+/calmodulin-dependent protein kinase IIα clusters are associated with stable lipid rafts and their formation traps PSD-95. J Neurochem 2008;104: 596–610.

[111] Weick JP, Groth RD, Isaksen AL, Mermelstein PG. Interactions with PDZ proteins are required for L-type calcium channels to activate cAMP response element-binding protein-dependent gene expression. J Neurosci 2003;23: 3446–3456.

[112] Zhang H, Maximov A, Fu Y, Xu F, Tang TS, Tkatch T, Surmeier DJ, Bezprozvanny I. Association of CaV1.3 L-type calcium channels with Shank. J Neurosci 2005;25: 1037-1049.

[113] Prybylowski K, Chang K, Sans N, Kan L, Vicini S, Wenthold RJ. The synaptic localization of NR2B-containing NMDA receptors is controlled by interactions with PDZ proteins and AP-2. Neuron 2005;47: 845-857.

[114] Hering H, Lin C-C, Sheng M. Lipid Rafts in the Maintenance of Synapses, Dendritic Spines, and Surface AMPA Receptor Stability. J Neurosci 2003;23: 3262–3271.

[115] Besshoh S, Chen S, Brown IR, Gurd JW. Developmental Changes in the Association of NMDA Receptors With Lipid Rafts. J Neurosci Res 2007;85:1876–1883.

[116] Delínte-Ramirez I, Salcedo-Tello P, Bermudez-Rattoni F. Spatial memory formation induces recruitment of NMDA receptor and PSD-95 to synaptic lípid rafts. J Neurochem 2008;106: 1658–1668.

[117] Marques-da-Silva D, Gutierrez-Merino C. L-type voltage-operated calcium channels, N-methyl-D-aspartate receptors and neuronal nitric-oxide synthase form a calcium/

redox nano-transducer within lipid rafts. Biochem Biophys Res Commun 2012;420: 257-262.

[118] Delinte-Ramirez I, Fernández E, Bayés A, Kicsi E, Komiyama NH, Grant SGN. In Vivo Composition of NMDA Receptor Signaling Complexes Differs between Membrane Subdomains and Is Modulated by PSD-95 and PSD-93. J Neurosci 2010;30: 8162– 8170.

[119] Hou Q, Huang Y, Amato S, Snyder SH, Huganir RL, Man HY. Regulation of AMPA receptor localization in lipid rafts. Mol Cell Neurosci 2008;38: 213-223.

[120] Keith DJ, Sanderson JL, Gibson ES, Woolfrey KM, Robertson HR, Olszewski K, Kang R, El-Husseini A, Dell'acqua ML. Palmitoylation of A-kinase anchoring protein 79/150 regulates dendritic endosomal targeting and synaptic plasticity mechanisms. J Neurosci 2012;32: 7119-7136.

[121] Sepúlveda MR, Berrocal-Carrillo M, Gasset M, Mata AM. The plasma membrane Ca2+-ATPase isoform 4 is localized in lipid rafts of cerebellum synaptic plasma membranes. J Biol Chem 2006;281: 447-453.

[122] Jiang L, Fernandes D, Mehta N, Bean JL, Michaelis ML, Zaidi A. Partitioning of the plasma membrane Ca2+-ATPase into lipid rafts in primary neurons: effects of cholesterol depletion. J Neurochem 2007;102: 378–388.

[123] Vorherr T, Kessler T, Hofmann F, Carafoli E. The calmodulin-binding domain mediates the self-association of the plasma membrane Ca2+ pump. J Biol Chem 1991;266: 22–27.

[124] Kuszczak I, Samson SE, Pande J, Shen DQ, Grover AK. Sodium–calcium exchanger and lipid rafts in pig coronary artery smooth muscle. Biochim Biophys Acta 2011;1808: 589–596.

[125] Teubl M, Groschner K, Kohlwein SD, Mayer B, Schmidt K. Na+/Ca2+ exchange facilitates Ca2+-dependent activation of endothelial nitric-oxide synthase. J Biol Chem 1999;274: 29529-29535.

[126] Bossuyt J, Taylor BE, James-Kracke M, Hale CC. Evidence for cardiac sodium-calcium exchanger association with caveolin-3. FEBS Lett 2002;511: 113-117.

[127] Sato Y, Sagami I, Shimizu T. Identification of Caveolin-1-interacting Sites in Neuronal Nitric-oxide Synthase. J Biol Chem 2004;279: 8827–8836.

[128] Venema VJ, Ju H, Zou R, Venema RC. Interaction of neuronal nitric-oxide synthase with caveolin-3 in skeletal muscle. Identification of a novel caveolin scaffolding/ inhibitory domain. J Biol Chem 1997;272: 28187–28190.

[129] Samhan-Arias AK, Martin-Romero FJ, Gutierrez-Merino C. Kaempferol blocks oxidative stress in cerebellar granule cells and reveals a key role for the plasma membrane

NADH oxidase activity in the commitment of apoptosis. Free Radic Biol Med 2004;37: 48-61.

[130] Samhan-Arias AK, Garcia-Bereguiain MA, Martin-Romero FJ, Gutierrez-Merino C. Clustering of plasma membrane-bound cytochrome b5 reductase within 'lipid rafts' microdomains of the neuronal plasma membrane. Mol Cell Neurosci 2009;40: 14–26.

[131] Samhan-Arias AK, Marques-da-Silva D, Yanamala N, Gutierrez-Merino C. Stimulation and clustering of cytochrome b(5) reductase in caveolin-rich lipid microdomains is an early event in oxidative stress-mediated apoptosis of cerebellar granule neurons. J Proteomics 2012;75: 2934-2949.

[132] Tiago T, Aureliano M, Gutierrez-Merino C. Effects of reactive oxygen and nitrogen species on actomyosin and their implications for muscle contractility. In: Gutierrez-Merino C., Leeuwenburgh C. (eds.) Free Radicals in Biology and Medicine. Kerala: Research Signpost; 2008. p. 131-149.

[133] Brenman JE, Bredt DS. Synaptic signalling by nitric-oxide. Curr Opin Neurobiol 1997;7: 374–378.

[134] Bonfoco E, Leist M, Zhivotovsky B, Orrenius S, Lipton SA, Nicotera P. Cytoskeletal breakdown and apoptosis elicited by NO donors in cerebellar granule cells require NMDA receptor activation. J Neurochem 1996;67: 2484–2493.

[135] Leach RN, Desai JC, Orchard CH. Effect of cytoskeleton disruptors on L-type Ca channel distribution in rat ventricular myocytes. Cell Calcium 2005;38: 515-526.

[136] Gutierrez-Merino C. Redox modulation of neuronal calcium homeostasis and its deregulation by reactive oxygen species. In: Gutierrez-Merino C., Leeuwenburgh C. (eds.) Free Radicals in Biology and Medicine. Kerala: Research Signpost; 2008. p. 67-101.

[137] Hidalgo C, Donoso P. Crosstalk between calcium and redox signalling: from molecular mechanisms to health implications. Antioxid Redox Signal 2008;10: 1275-1312.

[138] Garcia-Bereguiain MA, Samhan-Arias AK, Martin-Romero FJ, Gutierrez-Merino C. Hydrogen sulfide raises cytosolic calcium in neurons through activation of L-type Ca2+ channels. Antioxid Redox Signal 2008;10: 31-42.

[139] Orrenius S, McConkey DJ, Bellomo G, Nicotera P. Role of Ca2+ in toxic cell killing. Trends Pharmacol Sci 1989;10: 281-285.

[140] Triffaró JM, Vitale ML. Cytoskeleton dynamics during neurotransmitter release. Trends Neurosci 1993;16: 466-472.

[141] Benowitz LI, Routtenberg A. GAP-43: an intrinsic determinant of neuronal development and plasticity. Trends Neurosci 1997;20: 84-91.

[142] Bizat N, Hermel J-M, Boyer F, Jacquard C, Créminon C, Ouary S, Escartin C, Hantraye P, Krajewski S, Brouillet E. Calpain Is a Major Cell Death Effector in Selective

Striatal Degeneration Induced In Vivo by 3-Nitropropionate: Implications for Huntington's Disease. J Neurosci 2003;23: 5020-5030.

[143] Volbracht C, Chua BT, Ng CP, Bahr BA, Hong W, Li P. The critical role of calpain versus caspase activation in excitotoxic injury induced by nitric oxide. J Neurochem 2005;93: 1280-1292.

[144] Lagoa R, Lopez-Sanchez C, Samhan-Arias AK, Gañan CM, Garcia-Martinez V, Gutierrez-Merino C. Kaempferol protects against rat striatal degeneration induced by 3-nitropropionic acid. J Neurochem 2009;111: 473-487.

[145] Valencia A, Morán J. Role of oxidative stress in the apoptotic cell death of cultured cerebellar granule cells. J Neurosci Res 2001;64: 284–297.

[146] van Damme P, Dewil M, Robberecht W, van den Bosch L. Excitotoxicity and amyotrophic lateral sclerosis. Neurodegener Dis 2005;2: 147-159.

[147] Thibault O, Gant JC, Landfield PW. Expansion of the calcium hypothesis of brain aging and Alzheimer's disease: minding the store. Aging Cell 2007;6: 307-317.

[148] Marx J. Alzheimer's disease. Fresh evidence points to an old suspect: calcium. Science 2007;318: 384-385.

[149] Mattson MP. Calcium and neurodegeneration. Aging Cell2007; 6: 337-350.

[150] Surmeier DJ. Calcium, ageing, and neuronal vulnerability in Parkinson's disease. Lancet Neurol 2007;6: 933-938.

[151] Ionov ID. Survey of ALS-associated factors potentially promoting Ca2+ overload of motor neurons. Amyotroph Lateral Scler 2007;8: 260-265.

[152] Craft JM, Watterson DM, Marks A, Van Eldik LJ. Enhanced susceptibility of S-100B transgenic mice to neuroinflammation and neuronal dysfunction induced by intracerebroventricular infusion of human beta-amyloid. Glia 2005;51: 209-216.

[153] Vesce S, Rossi D, Brambilla L, Volterra A. Glutamate release from astrocytes in physiological conditions and in neurodegenerative disorders characterized by neuroinflammation. Int Rev Neurobiol 2007;82: 57-71.

[154] Farber JL. The role of calcium ions in toxic cell injury. Environ Health Perspect 1990;84: 107-111.

[155] Mao GD, Poznansky MJ. Electron spin resonance study on the permeability of superoxide radicals in lipid bilayers and biological membranes. FEBS Lett 1992;305: 233-236.

[156] Bedard K, Krause KH. The NOX family of ROS-generating NADPH oxidases: physiology and pathophysiology. Physiol Rev 2007;87: 245-313.

[157] Martin-Romero FJ, Gutierrez-Martin Y, Henao F, Gutierrez-Merino C. The NADH oxidase activity of the plasma membrane of synaptosomes is a major source of superoxide anion and is inhibited by peroxynitrite. J Neurochem 2002;82: 604–614.

[158] Samhan-Arias AK, Duarte RO, Martin-Romero FJ, Moura JJG, Gutierrez-Merino C. Reduction of ascorbate free radical by the plasma membrane of synaptic terminals from rat brain. Arch Biochem Biophys 2008;469: 243–254.

[159] Herrero A, Barja G. Localization of the site of oxygen radical generation inside the complex I of heart and nonsynaptic brain mammalian mitochondria. J Bioenerg Biomembr 2000;32: 609-615.

[160] Zimmerman BJ, Granger DN. Mechanisms of reperfusion injury. Am J Med Sci 1994;307: 284-292.

[161] Iadecola C. Bright and dark sides of nitric oxide in ischemic brain injury. Trends Neurosci 1997;20: 132-139.

[162] Szabo C, Ischiropoulos H, Radi R. Peroxynitrite: biochemistry, pathophysiology and development of therapeutics. Nat Rev Drug Discov 2007;6: 662-680.

[163] Huie RE, Padmaja S. The reaction of NO with superoxide. Free Radic Res Commun 1993;18: 195-199.

[164] van der Veen RC, Hinton DR, Incardonna F, Hofman FM. Extensive peroxynitrite activity during progressive stages of central nervous system inflammation. J Neuroimmunol 1997;77: 1-7.

[165] Liu D, Ling X, Wen J, Liu J. The role of reactive nitrogen species in secondary spinal cord injury: formation of nitric oxide, peroxynitrite, and nitrated protein. J Neurochem 2000;75: 2144-2154.

[166] Beal MF. Energetics in the pathogenesis of neurodegenerative diseases. Trends Neurosci. 2000;23: 298–304.

[167] Beal MF. Oxidatively modified proteins in aging and disease. Free Radic Biol Med 2002;32: 797-803.

[168] Murphy MP, Packer MA, Scarlett JL, Martin SW. Peroxynitrite: a biologically significant oxidant. General Pharmacology 1998;31: 179–186.

[169] Bolaños JP, Almeida A, Stewart V, Peuchen S, Land JM, Clark JB, Heales SJ. Nitric oxide-mediated mitochondrial damage in the brain: mechanisms and implications for neurodegenerative diseases. J Neurochem 1997;68: 2227-2240.

[170] Olanow CW. A radical hypothesis for neurodegeneration. Trends Neurosci 1993;16: 439-444.

[171] Espinosa-Garcia J, Gutierrez-Merino C. The Trapping of the OH Radical by Coenzyme Q. A Theoretical and Experimental Study. J Phys Chem A 2003;107: 9712-9723.

[172] Spencer JP, Jenner A, Aruoma OI, Cross CE, Wu R, Halliwell B. Oxidative DNA damage in human respiratory tract epithelial cells. Time course in relation to DNA strand breakage. Biochem Biophys Res Commun 1996;224: 17-22.

[173] Bao F, Liu D. Hydroxyl radicals generated in the rat spinal cord at the level produced by impact injury induce cell death by necrosis and apoptosis: protection by a metalloporphyrin. Neuroscience 2004:126: 285-295.

[174] Andrus PK, Fleck TJ, Gurney ME, Hall ED. Protein oxidative damage in a transgenic mouse model of familial amyotrophic lateral sclerosis. J Neurochem 1998;71: 2041-2048.

[175] Li SW, Lin TS, Minteer S, Burke WJ. 3,4-Dihydroxyphenylacetaldehyde and hydrogen peroxide generate a hydroxyl radical: possible role in Parkinson's disease pathogenesis. Brain Res Mol Brain Res 2001;93: 1-7.

[176] Sugimoto K, Iadecola C. Delayed effect of administration of COX-2 inhibitor in mice with acute cerebral ischemia. Brain Res 2003;960: 273-276.

[177] Teismann P, Tieu K, Choi DK, Wu DC, Naini A, Hunot S, Vila M, Jackson-Lewis V, Przedborski S. Cyclooxygenase-2 is instrumental in Parkinson's disease neurodegeneration. Proc Natl Acad Sci U S A 2003;100: 5473-5478.

[178] Mattson MP. Modification of ion homeostasis by lipid peroxidation: roles in neuronal degeneration and adaptive plasticity. Trends Neurosci 1998;21: 53-57.

[179] Sharma SS, Kaundal RK. Neuroprotective effects of 6-hydroxy-2,5,7,8-tetramethylchroman-2-carboxylic acid (Trolox), an antioxidant in middle cerebral artery occlusion induced focal cerebral ischemia in rats. Neurol Res 2007;29: 304-309.

[180] Bazan NG. Synaptic signaling by lipids in the life and death of neurons. Mol Neurobiol 2005;31: 219-230.

[181] Scragg JL, Fearon IM, Boyle JP, Ball SG, Varadi G, Peers C. Alzheimer's amyloid peptides mediate hypoxic up-regulation of L-type Ca2+ channels. FASEB J 2005;19: 150-152.

[182] Arien H, Wiser O, Arkin IT, Leonov H, Atlas D. Syntaxin 1A modulates the voltage-gated L-type calcium channel (Ca(v)1.2) in a cooperative manner. J Biol Chem 2003;278: 29231-29239.

[183] Koch SE, Bodi I, Schwartz A, Varadi G. Architecture of Ca(2+) channel pore-lining segments revealed by covalent modification of substituted cysteines. J Biol Chem 2000;275: 34493-34500.

[184] Nakajima M, Miura M, Aosaki T, Shirasawa T. Deficiency of presenilin-1 increases calcium-dependent vulnerability of neurons to oxidative stress in vitro. J Neurochem 2001;78: 807-814.

[185] Hudasek K, Brown ST, Fearon IM. H2O2 regulates recombinant Ca2+ channel alpha1C subunits but does not mediate their sensitivity to acute hypoxia. Biochem Biophys Res Commun 2004;318: 135-141.

[186] Willmott NJ, Wong K, Strong AJ. Intercellular Ca(2+) waves in rat hippocampal slice and dissociated glial-neuron cultures mediated by nitric oxide. FEBS Lett 2000;487: 239-247.

[187] Grassi C, D'Ascenzo M, Azzena GB. Modulation of Ca(v)1 and Ca(v)2.2 channels induced by nitric oxide via cGMP-dependent protein kinase. Neurochem Int 2004;45: 885-893.

[188] Ohkuma S, Katsura M, Higo A, Shirotani K, Hara A, Tarumi C, Ohgi T. Peroxynitrite affects Ca2+ influx through voltage-dependent calcium channels. J Neurochem 2001;76: 341-350.

[189] Shirotani K, Katsura M, Higo A, Takesue M, Mohri Y, Shuto K, Tarumi C, Ohkuma S. Suppression of Ca2+ influx through L-type voltage-dependent calcium channels by hydroxyl radical in mouse cerebral cortical neurons. Mol Brain Res 2001;92: 12-18.

[190] Mak IT, Zhang J, Weglicki WB. Protective effects of dihydropyridine Ca-blockers against endothelial cell oxidative injury due to combined nitric oxide and superoxide. Pharmacological Res 2002;45: 27-33.

[191] Yagami T, Ueda K, Asakura K, Nakazato H, Hata S, Kuroda T, Sakaeda T, Sakaguchi G, Itoh N, Hashimoto Y, Hori Y. Human group IIA secretory phospholipase A2 potentiates Ca2+ influx through L-type voltage-sensitive Ca2+ channels in cultured rat cortical neurons. J Neurochem 2003;85: 749-758.

[192] Lu C, Chan SL, Fu W, Mattson MP. The lipid peroxidation product 4-hydroxynonenal facilitates opening of voltage-dependent Ca2+ channels in neurons by increasing protein tyrosine phosphorylation. J Biol Chem 2002;277: 24368-24375.

[193] Peng S, Hajela RK, Atchison WD. Characteristics of block by Pb2+ of function of human neuronal L-, N- and R-type Ca2+ channels transiently expressed in human embryonic kidney 293 cells. Mol Pharmacol 2002;62: 1418-1430.

[194] Pall ML. NMDA sensitization and stimulation by peroxynitrite, nitric oxide, and organic solvents as the mechanism of chemical sensitivity in multiple chemical sensitivity. FASEB J 2002;16: 1407-1417.

[195] Fonnum F, Lock EA. The contributions of excitotoxicity, glutathione depletion and DNA repair in chemically induced injury to neurones: exemplified with toxic effects on cerebellar granule cells. J Neurochem 2004;88: 513-31.

[196] Cheung NS, Peng ZF, Chen MJ, Moore PK, Whiteman M. Hydrogen sulfide induced neuronal death occurs via glutamate receptor and is associated with calpain activation and lysosomal rupture in mouse primary cortical neurons. Neuropharmacology 2007;53: 505-514.

[197] Aizenman E, Lipton SA, Loring RH. Selective modulation of NMDA responses by reduction and oxidation. Neuron 1989;2: 1257-1263.

[198] Levy DI, Sucher NJ, Lipton SA. Redox modulation of NMDA receptor-mediated toxicity in mammalian central neurons. Neurosci Lett 1990;110: 291-296.

[199] Moriyoshi K, Masu M, Ishii T, Shigemoto R, Mizuno N, Nakanishi S. Molecular cloning and characterization of the rat NMDA receptor. Nature 1991;354: 31-37.

[200] Sullivan JM, Traynelis SF, Chen HS, Escobar W, Heinemann SF, Lipton SA. Identification of two cysteine residues that are required for redox modulation of the NMDA subtype of glutamate receptor. Neuron 1994;13: 929-936.

[201] Brimecombe JC, Potthoff WK, Aizenman E. A critical role of the N-methyl-D-aspartate (NMDA) receptor subunit (NR) 2A in the expression of redox sensitivity of NR1/NR2A recombinant NMDA receptors. J Pharmacol Exp Ther 1999;291: 785-792.

[202] Sanchez RM, Wang C, Gardner G, Orlando L, Tauck DL, Rosenberg PA, Aizenman E, Jensen FE. Novel role for the NMDA receptor redox modulatory site in the pathophysiology of seizures. J Neurosci 2000;20: 2409-2417.

[203] Lei SZ, Pan ZH, Aggarwal SK, Chen HS, Hartman J, Sucher NJ, Lipton SA. Effect of nitric oxide production on the redox modulatory site of the NMDA receptor-channel complex. Neuron 1992;8: 1087-1099.

[204] Moore PK, Bhatia M, Moochhala S. Hydrogen sulfide: from the smell of the past to the mediator of the future? Trends Pharmacol Sci 2003;24: 609-611.

[205] Qu K, Chen CP, Halliwell B, Moore PK, Wong PT. Hydrogen sulfide is a mediator of cerebral ischemic damage. Stroke 2006;37: 889-893.

[206] Di Stasi AMM, Mallozzi C, Macchia G, Maura G, Petrucci TC, Minetti M. Peroxynitrite affects exocytosis and SNARE complex formation and induces tyrosine nitration of synaptic proteins. J Neurochem 2002;82: 420-429.

[207] Trotti D, Rossi D, Gjesdal O, Levy LM, Racagni G, Danbolt NC, Volterra A. Peroxynitrite inhibits glutamate transporter subtypes. J Biol Chem 1996;271: 5976-5979.

[208] Lin LH, Talman WT. Colocalization of GluR1 and neuronal nitric oxide synthase in rat nucleus tractus solitarii neurons. Neuroscience 2001;106: 801-809.

[209] Trackey JL, Uliasz TF, Hewett SJ. SIN-1-induced cytotoxicity in mixed cortical cell culture: peroxynitrite-dependent and –independent induction of excitotoxic cell death. J Neurochem 2001;79: 445–455.

[210] Abele R, Lampinen M, Keinanen K, Madden DR. Disulfide bonding and cysteine accessibility in the alpha-amino-3-hydroxy-5-methylisoxazole-4-propionic acid receptor subunit GluRD. Implications for redox modulation of glutamate receptors. J Biol Chem 1998;273: 25132-25138.

[211] Mason HS, Bourke S, Kemp PJ. Selective modulation of ligand-gated P2X purinoceptor channels by acute hypoxia is mediated by reactive oxygen species. Mol Pharmacol 2004;66: 1525-1535.

[212] Sayers LG, Brown GR, Michell RH, Michelangeli F. The effects of thimerosal on calcium uptake and inositol 1,4,5-trisphosphate-induced calcium release in cerebellar microsomes. Biochem J 1993;289: 883-887.

[213] Takahashi A, Mikami M, Yang J. Hydrogen peroxide increases GABAergic mIPSC through presynaptic release of calcium from IP3 receptor-sensitive stores in spinal cord substantia gelatinosa neurons. Eur J Neurosci 2007;25: 705-716.

[214] Hilly M, Pietri-Rouxel F, Coquil JF, Guy M, Mauger JP. Thiol reagents increase the affinity of the inositol 1,4,5-trisphosphate receptor. J Biol Chem 1993;268: 16488-16494.

[215] Lopez-Colome AM, Lee I. Pharmacological characterization of inositol-1,4,5,-trisphosphate binding to membranes from retina and retinal cultures. J Neurosci Res 1996;44: 149-156.

[216] Joseph SK, Nakao SK, Sukumvanich S. Reactivity of free thiol groups in type-I inositol trisphosphate receptors. Biochem J 2006;393: 575-582.

[217] Higo T, Hattori M, Nakamura T, Natsume T, Michikawa T, Mikoshiba K. Subtype-specific and ER lumenal environment-dependent regulation of inositol 1,4,5-trisphosphate receptor type 1 by ERp44. Cell 2005;120: 85-98.

[218] Renard-Rooney DC, Joseph SK, Seitz MB, Thomas AP. Effect of oxidized glutathione and temperature on inositol 1,4,5-trisphosphate binding in permeabilized hepatocytes. Biochem J 1995;310: 185-192.

[219] Furuichi T, Furutama D, Hakamata Y, Nakai J, Takeshima H, Mikoshiba K. Multiple types of ryanodine receptor/Ca2+ release channels are differentially expressed in rabbit brain. J Neurosci 1994;14: 4794-4805.

[220] Mori F, Fukaya M, Abe H, Wakabayashi K, Watanabe M. Developmental changes in expression of the three ryanodine receptor mRNAs in the mouse brain. Neuroscience Lett 2000;285: 57-60.

[221] Waring P. Redox active calcium ion channels and cell death. Arch Biochem Biophys 2005;434: 33-42.

[222] Stoyanovsky D, Murphy T, Anno PR, Kim YM, Salama G. Nitric oxide activates skeletal and cardiac ryanodine receptors. Cell Calcium 1997;21: 19-29.

[223] Xu L, Eu JP, Meissner G, Stamler JS. Activation of the cardiac calcium release channel (ryanodine receptor) by poly-S-nitrosylation. Science 1998;279: 234-237.

[224] Anzai K, Ogawa K, Ozawa T, Yamamoto H. Oxidative modification of ion channel activity of ryanodine receptor. Antioxid Redox Signal 2000;2: 35-40.

[225] Aracena-Parks P, Goonasekera SA, Gilman CP, Dirksen RT, Hidalgo C, Hamilton SL. Identification of cysteines involved in S-nitrosylation, S-glutathionylation, and oxidation to disulfides in ryanodine receptor type 1. J Biol Chem 2006;281: 40354-40368.

[226] Eu JP, Sun J, Xu L, Stamler JS, Meissner G. The skeletal muscle calcium release channel: coupled O2 sensor and NO signaling functions. Cell 2000;102: 499-509.

[227] Sun J, Xin C, Eu JP, Stamler JS, Meissner G. Cysteine-3635 is responsible for skeletal muscle ryanodine receptor modulation by NO. Proc Natl Acad Sci USA 2001;98: 11158-11162.

[228] Favero TG, Zable AC, Abramson JJ. Hydrogen peroxide stimulates the Ca2+ release channel from skeletal muscle sarcoplasmic reticulum. J Biol Chem 1995;270: 25557-25563.

[229] Lehotsky J, Kaplan P, Matejovicova M, Murin R, Racay P, Raeymaekers L. Ion transport systems as targets of free radicals during ischemia reperfusion injury. Gen Physiol Biophys 2002;21: 31-37.

[230] Kelliher M, Fastbom J, Cowburn RF, Bonkale W, Ohm TG, Ravid R, Sorrentino V, O'Neill C. Alterations in the ryanodine receptor calcium release channel correlate with Alzheimer's disease neurofibrillary and beta-amyloid pathologies. Neuroscience 1999;92: 499-513.

[231] Lu YF, Hawkins RD. Ryanodine receptors contribute to cGMP-induced late-phase LTP and CREB phosphorylation in the hippocampus. J Neurophysiol 2002;88: 1270-1278.

[232] Kemmerling U, Munoz P, Muller M, Sanchez G, Aylwin ML, Klann E, Carrasco MA, Hidalgo C. Calcium release by ryanodine receptors mediates hydrogen peroxide-induced activation of ERK and CREB phosphorylation in N2a cells and hippocampal neurons. Cell Calcium 2007;41: 491-502.

[233] Grover AK, Samson SE, Misquitta CM. Sarco(endo)plasmic reticulum Ca2+ pump isoform SERCA3 is more resistant than SERCA2b to peroxide. Am J Physiol 1997;273: C420-C425.

[234] Barnes KA, Samson SE, Grover AK. Sarco/endoplasmic reticulum Ca2+-pump isoform SERCA3a is more resistant to superoxide damage than SERCA2b. Mol Cell Biochem 2000;203: 17-21.

[235] Grover AK, Kwan CY, Samson SE. Effects of peroxynitrite on sarco/endoplasmic reticulum Ca2+ pump isoforms SERCA2b and SERCA3a. Am J Physiol Cell Physiol 2003;285: C1537-C1543.

[236] Viner RI, Ferrington DA, Williams TD, Bigelow DJ, Schoneich C. Protein modification during biological aging: selective tyrosine nitration of the SERCA2a isoform of the sarcoplasmic reticulum Ca2+-ATPase in skeletal muscle. Biochem J 1999;340: 657-669.

[237] Doutheil J, Althausen S, Treiman M, Paschen W. Effect of nitric oxide on endoplasmic reticulum calcium homeostasis, protein synthesis and energy metabolism. Cell Calcium 2000;27: 107-115.

[238] Zhang K, Kaufman RJ. The unfolded protein response: a stress signaling pathway critical for health and disease. Neurology 2006;66: S102-S109.

[239] Zatti G, Burgo A, Giacomello M, Barbiero L, Ghidoni R, Sinigaglia G, Florean C, Bagnoli S, Binetti G, Sorbi S, Pizzo P, Fasolato C. Presenilin mutations linked to familial Alzheimer's disease reduce endoplasmic reticulum and Golgi apparatus calcium levels. Cell Calcium 2006;39: 539-550.

[240] Tu H, Nelson O, Bezprozvanny A, Wang Z, Lee SF, Hao YH, Serneels L, De Strooper B, Yu G, Bezprozvanny I. Presenilins form ER Ca2+ leak channels, a function disrupted by familial Alzheimer's disease-linked mutations. Cell 2006;126: 981-93.

[241] Cassarino DS, Bennett JPJr. An evaluation of the role of mitochondria in neurodegenerative diseases: mitochondrial mutations and oxidative pathology, protective nuclear responses, and cell death in neurodegeneration. Brain Res Rev 1999;29: 1-25.

[242] Fiskum G. Mitochondrial participation in ischemic and traumatic neural cell death. J Neurotrauma 2000;17: 843-855.

[243] Stout AK, Raphael HM, Kanterewicz BI, Klann E, Reynolds IJ. Glutamate-induced neuron death requires mitochondrial calcium uptake. Nature Neurosci 1998;1: 366-373.

[244] Ferrand-Drake M, Zhu C, Gido G, Hansen AJ, Karlsson JO, Bahr BA, Zamzami N, Kroemer G, Chan PH, Wieloch T, Blomgren K. Cyclosporin A prevents calpain activation despite increased intracellular calcium concentrations, as well as translocation of apoptosis-inducing factor, cytochrome c and caspase-3 activation in neurons exposed to transient hypoglycemia. J Neurochem 2003;85: 1431-1442.

[245] Whiteman M, Armstrong JS, Cheung NS, Siau JL, Rose P, Schantz JT, Jones DP, Halliwell B. Peroxynitrite mediates calcium-dependent mitochondrial dysfunction and cell death via activation of calpains. FASEB J 2004;18: 1395-1397.

[246] Rosenstock TR, Carvalho AC, Jurkiewicz A, Frussa-Filho R, Smaili SS. Mitochondrial calcium, oxidative stress and apoptosis in a neurodegenerative disease model induced by 3-nitropropionic acid. J Neurochem 2004;88: 1220-1228.

[247] Yang KT, Pan SF, Chien CL, Hsu SM, Tseng YZ, Wang SM, Wu ML. Mitochondrial Na+ overload is caused by oxidative stress and leads to activation of the caspase 3-dependent apoptotic machinery. FASEB J 2004;18: 1442-1444.

[248] Michaelis ML, Foster CT, Jayawickreme C. Regulation of calcium levels in brain tissue from adult and aged rats. Mech Ageing Dev 1992;62: 291-306.

[249] Zaidi A, Gao J, Squier TC, Michaelis ML. Age-related decrease in brain synaptic membrane Ca2+-ATPase in F344/BNF1 rats. Neurobiol Aging 1998;19: 487-495.

[250] Rohn TT, Hinds TR, Vincenzi FF. Inhibition of Ca2+-pump ATPase and the Na+/K+-pump ATPase by iron-generated free radicals. Protection by 6,7-dimethyl-2,4-DI-1-pyrrolidinyl-7H-pyrrolo[2,3-d] pyrimidine sulfate (U-89843D), a potent, novel, antioxidant/free radical scavenger. Biochem Pharmacol 1996;51: 471-476.

[251] Zaidi A, Michaelis ML. Effects of reactive oxygen species on brain synaptic plasma membrane Ca2+-ATPase. Free Radic Biol Med 1999;27: 810-821.

[252] Gutierrez-Martin Y, Martin-Romero FJ, Henao F, Gutierrez-Merino C. Synaptosomal plasma membrane Ca2+ pump activity inhibition by repetitive micromolar ONOO-pulses. Free Radic Biol Med 2002;32: 46-55.

[253] Zaidi A, Barron L, Sharov VS, Schoneich C, Michaelis EK, Michaelis ML. Oxidative inactivation of purified plasma membrane Ca2+-ATPase by hydrogen peroxide and protection by calmodulin. Biochemistry 2003;42: 12001-12010.

[254] Mark RJ, Hensley K, Butterfield DA, Mattson MP. Amyloid beta-peptide impairs ion-motive ATPase activities: evidence for a role in loss of neuronal Ca2+ homeostasis and cell death. J. Neurosci 1995;15: 6239-6249.

[255] Huschenbett J, Zaidi A, Michaelis ML. Sensitivity of the synaptic membrane Na+/Ca2+ exchanger and the expressed NCX1 isoform to reactive oxygen species. Biochim Biophys Acta 1998;1374: 34-46.

[256] Eigel BN, Gursahani H, Hadley RW. ROS are required for rapid reactivation of Na+/Ca2+ exchanger in hypoxic reoxygenated guinea pig ventricular myocytes. Am J Physiol Heart Circ Physiol 2004;286: H955-H963.

[257] Goldhaber JI. Free radicals enhance Na+/Ca2+ exchange in ventricular myocytes. Am J Physiol 1996;271: H823-H833.

[258] Parekh AB. Ca2+ microdomains near plasma membrane Ca2+ channels: impact on cell function. J Physiol 2008;586: 3043–3054.

[259] Neher E. Vesicle pools and Ca2+ microdomains: new tools for understanding their roles in neurotransmitter release. Neuron 1998;20: 389–399.

[260] Neher E. Usefulness and limitations of linear approximations to the understanding of Ca2+ signals. Cell Calcium 1998;24: 345–357.

[261] Samhan-Arias AK, Garcia-Bereguiain MA, Martin-Romero FJ, Gutierrez-Merino C. Regionalization of plasma membrane-bound flavoproteins of cerebellar granule neurons in culture by fluorescence energy transfer imaging. J Fluorescence 2006;16: 393–401.

[262] Nunez L, Sanchez A, Fonteriz RI, Garcia-Sancho J. Mechanisms for synchronous calcium oscillations in cultured rat cerebellar neurons. Eur J Neurosci 1996;8: 192–201.

[263] Wang X, Gruenstein EI. Mechanism of synchronized Ca2+ oscillations in cortical neurons. Brain Res 1997;767:239-249.

[264] Huang L, Liu Y, Zhang P, Kang R, Liu Y, Li X, Bo L, Dong Z. In vitro dose-dependent inhibition of the intracellular spontaneous calcium oscillations in developing hippocampal neurons by ketamine. PLoS One 2013;8(3): e59804.

[265] Yi Y-H, Ho P-Y, Chen T-W, Lin W-J, Gukassyan V, Tsai T-H, Wang D-W, Lew T-S, Tang C-Y, Lo SL, Chen T-Y, Kao F-J, Lin C-H. Membrane Targeting and Coupling of NHE1-IntegrinαIIbβ3-NCX1 by Lipid Rafts following Integrin-Ligand Interactions Trigger Ca2+ Oscillations. J Biol Chem 2009;284: 3855–3864.

[266] Heizmann CW, Braun K. Changes in Ca(2+)-binding proteins in human neurodegenerative disorders. Trends in Neurosci 1992;15: 259-264.

[267] Shaw PJ, Eggett CJ. Molecular factors underlying selective vulnerability of motor neurons to neurodegeneration in amyotrophic lateral sclerosis. J. Neurol 2000;247: I17-I27.

[268] Beers DR, Ho BK, Siklos L, Alexianu ME, Mosier DR, Mohamed AH, Otsuka Y, Kozovska ME, McAlhany RE, Smith RG, Appel SH. Parvalbumin overexpression alters immune-mediated increases in intracellular calcium, and delays disease onset in a transgenic model of familial amyotrophic lateral sclerosis. J. Neurochem 2001;79: 499-509.

[269] Bigelow DJ, Squier TC. Redox modulation of cellular signaling and metabolism through reversible oxidation of methionine sensors in calcium regulatory proteins. Biochem Biophys Acta 2005;1703: 121-134.

[270] Bahler M, Rhoads A. Calmodulin signaling via the IQ motif. FEBS Lett 2002;513: 107-113.

[271] Xia Z, Storm DR. The role of calmodulin as a signal integrator for synaptic plasticity. Nat Rev Neurosci 2005;6: 267-276.

[272] Ferri A, Nencini M, Battistini S, Giannini F, Siciliano G, Casali C, Damiano MG, Ceroni M, Chio A, Rotilio G, Carri MT. Activity of protein phosphatase calcineurin is decreased in sporadic and familial amyotrophic lateral sclerosispatients. J Neurochem 2004;90: 1237-1242.

[273] Yao Y, Yin D, Jas GS, Kuczer K, Williams TD, Schoneich C, Squier TC. Oxidative modification of a carboxyl-terminal vicinal methionine in calmodulin by hydrogen peroxide inhibits calmodulin-dependent activation of the plasma membrane Ca-ATPase. Biochemistry 1996;35: 2767-2787.

[274] Gao J, Yin D, Yao Y, Williams TD, Squier TC. Progressive decline in the ability of calmodulin isolated from aged brain to activate the plasma membrane Ca-ATPase. Biochemistry 1998;37: 9536-9548.

[275] Bartlett RK, Bieber Urbauer RJ, Anbanandam A, Smallwood HS, Urbauer JL, Squier TC. Oxidation of Met144 and Met145 in calmodulin blocks calmodulin dependent activation of the plasma membrane Ca-ATPase. Biochemistry 2003;42: 3231-3238.

[276] Gonzalez-Albo MC, Elston GN, DeFelipe J. The human temporal cortex: characterization of neurons expressing nitric oxide synthase, neuropeptides and calcium-binding proteins, and their glutamate receptor subunit profiles. Cereb Cortex 2001;11: 1170-1181.

[277] Jinno S, Kosaka T. Patterns of expression of calcium binding proteins and neuronal nitric oxide synthase in different populations of hippocampal GABAergic neurons in mice. J Comp Neurol 2002;449: 1-25.

[278] Kowianski P, Morys JM, Wojcik S, Dziewiatkowski J, Luczynska A, Spodnik E, Timmermans JP, Morys J. Neuropeptide-containing neurons in the endopiriform region of the rat: morphology and colocalization with calcium-binding proteins and nitric oxide synthase. Brain Res 2004;996: 97-110.

[279] Lee JE, Jeon CJ. Immunocytochemical localization of nitric oxide synthase-containing neurons in mouse and rabbit visual cortex and co-localization with calcium-binding proteins. Mol Cells 2005;19: 408-417.

[280] Di Leva F, Domi T, Fedrizzi L, Lim D, Carafoli E. The plasma membrane Ca2+ ATPase of animal cells: structure, function and regulation. Arch Biochem Biophys 2008;476:65-74.

2

Synaptic Soluble and Membrane-Bound Choline Acetyltransferase as a Marker of Cholinergic Function In Vitro and In Vivo

E.I. Zakharova and A.M. Dudchenko

1. Introduction

1.1. Synaptosomes — Definition, a bit of history

The synaptosome is the presynaptic part of the nerve ending with, as a rule, a postsynaptic membrane in the region of the junction of the pre- and postsynaptic membranes that remains with the presynapse during homogenization and centrifugation. The presynaptic part of the synaptosome is a membrane-bound structure with a preserved cytoplasm (synaptoplasm), synaptic vesicles, mitochondria and some other cellular components. The term *synaptosome* was adopted by V.P. Whittaker and coworkers [1]. Together, V.P. Whittaker and C.O. Hebb first isolated and identified nerve endings in nervous tissue [2].

Subcellular fractionation emerged in the 1930s and 1940s and has since established itself as a major technique in experimental biology. The first attempts at the fractionation of nervous tissue were made in the early 1950s. A few years later, the fraction of synaptosomes was successful, using discontinuous sucrose-density gradient centrifugation [2-4]. After this, researchers achieved the preparation of the synaptic components, including the synaptic membranes, synaptoplasm, synaptic vesicles [1, 5, 6] (Figure 1) and membrane junction complex [7, 8]. These studies were a powerful impetus for investigations into the biochemistry of synapses and in the development of new methods of synaptic fractionation. Synaptosomes, as nerve endings, are heterogeneous in density, size and mediator specificity. Therefore, a number of the methods were developed for separating the synaptosomal fraction into two fractions [4], as well as into many fractions using a continuous sucrose-density linear gradient [9-11]. Among the many publications at this time, two books stand out. In the first one, D.J. Jones recounts the story of subcellular fractionation techniques, and presents the entire set of modern synaptic and subsynaptic fractionation techniques and data about the ultrastructure of synaptosomes and synaptic components, their sedimentary characteristics and biomarkers [12]. In the second one, R.N. Glebov is focused on the achievements of that time in the field of the functional neurochemistry of synapses, their molecular structure as well as on the metabolism and biochemistry of "classic" neurotransmitters and on the concepts of mediator secretion [13].

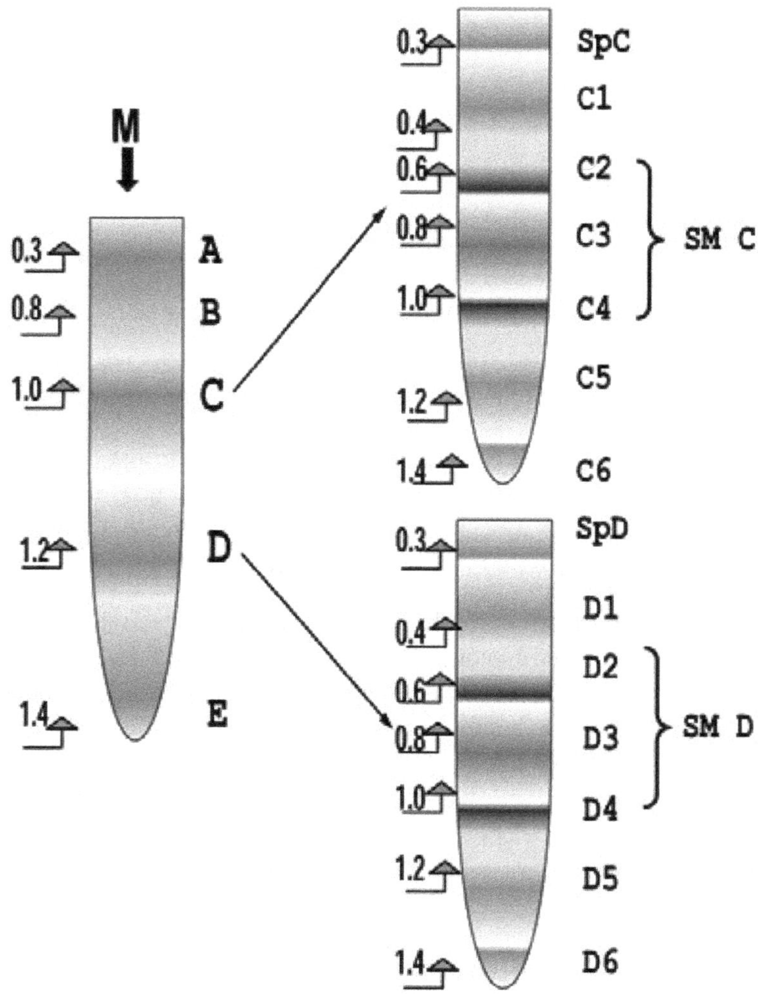

To the left of the tubes are marked the density of sucrose layers (in moles). Fractions obtained from crude mitochondrion fraction (by the method of De Robertis et al., 1962): myelin (A), neuronal and glial membrane and possibly small synaptosomes (B), light (C) and heavy (D) synaptosomes, cell mitochondria (E). Subsynaptic fractions obtained from light and heavy synaptosomes fractions (by the method of Whittaker et al., 1964): synaptoplasm (Sp), synaptic vesicles (1), synaptic membranes (2, 3, 4), non-disrupted synaptosomes (5), synaptic mitochondria (6).

Figure 1. Scheme of distribution of the fractions and subfractions of synaptosomes in discontinuous sucrose-density gradients.

2. Synaptosomes as an object of study in vitro and in vivo

Since these techniques were developed, new technologies in brain research have emerged. However, synaptosomes and their components remain a unique object of study. The reasons for this are as follows:

- the synapse is a unique structure specialized in the chemical transmission of nerve signals (chemical synapses are mainly in the mammalian brain).
- the synapse is always at the center of concepts about the adaptive properties of nervous tissue, such as learning and memory.
- the synapse is the most dynamic and labile structure of the nerve cell, and is an indicator of the reaction of the neuron to external stimuli.
- the synapse is an inherent structure of the neuron only.

It is now known that neurotransmitters and their key metabolic enzymes exist in some non-neuronal mammalian and human cells, including some cells of the neuroglia and vascular endothelium, epithelium and blood. In these cells, neurotransmitters perform specialized functions such as proliferation, differentiation, migration, organization of the cytoskeleton, cell-cell contact, secretion and transport of ions and water, blood-brain barrier maintenance and anti-inflammatory functions [14-17]. So, synaptomoses are the only object of molecular and biochemical studies that guarantees the investigation of neuronal function. Therefore, new technologies for the isolation of synaptosomes and their components continue to be developed, consistent with the purpose of science [18-20].

Using synaptosomes, one may study in vitro the molecular mechanisms of neurotransmitter secretion and the metabolism of neurotransmitter systems using the entire complexity of the molecular processes or using models of functional or pathological conditions in vitro and ex vivo.

Studies on synaptosomes in vivo are rarer but they are not less important. The brain is a very complicated organ in which a neuron exists in a permanent relationship with many other neurons. These interactions occur mainly through synapses. It is important not to forget about the signaling molecules that come into the brain through the blood, cerebrospinal fluid and intracellular matrix. The functional response of presynapses reflects the integrated response of the neuron to a stimulus. Therefore, it is important to know whether the patterns of synaptic functions are identical in vitro and in vivo.

In vivo models are used to investigate effects on the entire organism such as learning models and models of adapting and neuropathology. Then, the synaptosomes or subsynaptic components from the brain structures can be isolated. It is usually impossible to analyze the totality of the synaptic molecular and metabolic processes in these studies. The synaptic reaction is measured by the synaptic key indicators identified in studies in vitro. It is important that the biochemical methods allow the estimation of very fine metabolic and functional changes in synapses. The connection between nervous system function and synaptic processes has been investigated this way. It is possible to research the reaction of certain brain structures and even certain neuronal populations to external influences. Using neuromediators as markers, one can identify the participation of neuromediator systems in the mechanisms of various brain functions.

Furthermore, the in vivo study of synaptosomes has additional scope. Using biochemical parameters, not only metabolic changes can be evaluated, but also quantitative (synaptogenesis, reduction, degeneration) and morpho-structural (transformation) reorganizations in the synaptic pool. This is possible in comparative studies on the synaptic membrane and synaptoplasm subfractions. Subfractions of synaptic membranes and the synaptoplasm are the largest integral parts of the presynapse. Therefore, a correlation between the biochemical membrane (m) and cytosolic (c) biochemical parameters may reflect the reaction of the presynapse as a structural unit.

3. Natural markers of the neuronal systems

Neurotransmitters and some molecules of neurotransmitter metabolism are used as neuronal markers. These are natural indicators of functionally specialized brain systems, given to us by nature. Therefore, neuronal markers are widely used in biochemical studies, both in vitro and in vivo.

Neurotransmitter systems are named based on the main transmitter (glutamatergic, GABAergic, dopaminergic, etc.). Each mediator system consists of several neuronal populations. The neuronal populations in the brain are distributed topographically. Depending on the locus in the brain, neurons form specific neuronal connections using a specific combination of receptors. Moreover, these neurons can have specific metabolism dependent on their functional destination. Therefore, topography determines their metabolic and functional effects. Additionally, different neuronal populations often express comediators. These comediators influence the effects of mediators and metabolic pathways of the neuron in certain ways. It seems that future prospects in the study of brain function will be the investigation of the functional, metabolic and molecular features of distinct neuronal populations. It is necessary to understand the true mechanisms of the regulation, maintenance and recovery of brain functions. It should be noted that studies on synaptic fraction levels were carried out along these lines from the beginning [4, 18, 21-31].

In particular, regarding the cholinergic brain system, studies on this neurotransmitter system have been performed on synaptic fractions in vitro and in vivo. This review will present data from investigations into the molecular properties and metabolic and functional characteristics of cytosolic (c) and membrane-bound (m) choline acetyltransferase (ChAT) and of the use of cChAT and mChAT as cholinergic markers to establish brain function mechanisms. For the sake of completeness regarding modern notion, the characteristics of the molecular forms of ChAT will be presented using data from tissue cultures as well.

But first, a brief description of the cholinergic brain system.

4. Cholinergic brain system, cholinergic neuronal populations and their importance in health and disease

Cholinergic neurons use the classical neurotransmitter acetylcholine (ACh). ACh is a famous mediator. It was the first neurotransmitter discovered, by Otto Loewy in 1921-1926, and it proved the validity of the chemical nature of nervous communication [32]. ACh was quantified in P. Fatt's and B. Katz's experiments when the quantum nature of chemical neurotransmission was discovered [33]. S.O. Hebb and V.P. Whittaker used ACh and ChAT as indicators when they searched for and found subneuronal structures (synaptosomes) which accumulate mediators [2]. ACh was the first among the neuromediators found in the non-neuronal cells of mammals [34]. It would perhaps be helpful to add that ACh is also called "gentleman number one", for its non-neuronal function as well. It is clear that ACh is the most thoroughly examined neurotransmitter.

4.1. Metabolism of acetylcholine

ACh is an ester of acetic acid and choline with the chemical formula $CH_3COO(CH_2)_2N+(CH_3)_3$ and systematic name 2-acetoxy-N,N,N-trimethylethanaminium.The cycle of ACh synthesis, storage, release and degradation has been well-characterized at the cellular and molecular levels [26, 35, 36]. Briefly (Figure 2), ACh is synthesized in the cytoplasm of cholinergic neurons from the precursors choline and acetyl-coenzyme A by the enzyme choline acetyltransferase (ChAT), and is then taken up into synaptic vesicles for storage by the vesicular acetylcholine transporter (VAChT). Depolarization of the nerve terminal causes the fusion of synaptic vesicles with the presynaptic membrane at specialized release sites called active zones (named the junction complex in the subsynaptic fraction). Depositing and releasing ACh is a calcium-dependent process that involves the coordinated actions of many presynaptic proteins [26, 37]. When vesicles are linked up with the presynaptic membrane, ACh diffuses into the synaptic cleft where it can bind to subtypes of nicotinic and muscarinic receptors located on both post- and presynaptic membranes. ACh signaling is terminated by its diffusion away from the synaptic cleft and by its rapid hydrolysis into choline and acetate by acetylcholinesterase (AChE). The choline derived from ACh hydrolysis is recycled into the presynaptic terminal by the sodium-dependent high-affinity choline transporter (CHT) for resynthesis of ACh. After secretion of ACh, synaptic vesicles are recycled and are refilled with the neurotransmitter for another round of the depolarization-induced release. It should be noted that the details of the molecular mechanism of the regulation of these processes in both health and disease are lacking.

4.2. Topography and functions of cholinergic neuronal populations

Knowledge of the topography of mediator systems is basic for neurobiologists. The topography of the populations of cholinergic neurons and their projections has been studied in detail. ChAT has long been used as a marker of cholinergic structures in immunohistochemical studies. Initially, AChE was used as the cholinergic marker, but it was found that AChE coincides with ChAT only partially [38]. Later, colocalization of AChE was revealed in non-

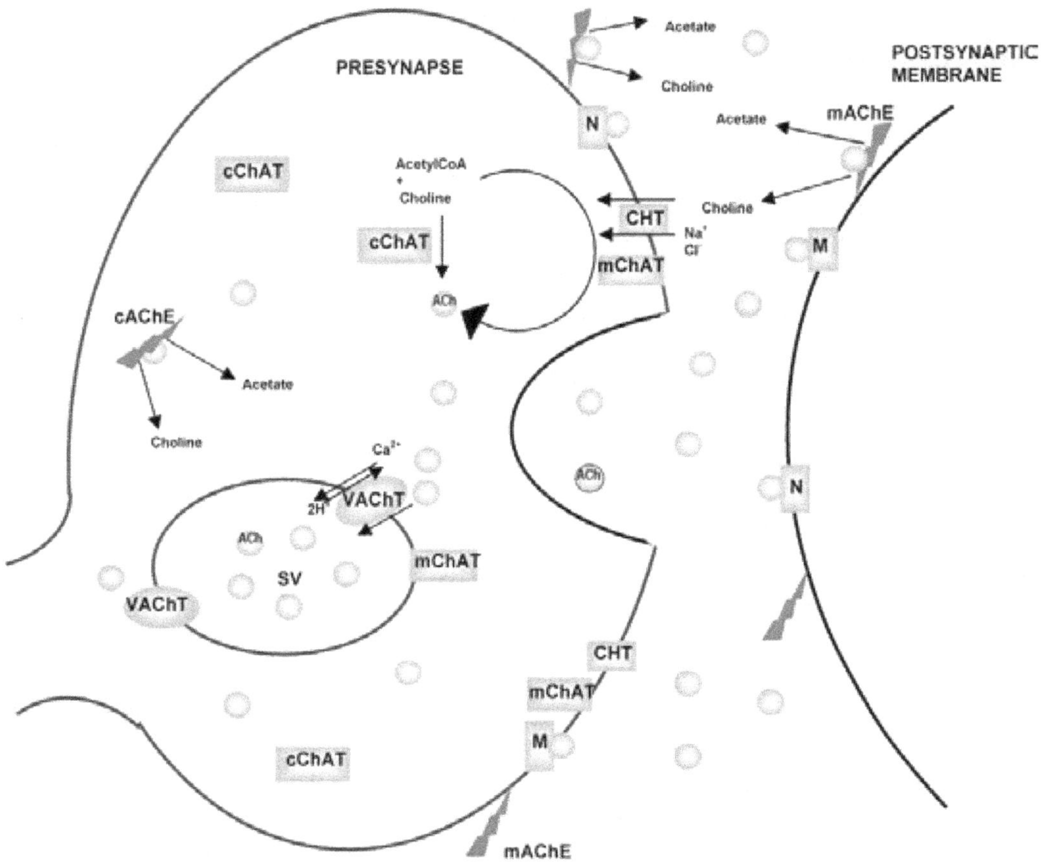

The idea of the scheme is taken from Black and Rylett [Black & Rylett, 2011]. Abbreviations: Presynapse, presynaptic part of nerve ending; SV, synaptic vesicle; ACh, acetylcholine; AcetylCo-A, acetylCoenzyme-A; cChAT and mChAT, cytoplasmic and membrane-bound choline acetyltransferase correspondingly; mAChE and cAChE, membrane-bound (extracellular isoform) and cytoplasmic acetylcholinesterase correspondingly; CHT, sodium-dependent, high-affinity choline transporter; M, muscarinic receptor; N, nicotinic receptor; VAChT, vesicular ACh transporter.
Some details of molecular mechanisms of the regulation of these processes are set out in sub-chapter 4.1.

Figure 2. Mechanisms involved in the synthesis, storage, release and degradation of ACh at the cholinergic synapse.

cholinergic neurons. For example, 36% of AChE-positive cells are GABA-immunoreactive [39]. VAChT, discovered after ChAT, is also used as a marker [40]. However, some discrepancies between VAChT and ChAT have been found [41].

Cholinergic neurons innervate almost all areas of the nervous system, both the central and peripheral systems. These areas can be innervated by either extrinsic projective neurons or by intrinsic interneurons. A very famous and major group of cholinergic projective neurons is found in the basal forebrain, which is comprised the nucleus basalis magnocellularis, also called the Meynert nucleus in primates and humans (a large bundle of cholinergic neurons encompassing the magnocellular preoptic nucleus, substantia innominata and globus pallidus), the medial septal nucleus and the vertical limb nucleus of the diagonal band of Broca.

The cortex, amygdaloid complex, hippocampus and olfactory bulb receive their cholinergic innervation principally from cholinergic projection neurons of the basal forebrain [40-49]. It is known that basal forebrain cholinergic projective neurons play a role in attention, learning, memory and consciousness. Another group of cholinergic projective neurons is found in the upper brainstem, which is comprised the pedunculopontine nucleus of the pontomesencephalic reticular formation and within the laterodorsal tegmental gray of the periventricular area. The thalamus and medulla receive their cholinergic innervation principally from cholinergic projection neurons of these brainstem nuclei. These neurons also present a minor component of the corticopetal cholinergic innervation of the frontal and visual cortical areas [43, 49-51]. The cholinergic projective neurons of the mesopontine region play a role in the primary treatment of some sensory information and memory (in the thalamus) and, hypothetically, in the central mechanisms regulating respiration and blood circulation (in the medulla). All immunohistochemical studies indicate the topographical arrangement of cholinergic projections. On the basis of connectivity patterns, M.M. Mesulam and coworkers proposed that the central cholinergic projective neurons to subdivide into six major sectors designated Ch1-Ch6 [43]. Moreover, the rostrocaudal and layerwise topographical arrangement of the cholinergic projections is indicated in the cerebral cortex [44-46, 48].

The most famous cholinergic interneurons are localized in the striatum, and they are involved in motor function and cognition [49]. As well, cholinergic interneurons have been detected in the cerebral cortex [46, 48, 52] and in the hippocampus [53-55]. Cortical and hippocampal interneurons perform associative functions and are presumably involved in learning and memory. Numerous electrophysiological studies have indicated this, but regarding cholinergic cortical and hippocampal neurons, such data are absent. In the human cerebral cortex, ChAT-immunoreactivity was found in some of the giant Betz and Meynert's pyramidal neurons [56].Cortical pyramidal neurons carry out motor functions. The medullar reticular formation has ChAT-positive neurons and their participation in the respiratory center is assumed [50].

Finally, ACh as a neurotransmitter is widely presented in the peripheral nerve system [40, 49, 57]. Acetylcholine is one of many neurotransmitters in the autonomic nervous system and is the only neurotransmitter used in the motor division of the somatic nervous system. The parasympathetic motoneurons of as the cranial nuclei of the caudal brainstem and postganglionic neurons and preganglionic sympathetic motoneurons of the spinal cord nuclei are ChAT- and VAChT-positive. Their efferents innervate all vegetative organs and glands, parasympathetic directly and sympathetic indirectly. ChAT- and VAChT-immunoreactivity has also been detected in the cell bodies of the spinal nerve motor neurons as well as in their axons and the endplates of the skeletal muscles.

It was found recently that the vagus (parasympathetic) nerve, involved in the control of heart rate, bronchomotor tone, hormone secretion and gastrointestinal motility, is also an immunomodulator. Its stimulation attenuates the production of proinflammatory cytokines and inhibits the inflammatory process via the $\alpha 7$ nicotinic acetylcholine receptor [58, 59]. It is possible that these studies are beginning to describe a new function of the cholinergic nerve system.

4.3. Comediators and other neuroactive components in some cholinergic neuronal populations

The functional effects of ACh are unique to each cholinergic population due to its targets and chemical composition. As a whole, ACh functions more often as a modulator in the central nervous system and as a mediator in the peripheral nervous system. Some populations of cholinergic neurons co-express vasoactive intestinal peptide (VIP) or/and nitric oxide (NO) or substance P. VIP has been found in cholinergic interneurons of the cortex [48, 60, 61] and in the parasympathetic efferents to the airways [62, 63]. Substance P is present in the majority of projections to the medial frontal cortex from ChAT-positive neurons in the midbrain [48]. ChAT-VIP-, NO synthase-ChAT- and NO synthase-ChAT-VIP-immunoreactive ganglionic cells have been detected in the sphenopalatine ganglia [64, 65].

All three substances as well as ACh are well-known vasodilators. Therefore, their co-localization with ACh is connected in the first place with blood flow regulation. The vasodilator action of ACh on the vessels of the vegetative organs was one of its first described effects [66]. With respect to cerebral vessels, it was detected in (1) direct contacts with small cortical vessels with vasodilator effects of the cholinergic projective neurons and interneurons, including ACh-VIP-containing interneurons [61, 67-69]; (2) ACh-, NO-ACh- and rarely ACh-VIP- containing fibers innervate the middle cerebral arteries composed of perivascular nerves of the sphenopalatine ganglia [64]; (3) ACh induces both direct vasodilation and atypical constriction in the internal cerebral arteries [64, 70, 71]; (4) brainstem ACh indirectly induces, via the stimulation of the dorsal facial area neurons of the medulla, a vasodilator effect in the common carotid and the internal cerebral arteries [72, 73].

The third vesicular glutamate transporter (VGLUT3) is present in a subset of cholinergic projective neurons in the basal forebrain and in cholinergic interneurons in the striatum [74]. It should be noted that both these cholinergic populations have similar large neurons. VGLUT3 is one of three transporter isoforms that fills synaptic vesicles with glutamate; however, VGLUT3 is also expressed in neurons and brain regions that were not previously thought to use glutamate as a neurotransmitter. It is possible that VGLUT3, because of its ionic balance, helps to load synaptic vesicles with ACh. In addition, the cholinergic projective neurons of the basal forebrain express the nerve growth factor (NGF) receptor [75, 76]. Basal forebrain neurons are trophically responsive to NGF. Neurotrophin is important for the development and maintenance of the basal forebrain cholinergic phenotype. In these neurons, NGF markedly increases ACh synthesis, content and release [77, 78].

4.4. Cholinergic functions and brain diseases

The brain cholinergic system is of permanent interest for neuroscientists because of its important role in cognitive, attention and motor functions. Dysfunction of cholinergic neurotransmission in the central nervous system is revealed in a number of neurological disorders. Dysfunction and degeneration of the cortical and hippocampal cholinergic projections from the basal forebrain nuclei is the basis of the pathogenesis of diseases such as Alzheimer's disease and Lewy body dementia, as well as diseases with other etiologies such as schizophrenia, Parkinson's disease and cerebral ischemia, in some cases aggravated by cognitive impairment [79-88]. The leading role of cholinergic afferent dysfunction in the development of ischemic pathology was suggested by data on the sensitivity of cortical and hippocampal cholinergic projections to ischemic exposure and a correlation between the development of cholinergic dysfunction, the delayed death of pyramidal neurons and cognitive impairments in rodents [89-91]. Dysfunction of cholinergic interneurons of the striatum is partly responsible for involuntary movements in Harrington's disease [80, 92]. Low expression of ChAT in the cholinergic neurons of the motor nuclei of the spinal cord is a specific early sign of amyotrophic lateral sclerosis [80, 92]. Multiple abnormalities in cholinergic function in the motor nuclei of the spinal cord a responsible for congenital myasthenic syndrome [93].

4.4.1. Synaptic soluble and membrane-bound choline acetyltransferase and their participation in cholinergic function in vitro and in vivo

Choline acetyltransferase (ChAT, E.C. 2.3.1.6) is a key enzyme in ACh synthesis and a marker of cholinergic neurons. It catalyzes the transfer of an acetyl group from acetyl-CoA to choline to form ACh. Studies in recent decades have revealed (1) the significant role of ChAT in the regulation of ACh synthesis and secretion and (2) that disturbances in the catalytic properties of ChAT may be the origin of some neuropathologies.

5. Forms of ChAT

It has been shown that ChAT has both a hydrophilic (cChAT) and hydrophobic state (stationary mChAT) in nerve endings. It has also been shown that ChAT is able to translocate from the cytosol to the synaptic membrane and to turn reversibly into the hydrophobic state associated with the synaptic membrane by ionic links (ionic-bound mChAT) [92, 94-96]. All this presupposes the existence of multiple forms or isoforms of the enzyme. Also, differences in the optimum pH, substrate specificity, sensitivity to the selective inhibitor 4-(1-naphthyl) pyridine (NVP) and some other molecular characteristics of the synaptoplasm and synaptic membrane fractions indicated this [97-99].

Research has revealed only one ChAT gene that encodes the multiple forms and isoforms of the enzyme [80, 83]. High homology has been detected between ChAT gene nucleotide sequences in the mouse, rat, pig and human brains with differences in the 5'-noncoding region. Polymorphisms of ChAT mRNAs are due to alternate splicing and various use of at least of five non-coding exons in the promoter region of the gene [100].

Five types of mRNA have been isolated from the rat brain ChAT (R1/2-, N1/2- transcripts and M-) [101] and six types from the human brain (R1/2-, N1/2-, S- and M-transcripts) [83]. All five ChAT transcripts generate ChAT with a molecular weight of 69 kDa (ChAT-69). This is the major form of ChAT in the CNS. In addition, the human M and S transcripts generate minor forms of ChAT with a molecular weight of 82-83 kDa (ChAT-82) and 74 kDa (ChAT-74) [80, 83, 93, 100, 102, 103]. Also, ChAT-69 and ChAT-82 are subdivided into a number of isoforms with differences in the isoelectric point [104].

The cytoplasm and plasma membranes of cholinergic neurons express only ChAT-69 [80, 83, 100]. In the human brain, ChAT is also found in the cell nucleus. Initially, ChAT-82 was selectively found in the nucleus in some brain structures [82, 95, 104, 105] and, later, ChAT-69 was also found [83]. In rat ganglia in the central nervous system at the level of the medulla oblongata, ChAT is expressed with a molecular mass of about 50 kDa and is called peripheral ChAT (pChAT). pChAT also exhibits alternative splicing of the mRNA [106].

The physiological significance of such a large number of isoforms of ChAT is not clear at present. Also, the relationship between of ChAT-69 isoforms in subsynaptic compartments is not known. Polymorphisms in ChAT transcripts suggest that ChAT isoforms or transcripts may vary in stability or translation efficiency or may be differentially expressed in response to trophic or pathological factors. Thus pChAT is not expressed in cholinergic neurons of the parasympathetic dorsal motor nucleus of the vagus nerve and nucleus ambiguus in the medulla of intact rats but pChAT- positive neurons were detected in these nuclei after axotomy against the background of almost disappearance of ChAT-69-positive neurons [107]. Furthermore, targeting of the enzyme to the cell nucleus suggests that ChAT may be able to perform other functions in addition to its essential role of synthesizing ACh in nerve terminals [102].

6. Features of ChAT phosphorylation

It is known that the genome does not provide the variety in the protein forms presented in a cell. In this regard, the post-genomic protein modifications are of special significance. Phosphorylation is one of the most studied pathways of the post-translational influence on the molecular properties of enzymes. Covalent modifications to serine, threonine and tyrosine residues in protein molecules can dynamically change their physicochemical nature, as well as regulate protein function and interactions with cellular components. This has been shown for the key enzyme in the synthesis of dopamine (tyrosine hydroxylase) and serotonin (tryptophan hydroxylase) and for glutamate decarboxylases GAD65 and GAD67, two synthetic enzymes of gamma-aminobutyric acid (GABA) [108].

For a long time, ChAT was not related to rate-limiting enzymes on the basis of kinetic calculations. It was believed that the ChAT synthesis rate dependents only on fluctuations in the levels of the substrate and the product of the synthesis, although ChAT is not saturated by choline and acetyl-CoA in their physiological concentrations [35]. However, in recent decades, other intracellular factors have been revealed to regulate the activity of the enzyme. These data suggest an important regulatory role of ChAT in the synthesis and secretion of ACh [36, 82, 103, 108, 109]. It is assumed that the cause of several diseases is spontaneous point mutations in the molecule of ChAT or of its regulatory proteins which lead to dysregulation of the enzyme or to changes in its ability to communicate with regulatory factors [93, 108].

As a rule, the different effects of phosphorylation on synaptic soluble (hydrophilic) cChAT and membrane-bound (hydrophobic) mChAT occur even with non-specific stimulation by the substrates ATP or phosphorus (Pi). Increased ATP markedly affects the specific activity of mChAT compared with cChAT [37]. At rest, cChAT but not mChAT is phosphorylated in incubation medium enriched with Pi. Under these incubation conditions, veratridine depolarization selectively activated and dephosphorylated mChAT but had no influence on either the degree of phosphorylation nor the activity of cChAT. Removal of Ca^{2+} from the incubation medium significantly inhibited the phosphorylation of cChAT and the specific activity of mChAT [110].

It has been shown that, in vivo, ChAT exists as a phosphoprotein [36, 111]. In vitro, phosphatase inhibitors activate cChAT and mChAT a little, even under non-phosphorylation conditions (ATP absent in the incubation medium) [37]. ChAT is a substrate for certain protein kinases. The amino acid sequence of the enzyme suggests the existence of multiple sites for phosphorylation by protein kinases such as protein kinase C (PKC), α-Ca^{2+}/calmodulin-dependent protein kinase II (CaM2), casein kinase II (CK2) and some others [108]. ChAT-69 is phosphorylated by the serine/threonine kinases CK2, PKC and CaM2 [92, 95, 105, 112].

It should be noted that PKC and CaM2 are the well-known and important regulators of neuronal functions. CaM2 is an obligatory component of the cholinergic vesicular mechanism [37], and PKC plays an important role in the regulation of ChAT molecular properties [36]. The authors also make the conjecture that oxidative stress can alter the phosphorylation-dependent regulation of ChAT expression and ACh synthesis in the aging brain and in the early stages of vascular and Alzheimer's disease and related disorders. Both of these protein kinases interact with serine/threonine residues which the protein kinases use for ChAT phosphorylation [92, 95, 108, 112]. In different studies, PKC activated cChAT and mChAT with variable efficacy [37, 95, 104]. It has been shown that different protein kinase isoforms have distinct patterns and ChAT phosphorylation by PKC isoforms has a hierarchical construct [92, 95, 108, 112]. Thus, phosphorylation of Ser-476 had no effect on the molecular properties of ChAT but allows the possibility of phosphorylating other serine residues, such as Ser-440 and/or Ser-346/347 which are necessary to maintain the catalytic activity of ChAT under basal and stimulated conditions. Also, Ser-346/347 modulates ChAT phosphorylation at other amino acid residues, and Ser-440 initiates the translocation of soluble ChAT to the cellular membrane and the formation of ionic-bound ChAT.

CaM2 and its inhibitors selectively regulate mChAT activity without affecting the activity of cChAT [37]. These data were also confirmed indirectly by experiments with total ChAT (actually cChAT), in which CaM2 phosphorylated but did not activate the enzyme [104]. Further investigations showed that CaM2 activated total ChAT in terms of the combined phosphorylation of Thr-456 by CaM2 and of Ser-440 by PKC [112]. It is assumed that this PKC feature of the potentiation of CaM2 action in cholinergic projection neurons of the hippocampus and the cortex is dramatically implicated in the pathogenesis of Alzheimer's disease [112]. Likewise, PKC inactivation of Ser-440 phosphorylation is implicated in the pathogenesis of myasthenic syndrome in the motor nuclei of the spinal cord [94, 113].

7. Role of cChAT and mChAT in regulation of acetylcholine synthesis and secretion – In vitro studies

In neurons, the principal place of synthesis of ACh is in the nerve endings. ChAT has long been recognized as a cytoplasmic enzyme, even after its detection on synaptic membranes in the 1960s [1, 114]. Later, it was shown that ChAT exists as a structural membrane protein [95, 115-117]. The long-term study of the properties of synaptic soluble (c) and membrane-bound (m) ChAT in vitro has shown that the relationship between ChAT activity and the secretion of ACh depends on the compartmentalization of the enzyme.

7.1. Functional properties of synaptic cChAT

Soluble cChAT activity is the prevalent activity of synaptic ChAT. cChAT regulates the dynamic equilibrium between the synthesis and degradation of ACh in the resting state [35, 99, 118, 119]. Under physiological conditions, cChAT is activated during stimulation by depolarizing agents such as K^+ and/or veratridine [37, 120, 121]. Another regulator of the level of free cytosolic ACh is AChE, the enzyme that mediates ACh splitting. A close interaction takes place between cChAT and soluble cAChE [120]. Thus, in calcium-free medium conditions, the quantum release of ACh is blocked, the activity of cChAT is not changed and cAChE is activated and cleaves an abundance of ACh [120, 122].

From these experiments, it follows that non-quantum, Ca^{2+}-independent "leak" of acetylcholine and its decay products, choline and acetate, is in direct dependence on the ratio of the activity of these two cytosolic enzymes [120, 122, 123]. In these studies, (1) K^+ stimulation in calcium-free medium causes the release of cytosolic choline due to disruption of cytosolic ACh by cAChE and (2) veratridine stimulation can cause the release of both choline and cytosolic ACh. (3) In mAChE and cAChE inhibition conditions by a tertiary inhibitor such as paraoxon coming through the plasma membrane, the release of choline is blocked under veratridine stimulation in calcium-free medium and its extracellular level is decreased. Instead of choline, the release of cytosolic ACh is observed. (4) Under cChAT and mChAT inhibition conditions by the selective inhibitor NVP, cChAT is selectively activated and the release of newly synthesized ACh is increased directly from the cytosol under veratridine stimulation in physiological medium (in the presence of Ca^{2+}). (5) A similar output of ACh is observed under the same conditions in calcium-free medium.

The choline and ACh concentrations could increase by 40-60% in the extracellular medium in such a non-quantum manner. Choline is a selective agonist of α-7 subtype of ACh nicotinic receptors [65, 124]. Thus, the "leak" of cytosolic choline and/or ACh, as well as changes in their relationship in the extracellular environment may have independent signaling effects in intercellular interactions.

7.2. Functional properties of synaptic mChAT

The functional purpose of mChAT has long been unclear [80, 125]. Investigation of this problem was difficult in the absence of selective inhibitors of cChAT and mChAT. Their separation is possible only by subsynaptic fractionation in combination with methods that destroy the synaptosome. The contribution of mChAT to general ChAT activity is low, i.e. 4-15% [1, 94, 95, 97, 119]. Therefore, for a long time, it was assumed that the association of ChAT with neuronal membranes was an artifact as the result of synaptoplasm contamination [1, 35, 114].It has now been shown that mChAT exists (1) as stationary membrane protein [99, 115, 117] and (2) as ionic-bound mChAT, a reversible form of cytosolic ChAT [95, 126].

In vitro, mChAT like cChAT are activated in response to K^+ or veratridine stimulation in physiological medium [37, 110, 120, 121]. Compelling data have accumulated regarding the direct involvement of mChAT in the mechanisms of quantum secretion of acetylcholine. This is indicated by a number of ultrastructural and functional characteristics of the enzyme.

mChAT is localized to synaptic vesicles [127]. Its activity, unlike cChAT, depends on the specific factors of ACh transfer into the vesicles, VAChT and the proton gradient, and on CaM2 activity, which is the main kinase associated with synaptic vesicles [37]. Activation and inhibition of mChAT are fully coupled with the activation or, respectively, blockade of ACh quantum release [120].

The non-vesicular Ca^{2+}-dependent pathway of the quantum secretion of ACh has been revealed [128-131]. It was shown that this pathway provides fast secretion of ACh by a synaptic membrane structural protein [132] called mediatophore [128]. It was found that mediatophore is functional linked to ChAT [133]. This suggests that mChAT located on the synaptic membrane participates in the regulation of the quantum secretion of ACh, similar to vesicular mChAT. This agrees with the preferential sensitivity of mChAT to the functional state of CHT that is selectively localized to the neuronal membrane of cholinergic neurons [94, 134].

mChAT is selectively sensitive to the balance of ions. It is known that ions are important regulators of quantum neurotransmitter release and other transmembrane functions. Control of quantum ACh release is carried out by the interaction of the Ca^{2+} and H^+ balance (vesicular Ca^{2+}/H^+ antiporter), Zn^{2+} and K^+ (K^+ channels) [131, 135-138]. mChAT activity is selectively or preferably (1) inhibited in calcium-free medium [118, 120, 121], (2) is increased at a high concentration of Ca^{2+} and/or K^+ [37, 110, 121, 123, 139], (3) is dose-dependently inhibited by the intracellular concentration of Cl^- [118, 125] and increases in conditions of a high Cl^- concentration and chloride conductivity stimulation [125]. (5) Zn^{2+} regulates both pathways of the quantum secretion of ACh. High concentrations of Zn^{2+} block ACh release from vesicles and through mediatophore [135, 140]. Similarly, the direction of ChAT translocation depends on Zn^{2+} ions. Zn^{2+} blocks the "anchoring" of ChAT on the membrane [126]. The last argument indicates the involvement of ionic-bound mChAT in the quantum release of ACh.

So, the catalytic properties of cChAT and mChAT depend on phosphorylation and possibly on the type of splicing. Moreover, the specific activity of mChAT, unlike cChAT, also depends on the ionic environment and on other factors affecting the quantum secretion of ACh. The functional significance of mChAT is not nearly as clear as cChAT. The relationship between cChAT and mChAT and their dependence on external influences are poorly understood [138]. Nevertheless, it seems that the compartmentalization of the enzyme ensures the involvement of cChAT and mChAT in different functional-metabolic cycles, which may contribute to the fine regulation of the mediator actions of ACh.

8. cChAT and mChAT as markers of functional and structural reorganization in cholinergic nerve endings following external exposure — In vivo studies

The synaptosomal subfractions of the synaptic membranes and synaptoplasm of the cortex, hippocampus and some other rat brain structures are used for research in vivo cholinergic mechanisms of brain functions by biochemical methods (radiometric and spectrophotometric). Subsynaptic fractions gave according to the scheme shown in Figure 1. Respectively, mChAT and cChAT activity and the m-protein and c-protein content have been measured to estimate cholinergic function. In addition, in some experiments, mAChE and cAChE and Na^{+}/K^{+}-ATPase activity was measured. The Na^{+}/K^{+}-ATPase activity and content of synaptic proteins, as universal synaptic parameters, as well AChE activity were correlated with ChAT activity in those cases when the cholinergic reaction following exposure was dominant in the synaptosomal fraction. Generally, models of acute (3 hours) and chronic (11-14 days) brain ischemia (bilateral occlusion of the carotid arteries, the 2VO model) or acute hypobaric hypoxia with variable intensity (10% O_2, 60 min; 6.5% O_2, 15 min; 4.5% O_2, 1-3 minutes or 10-20 minutes) were used as the exposure methods.

8.1. Biochemical equivalents of activation and inhibition of cholinergic mediator function

In in vivo investigations, ChAT activity was found to be the most mobile parameter. So, ChAT has become the main landmark for analysis of the cholinergic reaction to exposure.

cChAT activation was observed under acute ischemia or hypoxia at all intensities [27, 29, 141]. mChAT or both mChAT and cChAT activation was revealed under acute and chronic ischemia and only in severe hypoxia (4.5% O_2) [27-29, 141]. When the activation of ChAT was observed (165-170%), extracellular mAChE (the predominant isoform of mAChE) was simultaneously activated [141]. cChAT activation positively correlated with the activation of Na^{+}/K^{+}-ATPase and negatively correlated with the decrease in the c-protein content [27]. All these reactions of the synaptic biochemical parameters and their combinations are regarded as the activation of cholinergic synaptic function, because they conform to the characteristics of synaptic activation.

Compared to cChAT, the selective activation of mChAT has been revealed (1) under equal experimental conditions (3 hours of ischemia) in rats less resistant to hypoxia [141], and (2) under hypoxic conditions with variable intensity only in severe hypoxia [27] and was not observed in the subcritical and moderate hypoxia (6.5% or 10% O_2) [27, 29]. A parallel study of the ultrastructure of the synapses in the cortex revealed the dependence of swelling synapses and synaptic mitochondria on the duration of severe hypoxia [27]. Taken together, these data suggest that the activation of mChAT in vivo occurs due to an imbalance of synaptic Ca2^{+}, while cChAT activation is apparently initiated in the natural physiological way, under neuronal influences [27].

The inhibitory reactions of ChAT under ischemic/hypoxic conditions were revealed as well. It was found that these conditions decrease cChAT or mChAT or both cChAT and mChAT activity [27-29, 141]. Also, a negative correlation has been found between cChAT activity and the c-protein content and a positive correlation has been found between mChAT activity and the m-protein content [27, 29, 141].

A parallel study of the ultrastructure of the synapses in the cortex revealed a significant decrease in the number of vesicles docked to the presynaptic active zone in the rat with a profound decrease in both cChAT and mChAT activity in acute hypoxia [27, 142].Taken together, these data suggest that such a decrease in ChAT activity in vivo may reflect the deep inhibition of cholinergic synaptic function as result of the superexcitation, the equivalent of the well-known "depression of neurons" in electrophysiology, i.e. reduced neuronal excitability due to the depletion of mediator substrates.

Selective inhibition of mChAT, as well as its activation, is likely a consequence of a disturbance in the ion balance. Based on the dominance of the hypoxic factors in these experiments, it is supposed that the decrease in mChAT activity is due to the accumulation of H^+ ions in the presynapses [27, 29]. It can be induced (1) by acidosis in the case of severe hypoxia and (2) by the weak increase in H^+ ion concentrations as the primary response to hypoxia in the case of moderate hypoxia (10% O_2). It has been shown that such primary H^+ ion accumulation is subthreshold for the initiation of cellular acidosis and can disrupt the function of the Ca^{2+}/H^+ antiporter [143].

Finally, cAChE activation has been detected under acute ischemia [141]. This is probably another means of regulating the abundance of free cytosolic ACh during the inhibition of ACh quantum transmission. The simultaneous increase in the c-protein content in the same synaptosomal fraction corroborates this supposition. It is well-known that numerous fibrillar synaptic proteins are soluble at rest and quickly form a structure under stimulation conditions.

So, the high reactivity as cChAT and mChAT and the peculiarities in the manifestation of ChAT (and AChE) activity according to the compartmentalization of the enzyme and to the experimental situation in vivo testify to the naturalness of functional properties cChAT and mChAT (and also c- and mAChE) revealed in vitro.

8.2. Biochemical equivalents of the quantitative changes in the cholinergic synaptic pool

The correlations in the activation or inhibition of cChAT and mChAT may reflect changes in a number of cholinergic synapses, namely synaptogenesis (the growth of new synapses) or their elimination, retraction or another means of reduction in the quantity of nerve endings. As was described above, the correlation between the biochemical synaptic membrane and cytosolic parameters may reflect the reaction of the presynapse as a structural unit. The most reliable criterion of the quantitative reorganization of cholinergic synapses is the positive correlation between ChAT activity and the c-protein content, since their functional changes have contrasting directionality.

A reduction in the number of presynapses was provoked by acute hypoxia of variable severity [27, 29]. It was shown by various methods, including non-invasive video technology, that a reduction in the number of synapses can occur within minutes or tens of minutes [144-148].

Sprouting as well as destruction with the swelling of neurons and their terminals, including cholinergic neurons, predominates in late brain ischemia or postischemic reoxygenation (over days and months) [149-152]. In biochemical studies, the activation of ChAT was observed in the majority of the synaptic subfractions of the cortex and hippocampus following chronic brain ischemia [28]. The correlated increase between mChAT activity and m-protein content could indicate synaptogenesis and hyperfunction of the cholinergic synapses, whereas the correlated increase between cChAT/mChAT activity and the c-protein content indicates synaptogenesis only.

8.3. Biochemical equivalents of the morpho- structural reorganization in the cholinergic synaptic pool

Under the influence of moderate hypoxia (10% of O_2, 60 min), an increase in the activity of cChAT and the c-protein content was observed in the "light" synaptosomes from the caudal structures of the brainstem [29]. This indicated an increase in quantity of the corresponding synapses; however, synaptogenesis was impossible in such a brief period. Additional analysis revealed a decrease in the activity of mChAT and the m-protein content in the "heavy" synaptosomal fraction of the same brain structures. This decrease in the "m" biochemical parameters in the "heavy" fraction negatively correlated with the increase in the corresponding "c" biochemical parameters in the "light" fraction.These data indicate the transformation of presynapses from one morphological type to another.

This phenomenon of the transformation of synapses was found in electron microscopic experiments during 90 minutes of severe hypoxia [144, 145]. It was shown that the change of a morphological type occurs due to the changes in the area, density and configuration of the network elements of the presynapses and in their configuration [153]. Almost all of these parameters can affect the density of the presynapses. Therefore, it is possible that some population of the cholinergic presynapses from the "heavy" synaptosomal fraction transformed into presynapses with the less density and was located in the "light" fraction of the sucrose density gradient. Apparently, this transformation resulted in a morphological type more resistant to hypoxia.

In such studies on synaptic subfractions in vivo, various cholinergic synaptic reactions have been revealed in response to hypoxic/ischemic exposures. The responsiveness of synaptic cChAT and mChAT allows the study of synaptic reactions depending on the exposure conditions, the functional specificity of different brain structures and neuronal populations. It was noticed that a reaction to the hypoxia had phase type of change in the course of intensification of hypoxic exposure [27]. As well a diversity of the plastic possibilities of the brain is detected. For example, under the same moderate hypobaric hypoxic conditions (10% O_2, 60 min) which initiated an increase in resistance to hypoxia, three alternative cholinergic adaptive pathways were obtained in the same brain structure (the caudal brainstem) in three different groups of rats. Transformation and activation of the presynapses was seen in one of the rat groups and the inhibition of cholinergic activity in different populations of presynapses (in the light or heavy synaptosomes) was seen in the other two groups [29]. The mechanisms behind this plastic diversity are unknown, although it is clear that it is associated with individual neuronal organization of brain functions.

8.4. Cholinergic organization of brain functions under normal conditions and patterns of adaptive reorganization under the influence of stress stimuli or pathological conditions

Synaptic ChAT activity can be used as an instrument to study the cholinergic mechanisms of brain functions in vivo. Biochemical (radiometric) methods to estimate synaptic ChAT activity are very sensitive and allow for assessing fine individual differences between experimental animals. In turn, this method allows for successful correlation analysis between ChAT activity and indicators of brain function and performance. Moreover, it is possible to study certain populations of cholinergic neurons using, for example, the synaptic fractions of the cortex and hippocampus.

As mentioned above, according to immunohistochemical data, both the cortex and the hippocampus have two basic sources of cholinergic innervation. The first major source is neuronal projections from the forebrain nuclei. The second minor source is interneurons (intrinsic neurons). The third source to the frontal and visual cortical areas from the mesopontine region is weak and biochemical methods can detect it only when the frontal or visual area is assessed separately. In these brain structures, ChAT activity was estimated in the fractions of the light and heavy synaptosomes (isolated as in [4]), and it appeared that these fractions both in the cortex and in the hippocampus differ in terms of functional activity. From this, it follows that in both brain structures, the cholinergic presynapses from different sources are isolated in different synaptosomal fractions during preparation in the sucrose density gradient.

Next, it was revealed that the ratio of ChAT activity in the light and heavy synaptosomal fractions corresponded to the ratio of the immunoreactivity of the enzyme in the projections and interneurons [46, 48, 52, 53, 154].This and some other data promoted the conclusion that, in the cortex and hippocampus, the presynapses of cholinergic projections from the forebrain nuclei accumulate mainly in the light synaptosomal fractions, whereas the presynapses of cholinergic interneurons accumulate mainly in the heavy synaptosomal fractions [27, 27, 155].

This differential approach was used to study rat and cat brain cholinergic synaptic organization of cognitive functions such as learning, different forms of memory and inherited abilities in some experimental situations. mChAT and cChAT activities of the light and heavy synaptosomes of the hippocampus and/or cortex were used as markers of forebrain projections and interneurons, respectively. These studies revealed some patterns in the relationship between cognitive functional mechanisms that have not been sufficiently analyzed or defined by any other methods.

Thus, under normal brain conditions, it was shown that (Figure 3, a):

1. Both the cholinergic projective systems and interneurons of the rat cortex and hippocampus are actively involved in learning and memory processes in the Morris water maze

model [28]. The presynapses of cholinergic interneurons in the cat temporal associative cortical area do not participate in inherited abilities for the analysis of images [25] but all of other associative cortical areas (frontal and parietal) active participated in cognitive processes [153].

2. The cholinergic system participates not only in the mechanisms of learning and working memory, which has been repeatedly observed [151, 157-160], but also in the mechanisms of long-term memory [28]. The involvement of cholinergic projective systems in the mechanisms of long-term memory is usually denied [161-164] or has been discussed in only a few studies [165-167].
3. Each form of memory has an individual cholinergic synaptic composition [28]. This conclusion agrees with the results of investigations into cholinergic and monoaminergic systems obtained in the Morris water maze and some other behavioral models [165, 168-170].
4. Cholinergic projective neurons and interneurons of the rat cortex and hippocampus can have both positive and negative connections with cognitive functions [28]. Identical results were obtained in all cat cortical areas except the temporal zone. Cholinergic projections in the temporal area had only negative connections with inherited cognitive functions. The number of cholinergic presynapses may be more than doubled in this brain area of cats with weak cognitive abilities as compared with cats with strong abilities [25]. Negative connections with cognitive functions are not specific for only the cholinergic system. In morphological research on hippocampal mossy fibers (glutamatergic) in the rat and mouse brain, feedback was also found between the quantity of synapses which mossy fibers create and learning [171].

Taken together, these data demonstrate that the cholinergic mechanisms of learning and memory are more complex than is currently perceived.

Stress and pathological stimuli initiate a considerable reorganization of the normal cholinergic synaptic connections in cognitive functions. As an illustration, it was revealed during chronic 2VO conditions in the Morris water maze models that [28] (Figure 3, b):

1. The majority of normal cholinergic connections are lost and new connections arise.
2. Cholinergic link was considerably reduced in mechanisms of cognitive functions and proportion of negative connections increased.
3. In addition to reduction, the structural isolation of cholinergic links in cognitive functions and performance takes place; cortical cholinergic influences are completely removed from spatial contextual functions as are hippocampal influences from spatially cued functions.

In general, cholinergic synaptic influences disappear in some forms of cognition. It is clear that the consequences of different exposures on the cholinergic composition of cognitive functions are individual; however, the itemized consequences of 2VO are general for other stress stimuli such as acute severe hypoxia (4.5% O_2, Figure 3, c) [141, 156] and changes in season from warm to cold [25] (Figure 4).

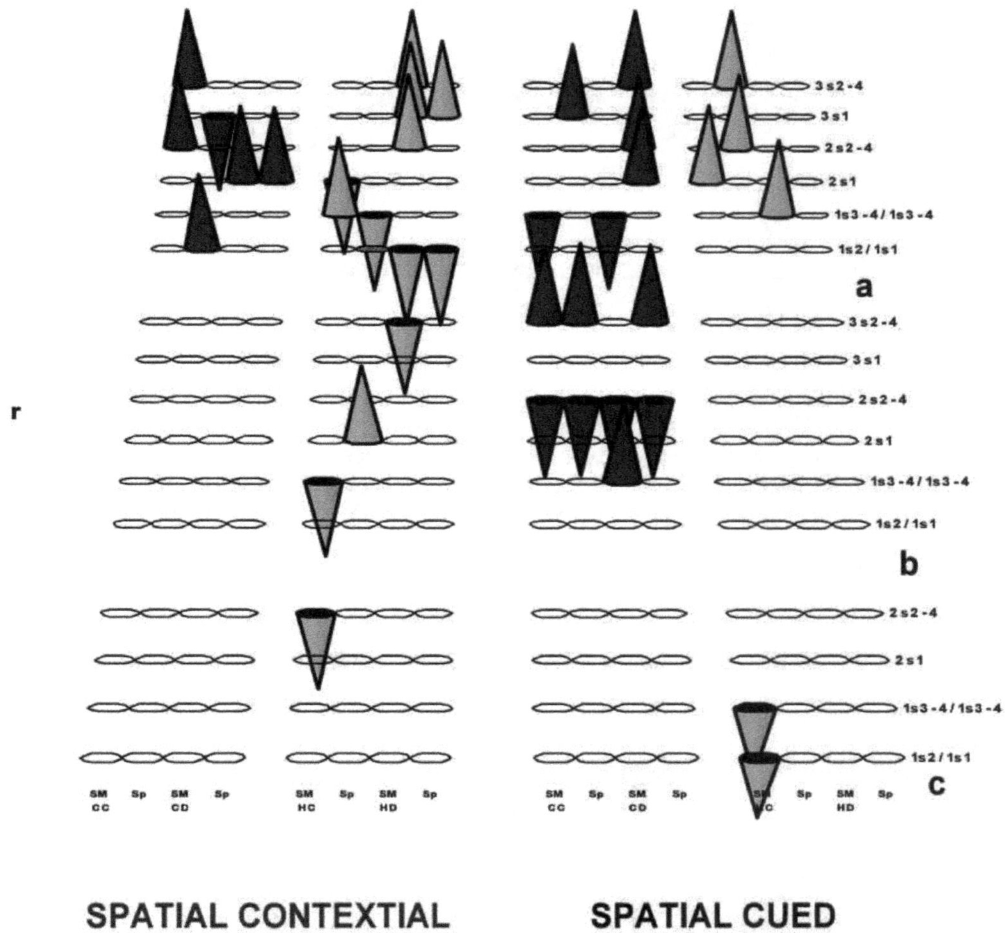

Abbreviations: 1s2(Contextual)/1s1 (Cued), the inherited abilities, the first non-casual attempt of making decision in the task (respectively, the second/ the first trial in the first session, "s " inclued in the abbreviations of the forms of cognition); 1s3-4 (Contextual)/1s2-4 (Cued), the working memory (averaged from the following trials in the first session); 2s2-4 and 3s2-4, the learning (average of trials in the second and the third sessions respectively); 2s1 and 3s1, the long-term memory (the first trials on the next days after the first and the second sessions of training respectively). SM and Sp, subfractions of the synaptic membranes and the synaptoplasm, respectively, of the cortical light (CL) and heavy synaptosomes (CH) and hippocampal light (HL) and heavy synaptosomes (HH).

Pyramids towards up indicate a positive correlation between behavioural performance and ChAT activity; inverted pyramidы indicate a negative correlation between behavioural performance and ChAT activity. In the rat groups n=4-7. Correlations between behavioural performance and ChAT activity are represented with only valid values and with the Bonferroni correction ($p<0.02$-0.001).

Figure 3. Values of *r*-criterion by the Pearson's test of behavioural performance and ChAT activity in rats in the Morris water maze in the spatial contextual and the spatial cued behavioural models under control (a, sham operated rats), ischaemic (b, 2VO operated rats) and one month after a single severe hypobaric hypoxia (c, sham operated rats) conditions.

It is logical to assume that the reduction in cholinergic links in cognitive mechanisms is a consequence of the degeneration of cholinergic fibers. However, the reverse was actually

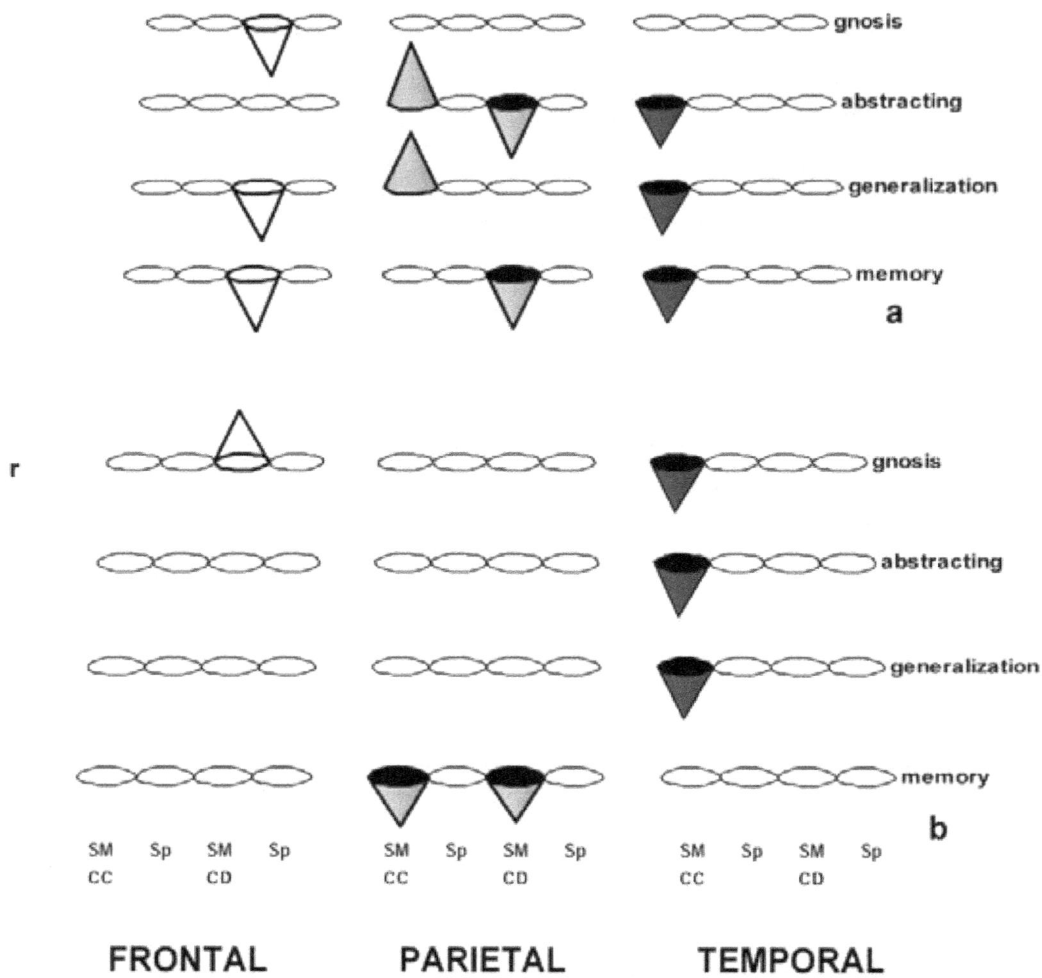

Abbreviations: SM, Sp, CL, CH, the same abbreviations of the subfractions as on Figure 3.
As on Figure 3, the pyramids towards up indicate a positive correlation between behavioural performance and ChAT activity; inverted pyramids indicate a negative correlation between behavioural performance and ChAT activity. In the cat groups n=6-8. Correlations behavioural performance and ChAT activity are represented with only valid values and with the Bonferroni correction (p<0.02-0.001).

Figure 4. Values of r-criterion by the Pearson's test of behavioural performance and ChAT activity in cats in the inherited abilities of generalisation, abstracting and gnosis of images tested on the basis of the food reflex (memory) in the summer (a) and winter (b).

observed. As was noted above, activation of ChAT was detected in the majority of the synaptic subfractions, and this may reflect cholinergic hyperfunction or synaptogenesis in the 2VO rat brain [28]. Moreover, ChAT activity showed a five- to ten-fold increase in the winter as compares with the summer in synaptic subfractions of both projection and interneurons in the temporal [25] as well in other cat cortical areas [156]. No quantitative distinctions in ChAT activity were found in the synaptic subfractions of the cortex and the hippocampus of rats in a month after a single acute hypoxic stress [156].

The new cholinergic connections with cognitive functions that arise after 2VO are not necessarily the consequence of degeneration or dysfunction in the presynapses of key cholinergic populations, i.e. these new connections could arise for other, indirect reasons. Therefore, it was assumed that noticeable weakening of cholinergic synaptic influences on cognitive processes is a consequence of adaptation. It seems that the cholinergic synaptic components of the highest brain structures, besides their participation in cognition, are necessary for the functions connected with survival under stress conditions.

At the same time, some cognitive functions were not affected by cholinergic reduction after 2VO [28]. All the more the inherited cognitive processes are preserved with annual seasonal cholinergic reorganization [25, 156]. From this, it was concluded that, during stress conditions, other mediator systems replace the cholinergic system in cognitive processes.

At least four questions follow from these data:

1. In what nervous functions are the cholinergic neuronal populations of the cortex and the hippocampus involved, both projective and intrinsic, for the maintenance of viability of an organism? Is it a function of regulation of the regional blood vessels or some other factor?
2. Why are cholinergic synaptic influences lost from cognitive mechanisms? Is it a negative dependence between vital and cognitive functions or low resistance of this neuronal population to stress conditions?
3. Is the structural isolation of cholinergic links in cognitive functions presumes a functional disbalance between the cortex and hippocampus? Is it a consequence of loss of cholinergic modulating influences?
4. What mediator systems mediate the execution of cognitive functions instead of the cholinergic system?

The answers to these questions are important for the restoration, maintenance and regulation of cognitive and vital brain functions under stress and pathological conditions.

9. Conclusion

The synapse is a unique and the most dynamic and labile structure specialized in the chemical transmission of nerve signals, an inherent structure of the neuron only.

Cholinergic system is essential constituent of the mammalian brain. Due to research using the synaptosomal and other synaptic fractions, knowledge behind the metabolism and secretory function of ACh and some new notion concerning the cholinergic mechanisms of cognitive functions under normal conditions and stress stimuli were gained. Today, however, accumulated data does not provide answers to the all questions as many more questions are asked. We have tried to outline some of the outstanding problems in the course of presenting the material.

The experimental cell physiology began to develop after the invention of the microscope by A. van Leeuwenhoek and his discoveries in the middle of the 17th century. Experimental synaptology began to develop after the invention of the electron microscope in the 1930s by M. Knoll and E. Ruska, ie three centuries later! Prior to this, researchers for the longest time, following two great neurohistologists, S. Ramón y Cajal and C. Golgi, in general could not reach a consensus, whether the brain is a cellular structure or syncytium? Only the electron microscope proved that a synapse exists.

Thus the science of the synapse is very young neuroscience.

Acknowledgements

We are grateful to all the mentors and colleagues, co-authors of our publications, especially to Prof. M.D. E.I. Mukhin, doctor of biology Z.I. Storozheva and Ph.D. M.Y. Monakov. Special thanks to Academician RAMS A.A. Kubatiev for supporting our research.

Author details

E.I. Zakharova and A.M. Dudchenko

*Address all correspondence to: zakharova-ei@yandex.ru

Institute of General Pathology and Pathophysiology, Russian Academy of Medical Sciences, Moscow, Russia

References

[1] Whittaker V P, Michaelson I A, Kirkland R J. The separation of synaptic vesicles from nerve-ending particles ('synaptosomes'). Biochemical Journal 1964; 90(2) 293-303.

[2] Hebb C O, Wh ittaker V P. Intracellular distributions of acetylcholine and choline acetylase. Journal of Physiology 1958; 142 (1) 187-196.

[3] Whittaker V P. The isolation and characterization of acetylcholine-containing particles from brain. Biochemical Journal 1959; 72, 694-706.

[4] De Robertis E, Pellegrino De Iraldi A, Rodrigues De Lores A G, Salganicoff L. Cholinergic and non-cholinergic nerve endings in rat brain. Journal of Nerochemistry 1962; 9, 23-35.

[5] Rodríguez de Lores A, Alberic M, De Robertis E. Ultrastructural and enzymic studies

of cholinergic and non-cholinergic synaptic membranes isolated from brain cortex. Journal of Nerochemistry 1967; 14(2) 215-225.

[6] Cotman C W, Matthews D A. Synaptic plasma membranes from rat brain synaptosomes: isolation and partial characterization. Biochimica et Biophysica Acta 1971; 249(2) 380-394.

[7] De Robertis E. Ultrastructure and cytochemistry of the synaptic region. The macromolecular components involved in nerve transmission are being studied. Science 1967; 156(3777) 907-914.

[8] Davis G A, Bloom F E. Isolation of synaptic junctional complexes from rat brain. Brain Research 1973; 62(1) 35-53.

[9] Balázs R, Dahl D, Harwood J R. Subcellular distribution of enzymes of glutamate metabolism in rat brain. Journal of Nerochemistry 1966; 13(10) 897-905.

[10] Whittaker V P. The morphology of fractions of rat forebrain synaptosomes separated on continuous sucrose density gradients. Biochemical Journal 1968; 106(2) 412-417.

[11] Fonnum F. The distribution of glutamate decarboxylase and aspartate transaminase in subcellular fractions of rat and guinea-pig brain. Biochemical Journal 1968; 106(2) 401–412.

[12] Jones D G. Synapses and synaptosomes: Morphological aspects. London and New York: Chapman and Hall; 1975.

[13] Glebov RN, Kryzhanovskii G N. [Functional biochemistry of synapses]. Moscow: Meditsina; 1978. Russian.

[14] Wessler I, Kirkpatrick C J, Racké K. The cholinergic 'pitfall': acetylcholine, a universal cell molecule in biological systems, including humans. Clinical and Experimental Pharmacology and Physiology 1999; 26(3) 198-205.

[15] Wessler I, Bittinger F, Kamin W, Zepp F, Meyer E, Schad A, Kirkpatrick C J. Dysfunction of the non-neuronal cholinergic system in the airways and blood cells of patients with cystic fibrosis. Life Sciences 2007; 80(24-25) 2253-2258..

[16] Brust P, Friedrich A, Krizbai I A, Bergmann R, Roux F, Ganapathy V, Johannsen B. Functional expression of the serotonin transporter in immortalized rat brain microvessel endothelial cells. Journal of Nerochemistry 2000; 74(3) 1241-1248.

[17] Kirkpatrick C J, Bittinger F, Unger R E, Kriegsmann J, Kilbinger H, Wessler I. The non-neuronal cholinergic system in the endothelium: evidence and possible pathobiological significance. Japan Journal of Pharmacology 2001; 85(1) 24-28.

[18] Gorini A, D'Angelo A, Villa R F. Energy Metabolism of Synaptosomal Subpopulations from Different Neuronal Systems of Rat Hippocampus: Effect of L-Acetylcarnitine Administration In Vivo. Neurochemical Research 1999; 24(5) 617-624.

[19] Sokolow S, Henkins K M, Williams I A, Vinters H V, Schmid I, Cole G M, Gylys K H. Isolation of synaptic terminals from Alzheimer's disease cortex. Cytometry Part A 2012; 81(3) 248-254. doi: 10.1002/cyto.a.22009. http://www.ncbi.nlm.nih.gov/pubmed/?term=Sokolow+S%2C+Henkins+K+M%2C+Williams+I+A%2C+Vinters+H+V%2C+Schmid+I%2C+Cole+G+M%2C+Gylys+K+H (accessed 2011 Dec 28).

[20] Ammons D, Manrrique J, Rampersad J. An apparatus to control and automate the formation of continuous density gradients. Analytical Biochemistry 2012; 427(2) 124-126. doi: 10.1016/j.ab.2012.05.012. http://www.ncbi.nlm.nih.gov/pubmed/?term=Ammons+D%2C+Manrrique+J (accessed 2012 May 22).

[21] Laverty R, Michaelson I A, Sharman D F, Whittaker V P. The subcellular localization of dopamine and acetylcholine in the dog caudate nucleus. British Journal of Pharmacology and Chemotherapy 1963; 21, 482-490.

[22] Mangan J L, Whittaker V P. The distribution of free amino acids in subcellular fractions of guinea-pig brain. Biochemical Journal 1966; 98(1) 128-137.

[23] Sheridan M N, Whittaker V P, Israël M. The subcellular fractionation of the electric organ of Torpedo. Zeitschrift für Zellforschung und Mikroskopische Anatomie 1966; 74(3) 293-307.

[24] Robinson M B. Examination of glutamate transporter heterogeneity using synaptosomal preparations. Methods in Enzymology 1998; 296, 189-202.

[25] Mukhin E I, Zakharova E I, Kikteva E A. Comparison of the cholinergic system in neocortical field Ep in cats with strong and weak cognitive abilities. Neuroscience of Behavioral and Physiology 2002; 32(4) 379-387.

[26] Whittaker V P. Some Currently Neglected Aspects of Cholinergic Function. Journal of Molecular Neuroscience 2010; 40(1-2) 7–11.

[27] Zakharova E I, Dudchenko A M, Svinov M M, Fedorova M M, Germanova E L. Cholinergic Systems of the Rat Brain and Neuronal Reorganization under Conditions of Acute Hypoxia. Neurochemical Journal 2010; 4(4) 290–303.

[28] Zakharova E I, Storozheva Z I, Dudchenko A M, Kubatiev A A. Chronic Cerebral Ischaemia Forms New Cholinergic Mechanisms of Learning and Memory. International Jornal of Alzheimers Disease 2010; 2010: 954589. doi: 10.4061/2010/954589. http://www.ncbi.nlm.nih.gov/pmc/articles/PMC3010649/ (accessed 2010 December 20).

[29] Zakharova E I, Germanova E L, Kopaladze R A, Dudchenko A. M. Central Cholinergic Systems in the Mechanisms of Hypoxic Preconditioning: Diverse Pathways of Synaptic Reorganization in Vivo. Neurochemical Journal 2013; 7(1) 45–55.

[30] Villa R F, Ferrari F, Gorini A. Effect of in vivo L-acetylcarnitine administration on ATP-ases enzyme systems of synaptic plasma membranes from rat cerebral cortex. Neurochemical Research 2011; 36(8) 1372-1382. doi: 10.1007/s11064-011-0462-x. http://www.ncbi.nlm.nih.gov/pubmed/21479591 (accessed 2011 Apr 9).

[31] Villa R F, Ferrari F, Gorini A. ATP-ases of synaptic plasma membranes in striatum: Enzymatic systems for synapses functionality by in vivo administration of l-acetyl-carnitine in relation to Parkinson's Disease. Neuroscience 2013; 248C, 414-426.

[32] Dale H. Transmission of Nervous Effects by Acetylcholine. Harvey Lecture, May 20, 1937. Bulletin of the New York Academy of Medicine 1937; 13(7) 379–396.

[33] Fatt P, Katz B. Spontaneous subthreshold activity at motor nerve endings. Journal of Physiology 1952; 117(1) 109-128.

[34] Chang H C, Gaddum J H. Choline esters in tissue extracts. Journal of Physiology 1933; 79(3) 255-285.

[35] Tuček S. Regulation of Acetylcholine Synthesis in the Brain. Journal of Nerochemistry 1985; 44(1) 11-24.

[36] Black S A G, Rylett R J. Impact of Oxidative - Nitrosative Stress on Cholinergic Presynaptic Function, In: De La Monte S. (Ed.) Alzheimer's Disease Pathogenesis-Core Concepts, Shifting Paradigms and Therapeutic Targets. InTech; 2011. p345-368.

[37] Sha D, Jin H, Kopke R D, Wu J Y. Choline acetyltransferase: regulation and coupling with protein kinase and vesicular acetylcholine transporter on synaptic vesicles. Neurochemical Research 2004; 29(1) 199-207.

[38] Levey A I, Wainer B H, Rye D B, Mufson E J, Mesulam M M. Choline acetyltransferase-immunoreactive neurons intrinsic to rodent cortex and distinction from acetylcholinesterase-positive neurons. Neuroscience 1984; 13(2) 341-453.

[39] Hallanger A E, Wainer B H, Rye D B. Colocalization of gamma-aminobutyric acid and acetylcholinesterase in rodent cortical neurons. Neuroscience 1986; 19(3) 763-769.

[40] Arvidsson U, Riedl M, Elde R, Meister B. Vesicular acetylcholine transporter (VAChT) protein: a novel and unique marker for cholinergic neurons in the central and peripheral nervous systems. Journal of Comparative Neurology and Psychology 1997; 378(4) 454-467.

[41] Ichikawa T, Ajiki K, Matsuura J, Misawa H. Localization of two cholinergic markers, choline acetyltransferase and vesicular acetylcholine transporter in the central nervous system of the rat: in situ hybridization histochemistry and immunohistochemistry. Journal of Chemical Neuroanatomy 1997; 13(1) 23-39.

[42] McKinney M, Coyle J T, Hedreen J C. Topographic analysis of the innervation of the rat neocortex and hippocampus by the basal forebrain cholinergic system. Journal of Comparative Neurology and Psychology 1983; 217(1) 103-121.

[43] Mesulam M M, Mufson E J, Wainer B H, Levey A I. Central cholinergic pathways in the rat: an overview based on an alternative nomenclature (Ch1-Ch6). Neuroscience 1983; 10(4) 1185-1201.

[44] Saper C B. Organization of cerebral cortical afferent systems in the rat. II. Magnocellular basal nucleus. Journal of Comparative Neurology and Psychology 1984; 222(3); 313-342.

[45] Woolf N J, Eckenstein F, Butcher L L. Cholinergic systems in the rat brain: I. projections to the limbic telencephalon. Brain Research Bulletin 1984; 13(6) 751-784.

[46] Houser C R, Crawford G D, Salvaterra P M, Vaughn J E. Immunocytochemical localization of choline acetyltransferase in rat cerebral cortex: a study of cholinergic neurons and synapses. Journal of Comparative Neurology and Psychology 1985; 234(1) 17-34.

[47] Anderson K J, Gibbs R B, Salvaterra P M, Cotman C W. Ultrastructural characterization of identified cholinergic neurons transplanted to the hippocampal formation of the rat. Journal of Comparative Neurology and Psychology 1986; 249(2) 279-292.

[48] Eckenstein F P, Baughman R W, Quinn J. An anatomical study of cholinergic innervation in rat cerebral cortex. Neuroscience 1988; 25(2) 457-474.

[49] Butcher L L, Oh J D, Woolf N J, Edwards R H, Roghani A. Organization of central cholinergic neurons revealed by combined in situ hybridization histochemistry and choline-O-acetyltransferase immunocytochemistry. Neurochemistry International 1992; 21(3) 429-445.

[50] Jones B E. Immunohistochemical study of choline acetyltransferase-immunoreactive processes and cells innervating the pontomedullary reticular formation in the rat. Journal of Comparative Neurology and Psychology 1990; 295(3) 485-514.

[51] Higo S, Matsuyama T, Kawamura S. Direct projections from the pedunculopontine and laterodorsal tegmental nuclei to area 17 of the visual cortex in the cat. Neuroscience Research 1996; 26(2) 109–118.

[52] Parnavelas J G, Kelly W, Franke E, Eckenstein F P. Cholinergic neurons and fibers in rat visual cortex. Journal of Neurocytology 1986; 15(3) 329-336.

[53] Matthews D A, Salvaterra P M, Crawford G D, Houser C R, Vaughn J E. An immunocytochemical study of choline acetyltransferase-containing neurons and axon terminals in normal and partially deafferented hippocampal formation. Brain Research 1987; 402(1) 30-43.

[54] Kanaya-Ida S, Ben Ari Y. Transient increase in the number of cholinergic neurons in the developing rat dentate gyrus. Neuroscience Letters 1989; 101(1) 23-28.

[55] Frotscher M, Vida I, Bender R. Evidence for the existence of non-GABAergic, cholinergic interneurons in the rodent hippocampus. Neuroscience 2000; 96(1) 27-31.

[56] Motavkin PA, Okhotin V E, Sulimov G Iu. [Cholinergic pyramidal Betz's and Meynert's neurons in human cerebral cortex]. Zhornal Nevropatologii i Psikhiatrii im. S.S. Korsakova 1990; 90(10) 14-16. Russian.

[57] Houser C R, Crawford G D, Barber R P, Salvaterra P M, Vaughn J E. Organization and morphological characteristics of cholinergic neurons: an immunocytochemical study with a monoclonal antibody to choline acetyltransferase. Brain Research 1983; 266(1) 97-119.

[58] De Jonge W J, Ulloa L. The alpha7 nicotinic acetylcholine receptor as a pharmacological target for inflammation. British Journal of Pharmacology 2007; 151(7) 915-929. http://www.ncbi.nlm.nih.gov/pubmed/17502850 (accessed 2007 May 14)

[59] Gallowitsch-Puerta M, Pavlov V A. Neuro-immune interactions via the cholinergic anti-inflammatory pathway. Life Sciences 2007; 80(24-25) 2325-2329. http://www.ncbi.nlm.nih.gov/pubmed/17289087 (accessed 2007 Jan 13).

[60] Miao F J, Lee T J. Cholinergic and VIPergic innervation in cerebral arteries: a sequential double-labeling immunohistochemical study. Journal of Cerebral Blood Flow and Metabolism 1990; 10(1) 32-37.

[61] Chédotal A, Cozzari C, Faure M P, Hartman B K, Hamel E. Distinct choline acetyltransferase (ChAT) and vasoactive intestinal polypeptide (VIP) bipolar neurons project to local blood vessels in the rat cerebral cortex. Brain Research 1994; 646(2) 181-193.

[62] Fischer A, Canning B J, Kummer W. Correlation of vasoactive intestinal peptide and nitric oxide synthase with choline acetyltransferase in the airway innervation. Annals of the New York Academy of Sciences 1996; 805, 717-722.

[63] Kc P, Mayer C A, Haxhiu M A. Chemical profile of vagal preganglionic motor cells innervating the airways in ferrets: the absence of noncholinergic neurons. Journal of Applied Physiology 2004; 97(4) 1508-1517.

[64] Yu J G, Kimura T, Chang X F, Lee T J. Segregation of VIPergic-nitric oxidergic and cholinergic-nitric oxidergic innervation in porcine middle cerebral arteries. Brain Research 1998; 801(1-2) 78-87.

[65] Si M L, Lee T J. Alpha7-nicotinic acetylcholine receptors on cerebral perivascular sympathetic nerves mediate choline-induced nitrergic neurogenic vasodilation. Circulation Research 2002; 91(1) 62-69.

[66] Mikhelson M Ya, Zeimal E V. [Achetylcholine]. Leningrad: Nauka; 1970. Russian.

[67] Dauphin F, Lacombe P, Sercombe R, Hamel E, Seylaz J. Hypercapnia and stimulation of the substantia innominata increase rat frontal cortical blood flow by different cholinergic mechanisms. Brain Research 1991; 553(1) 75-83.

[68] Vaucher E, Hamel E. Cholinergic basal forebrain neurons project to cortical microvessels in the rat: electron microscopic study with anterogradely transported Phaseolus vulgaris leucoagglutinin and choline acetyltransferase immunocytochemistry. Journal of Neuroscience 1995; 15(11) 7427-7441.

[69] Lacombe P, Sercombe R, Vaucher E, Seylaz J. Reduced cortical vasodilatory response to stimulation of the nucleus basalis of Meynert in the aged rat and evidence for a control of the cerebral circulation. Annals of the New York Academy of Sciences 1997; 826, 410-415.

[70] Miao F J, Lee T J. VIP-ergic and cholinergic innervations in internal carotid arteries of the cat and rat. Journal of Cardiovascular Pharmacology 1991; 18(3) 369-378.

[71] Dauphin F, Ting V, Payette P, Dennis M, Hamel E. Vasocontractile muscarinic M1 receptors in cat cerebral arteries: pharmacological identification and detection of mRNA. European Journal of Pharmacology 1991; 207(4) 319-327.

[72] Nakai M, Tamaki K, Ogata J, Matsui Y, Maeda M. Parasympathetic cerebrovasodilator center of the facial nerve. Circulation Research 1993; 72(2) 470-475.

[73] Kuo J S, Leung Y M, Lin N N, Lee T J, Gong C L. Nicotine stimulation of the medulla increases blood flow of the common carotid artery in cats. Autonomic Neurosience 2010; 152(1-2) 49-54. doi: 10.1016/j.autneu.2009.08.019. http://www.ncbi.nlm.nih.gov/pubmed/19767248 (accessed 2009 Sep 19).

[74] Commons K G, Serock M R. Coincidence of Neurokinin 1 Receptor with the Vesicular Glutamate Transporter 3 (VGLUT3) in the Rat Forebrain. Neuroscience Letters 2009; 464(3) 188–192. doi: 10.1016/j.neulet.2009.08.042. http://www.ncbi.nlm.nih.gov/pubmed/?term=Commons+K+G%2C+Serock+M+R (accessed 2009 Aug 21).

[75] Batchelor P E, Armstrong D M, Blaker S N, Gage F H. Nerve growth factor receptor and choline acetyltransferase colocalization in neurons within the rat forebrain: response to fimbria-fornix transection. Journal of Comparative Neurology and Psychology 1989; 284(2) 187-204.

[76] Schnitzler A C, Lopez-Coviella I, Blusztajn J K. Differential modulation of nerve growth factor receptor (p75) and cholinergic gene expression in purified p75-expressing and non-expressing basal forebrain neurons by BMP9. Brain Research 2008; 1246, 19–28. doi: 10.1016/j.brainres.2008.09.085. http://www.ncbi.nlm.nih.gov/pubmed/18952073 (accessed 2008 Oct 14).

[77] Auld D S, Mennicken F, Day J C, Quirion R. Neurotrophins differentially enhance acetylcholine release, acetylcholine content and choline acetyltransferase activity in basal forebrain neurons. Journal of Nerochemistry 2001; 77(1) 253-262.

[78] Pongrac J L, Rylett R J. Differential effects of nerve growth factor on expression of choline acetyltransferase and sodium-coupled choline transport in basal forebrain cholinergic neurons in culture. Journal of Nerochemistry 1996; 66(2) 804-810.

[79] Zakharov V V, Khatiashvily I T, Iakhno N N. [Dementia with Lewy bodies]. Neurologicheskii Journal 1998; (6) 7-11. http://memorylab.ru/for_specialists/nejrozabolevania/demencia_s_telcam/ Russian.

[80] Oda Y. Choline acetyltransferase: the structure, distribution and pathologic changes in the central nervous system. Pathology International 1999; 49(11) 921-937.

[81] Mosimann U P, McKeith I G. Dementia with Lewy bodies – diagnosis and treatment. Swiss Medical Weekly 2003; 133(9-10) 131-142.

[82] Dobransky T, Rylett R J. Functional regulation of choline acetyltransferase by phosphorylation. Neurochemical Research 2003; 28(3-4) 537-542.

[83] Gill S K, Ishak M, Dobransky T, Haroutunian V, Davis K L, Rylett R J. 82-kDa choline acetyltransferase is in nuclei of cholinergic neurons in human CNS and altered in aging and Alzheimer disease. Nerobiology of Aging 2007; 28(7) 1028-1040.

[84] Wang J, Zhang H Y, Tang X C. Cholinergic deficiency involved in vascular dementia: possible mechanism and strategy of treatment. Acta Pharmacologica Sinica 2009; 30(7) 879-888.

[85] Nardone R, De Blasi P, Seidl M, Höller Y, Caleri F, Tezzon F, Ladurner G, Golaszewski S, Trinka E. Cognitive function and cholinergic transmission in patients with subcortical vascular dementia and microbleeds: a TMS study. Journal Of neuronal Pransmission 2011; 118(9) 1349-1358.

[86] Rochester L, Yarnall A J, Baker M R, David R V, Lord S, Galna B, Burn D J. Cholinergic dysfunction contributes to gait disturbance in early Parkinson's disease. Brain 2012; 135(9) 2779-2788.

[87] Shin J, Choi S, Lee J E, Lee H S, Sohn Y H, Lee P H. Subcortical white matter hyperintensities within the cholinergic pathways of Parkinson's disease patients according to cognitive status. Journal of neurology, neurosurgery and psychiatry 2012; 83(3) 315-321.

[88] Yarnall A, Rochester L, Burn D J. Mild cognitive impairment in Parkinson's disease. Age Ageing 2013; 42(5) 567-576.

[89] Onodera H, Sato G, Kogure K. Quantitative autoradiographic analysis of muscarinic and adenosine A1 binding sites after transient forefrain ischemia in the gerbil. Brain Research 1987; 415(2) 309-322.

[90] Ogawa N, Haba K, Asanuma M, Mizukava K, Mori A. Super-delayed changes of muscarinic acetylcholine receptors in the gerbil hippocampus following transient ischemia. In: Kito S. et al. (Eds) Advances in Experimental Medicine and Biology Volume 287: Neuroreceptor Mechanisms in Brain. New York: Plenum Press; 1991. p343-347.

[91] Ishimaru H, Takahashi A, Ikarashi Y, Maruiama Y. NGF delays rather then prevents the colinergic terminal and delayed neuronal death in the hippocampus after ischemia. Brain Research 1998; 789(2) 194-200.

[92] Dobransky T, Doherty-Kirby A, Kim A R, Brewer D, Lajoie G, Rylett R J. Protein kinase-C isoforms differentially phosphorylate human choline acetyltransferase regulating its catalytic activity. Journal of Biological Chemistry 2004; 279(50) 52059-52068.

[93] Ohno K, Tsujino A, Brengman J M, Harper C M, Bajzer Z, Udd B, Beyring R, Robb S, Kirkham F J, Engel A G. Choline acetyltransferase mutations cause myasthenic syndrome associated with episodic apnea in humans. Proceedings of the National Academy of Sciences of the United States of America-Physical Sciences 2001; 98, 2017–2022.

[94] Rylett R J. Synaptosomal "membrane-bound" choline acetyltransferase is most sensitive to inhibition by choline mustard. Journal of Nerochemistry 1989; 52(3) 869-875.

[95] Dobransky T, Davis W L, Rylett R J. Functional Characterization of Phosphorylation of 69-kDa Human Choline Acetyltransferase at Serine 440 by Protein Kinase C. Journal of Biological Chemistry 2001; 276(25) 22244-22250.

[96] Pahud G, Medilanski J, Eder-Colli L. Cytosolic Choline Acetyltransferase Binds Specifically to Cholinergic Plasma Membrane of Rat Brain Synaptosomes to Generate Membrane-Bound Enzyme. Neurochemical Research 2003, 28(3-4) 543–549.

[97] Fonnum F, Malthe-Sorenssen D. Membrane affinities and subcellular distribution of the different molecular forms of choline acetyltransferase from rat. Journal of Nerochemistry 1973; 20(5) 1351-1359.

[98] Smith C P, Carroll P T. A comparison of solubilized and membrane bound forms of choline-O-acetyltransferase (EC 2.3.1.6) in mouse brain nerve endings. Brain Research 1980; 185(2) 363-371.

[99] Benishin C G, Carroll P T. Multiple forms of choline-O-acetyltransferase in mouse and rat brain: solubilization and characterization. Journal of Nerochemistry 1983; 41(4) 1030-1039.

[100] Misawa H, Matsuura J, Oda Y, Takahashi R, Deguchi T. Human choline acetyltransferase mRNAs with different 5_-region produce a 69-kDa major translation product. Molecular Brain Research 1997; 44, 323–433.

[101] Kengaku M, Misawa H, Deguchi T. Multiple mRNA species of choline acetyltransferase from rat spinal cord. Molecular Brain Research 1993; 18(1-2) 71-76.

[102] Kim A R, Rylett R J, Shiton B H. Substrate binding and catalytic mechanism of human choline acetyltransferase. Biochemistry 2006; 45(49) 14621-14631.

[103] Matsuo A, Bellier J P, Nishimura M, Yasuhara O, Saito N, Kimura H. Nuclear choline acetyltransferase activates transcription of a high-affinity choline transporter. Journal of Biological Chemistry 2011; 286(7) 5836-5845.

[104] Dobransky T, Davis W L, Xiao G H, Rylett R J. Expression, purification and characterization of recombinant human choline acetyltransferase: phosphorylation of the enzyme regulates catalytic activity. Biochemical Journal 2000; 349(1) 141-145.

[105] Resendes M C, Dobransky T, Ferguson S S G, Rylett R J. Nuclear localization of the 82-kDa form of human choline acetyltransferase. Journal of Biological Chemistry 1999; 274, 19417–19421.

[106] Tooyama I, Kimura H. A protein encoded by an alternative splice variant of choline acetyltransferase mRNA is localized preferentially in peripheral nerve cells and fibers. Journal of Chemical Neuroanatomy 2000; 17(4) 217-226.

[107] Saito A, Sato T, Okano H, Toyoda K, Bamba H, Kimura S, Bellier J P, Matsuo A, Kimura H, Hisa Y, Tooyama I. Axotomy alters alternative splicing of choline acetyltransferase in the rat dorsal motor nucleus of the vagus nerve. Journal of Comparative Neurology and Psychology 2009; 513(2) 237-248.

[108] Dobransky T, Rylett R J. Protein kinase C isoforms differentially phosphorylate human choline acetyltransferase regulating its catalytic activity. Journal of Nerochemistry 2005; 95(2) 305-313.

[109] Dobransky T, Rylett R J. A model for dynamic regulation of choline acetyltransferase by phosphorylation. Journal of Nerochemistry 2005; 95, 305–313.

[110] Schmidt B M, Rylett R J. Phosphorylation of rat brain choline acetyltransferase and its relationship to enzyme activity. Journal of Nerochemistry 1993; 61(5) 1774-1781.

[111] Bruce G, Hersh L B. The phosphorylation of choline acetyltransferase. Neurochemical Research 1989; 14(7) 613-620.

[112] Dobransky T, Brewer D, Lajoie G, Rylett R J. Phosphorylation of 69-kD choline acetyltransferase at threonine-456 in response to short-term exposure to amyloid-b peptide 1-42. Journal of Biological Chemistry 2003; 278(8) 5883–5893.

[113] Rylett R J, Goddard S, Lambro A. Regulation of expression of cholinergic neuronal phenotypic markers in neuroblastoma LA-N-2.. Journal of Nerochemistry 1993; 61, 1388–1397.

[114] Fonnum F. The 'compartmentation' of choline acetyltransferase within the synaptosome. Biochemical Journal 1967; 103(1) 262-270.

[115] Eder-Colli L, Briand P A, Dunant Y. Membrane-bound choline acetyltransferase of the torpedo has characteristics of an integral membrane protein and can be solubilized by proteolysis. Brain Research 1992; 573(2) 284-292.

[116] Pahud G, Salem N, Van de Goor J, Medilanski J, Pellegrinelli N, Eder-Colli L. Study of subcellular localization of membrane-bound choline acetyltransferase in Drosophila central nervous system and its association with membranes. European Journal of Neuroscience 1998; 10(5) 1644-1653.

[117] Pahud G, Pahud G, Eder-Colli L. Cytosolic Choline Acetyltransferase Binds Specifically to Cholinergic Plasma Membrane of Rat Brain Synaptosomes to Generate Membrane-Bound Enzyme. Neurochemical Research 2003; 28(3-4) 543–549.

[118] Schmidt B M, Rylett R J. Basal synthesis of acetylcholine in hippocampal synaptosomes is not dependent upon membrane-bound choline acetyltransferase activity. Neuroscience 1993; 54(3) 649–656.

[119] Salem N, Medilanski J, Pellegrinelli N, Eder-Colli L. Hydrophilic and amphiphilic forms of Drosophila choline acetyltransferase are encoded by a single mRNA. European Journal of Neuroscience 1994; 6(5) 737-745.

[120] Carroll P T, Badamchian M, Craig P, Lyness W H. Veratridine-induced breakdown of cytosolic acetylcholine in rat hippocampal minces: an intraterminal form of acetylcholinesterase or choline O-acetyltransferase? Brain Research 1986; 383(1-2) 83-99.

[121] Carroll P T. Veratridine-induced activation of choline-O-acetyltransferase activity in rat hippocampal tissue: relationship to the veratridine-induced release of acetylcholine. Brain Research 1986; 414(2) 401-404.

[122] Carroll P T, Benishin C G. Depolarization of mouse forebrain minces with veratridine and high K+: failure to stimulate the Ca2+ independent, spontaneous release of acetylcholine from the cytoplasm due to hydrolysis of the acetylcholine stored there. Brain Research 1984; 291(2) 261-272.

[123] Carroll P T. Evidence to suggest that extracellular acetate is accumulated by rat hippocampal cholinergic nerve terminals for acetylcholine formation and release. Brain Research 1997; 753(1) 47-55.

[124] Alkondon M, Pereira E F, Cortes W S, Maelicke A, Albuquerque E X. Choline is a selective agonist of alpha7 nicotinic acetylcholine receptors in the rat brain neurons. European Journal of Neuroscience 1997; 9, 2734-2742.

[125] Rylett R J, Schmidt B M. Regulation of the synthesis of acetylcholine. Progress in Braim Research 1993; 98, 161-166.

[126] Smith L K, Carroll PT. Membrane-bound choline-O-acetyltransferase in rat hippocampal tissue is anchored by glycosyl-phosphatidylinositol. Brain Research 1993; 605(1) 155-163.

[127] Carroll P T. Membrane-bound choline-O-acetyltransferase in rat hippocampal tissue is associated with synaptic vesicles. Brain Research 1994; 633(1-2) 112-118.

[128] Birman S, Israël M, Lesbats B, Morel N. Solubilization and partial purification of a presynaptic membrane protein ensuring calcium-dependent acetylcholine release from proteoliposomes. Journal of Nerochemistry 1986; 47(2) 433-444.

[129] Israël M, Lesbats B, Morel N, Manaranche R, Le Gal la Salle G. Is the acetylcholine releasing protein mediatophore present in rat brain? FEBS Letters 1988; 233(2) 421-426.

[130] Falk-Vairant J, Corrèges P, Eder-Colli L, Salem N, Roulet E, Bloc A, Meunier F, Lesbats B, Loctin F, Synguelakis M, Israel M, Dunant Y. Quantal acetylcholine release induced by mediatophore transfection. Proceedings of the National Academy of Sciences of the United States of America-Physical Sciences 1996; 93(11) 5203-5207.

[131] Dunant Y, Cordeiro J M, Gonçalves P P. Exocytosis, mediatophore, and vesicular Ca2+/H+ antiport in rapid neurotransmission. Annals of the New York Academy of Sciences 2009; 1152, 100-112.

[132] Dunant, Y.; Israël M. Neurotransmitter release at rapid synapses. (2000). Biochimie, Vol. 82, No. 4, pp. 289-302.

[133] Bloc A, Bugnard E, Dunant Y, Falk-Vairant J, Israël M, Loctin F, Roulet E. Acetylcholine synthesis and quantal release reconstituted by transfection of mediatophore and choline acetyltranferase cDNAs. European Journal of Neuroscience 1999; 11(5) 1523-1534.

[134] Black S A, Rylett R J. Choline transporter CHT regulation and function in cholinergic neurons. Central Nervous System Agents in Medicinal Chemistry 2012; 12(2) 114-121.

[135] Dunant Y, Loctin F, Vallée J P, Parducz A, Lesbats B, Israël M. Activation and desensitisation of acetylcholine release by zinc at Torpedo nerve terminals. Pflügers Archiv 1996; 432(5) 853-858.

[136] Bancila V, Nikonenko I, Dunant Y, Bloc A. Zinc inhibits glutamate release via activation of pre-synaptic K channels and reduces ischaemic damage in rat hippocampus. Journal of Nerochemistry 2004; 90(5) 1243-1250.

[137] Medvedeva Y V, Lin B, Shuttleworth C W, Weiss J,H. Intracellular Zn2+ accumulation contributes to synaptic failure, mitochondrial depolarization, and cell death in an acute slice oxygen-glucose deprivation model of ischemia. Journal of Neuroscience 2009; 29(4) 1105-1114.

[138] Cordeiro J M, Gonçalves P P, Dunant Y. Synaptic vesicles control the time course of neurotransmitter secretion via a Ca^{2+}/H+ antiport. Journal of Physiology 2011; 589(1) 149-167.

[139] Carroll P T. Evidence to suggest that cytosolic acetylcholine in rat hippocampal nerve terminals is not directly transferred into synaptic vesicles for release. Brain Research 1996; 725(1) 3-10.

[140] Parducz A, Corrèges P, Sors P, Dunant Y. Zinc blocks acetylcholine release but not vesicle fusion at the Torpedo nerve-electroplate junction. European Journal of Neuroscience 1997; 9(4) 732-738.

[141] Zakharova E I. Storojeva Z I, Germanova E L, Monakov M Y, Proshin A T, Dudchenko A M, Lukyanova L D. Characteristics of cholinergic and cognitive functions in rats with individual resistance to the cerebral ischemia. In: Lukyanova L., Takeda N. and Singal P.K. (Eds.) Adaptation Biology and Medicine Volume 5: Health Potentials. New Delhi: Narosa Publishing House Pvt. Ltd.; 2008. p122-141,

[142] Svinov M M, Zakharova E I, Kositsyn N S. Ultrastructure of synapses in cerebral cortex layer i in rats with low and high resistance to hypoxia. Biulleten eksperimentalnoi biologii i meditsini 2001; 131(5) 499-501.

[143] Samoilov M O. [Reaction of brain neurons to hypoxia]. Leningrad: Nauka; 1985. Russian.

[144] Semchenko V V, Stepanov S S. [Effect of hypoxia on the structure of the presynaptic grid of the interneuronal contacts of the rat neocortex]. Tsitologia 1985; 27(11) 1235-1239. Russian.

[145] Semchenko V V, Stepanov S S. [Electron microscopic cytochemical and morphometric study of the cerebral cortex synapses in postmortem autolysis]. Biulleten eksperimentalnoi biologii i meditsini 1986; 102(7) 100-102. Russian.

[146] Gallo G. RhoA-kinase coordinates F-actin organization and myosin II activity during semaphorin-3A-induced axon retraction. Journal of Cell Science 2006; 119(16) 3413-3423.

[147] Keck T, Scheuss V, Jacobsen R I, Wierenga C J, Eysel U T, Bonhoeffer T, Hübener M. Loss of sensory input causes rapid structural changes of inhibitory neurons in adult mouse visual cortex. Neuron 2011; 71(5) 869-882.

[148] Woods G F, Oh W C, Boudewyn L C, Mikula S K, Zito K. Loss of PSD-95 enrichment is not a prerequisite for spine retraction. Journal of Neuroscience 2011; 31(34) 12129-12138.

[149] Semchenko V V, Bogolepov N N, Stepanov S S, Maksimishin S V, Khizhnyak A S. Synaptic plasticity of the neocortex of white rats with diffuse-focal brain injuries. Neuroscience of Behavioral and Physiology 2006; 36(6) 613-618.

[150] Bueters T, Von Euler M, Bendel O, Von Euler G. Degeneration of newly formed CA1 neurons following global ischemia in the rat. Experimental Neurology 2008; 209(1) 114-124.

[151] Mufson E J, Counts S E, Perez S E, Ginsberg S D. Cholinergic system during the progression of Alzheimer's disease: therapeutic implications. Expert Reviews of Neurotherapeutics 2008; 8(11) 1703–1718.

[152]] Sun M K, Hongpaisan J, Nelson T J, Alkon D L. Poststroke neuronal rescue and synaptogenesis mediated in vivo by protein kinase C in adult brains. Proceedings of the National Academy of Sciences of the United States of America-Physical Sciences 2008; 105(36) 13620-13625.

[153] Semchenko V V, Stepanov S S. [The system of subsynaptic units as an universal system-organizing and regulating factor of brain synapses]. Biulleten eksperimentalnoi biologii i meditsini 1997; 124(7) 4-12. Russian.

[154] Rossor M N, Svendsen C, Hunt S P, Mountjoy C Q, Roth M, Iversen L L. The substantia innominata in Alzheimer's disease: an histochemical and biochemical study of cholinergic marker enzymes. Neuroscience Letters 1982; 28(2) 217-222.

[155] Zakharova E I, Dudchenko A M, Svinov M M. Ivanov D S. Ignatiev I V. [The comparative characteristics of the cholinergic systems in the brains of the low and high resistant to the oxygen deficit rats]. Neurokhimia 2001; 18(2) 119-131. Russian.

[156] Zakharova E I, Storozheva Z I, Mukhin E I, Dudchenko A M. [Regulation of cognitive functions: cholinergic mechanisms and their variability]. In: Falikman M.V. & Pechenkova E.V. (Eds.) Cognitive Science in Moscow: new researches. Moscow: Buki-Vedi; 2011. p120-124. Russian.

[157]] Ni J W, Matsumoto K, Li H B, Murakami Y, Watanabe H. Neuronal damage and decrease of central acetylcholine level following permanent occlusion of bilateral common carotid arteries in rat. Brain Research 1995; 673(2) 290-296.

[158] Watanabe H, Ni J W, Sakai Y, Matsumoto K, Murukami Y, Tohda M. Permanent occlusion of bilateral internal carotid arteries produces cognitive deficits in two learning behavior tasks. Nihon Shinkei Seishin Yakurigaku Zasshi 1996; 16(1) 19-24.

[159] Rogers D C, Hunter A J. Photothrombotic lesions of the rat cortex impair acquisition of the water maze. Pharmacology, Biochemistry and Behavior 1997; 56(4) 747-754.

[160] Higashi H, Meno J R, Marwaha A S, Winn H R. Hippocampal injury and neurobehavioral deficits following hyperglycemic cerebral ischemia: effect of theophylline and ZM 241385. Journal of Neurosurgery 2002; 96(1) 117-126.

[161] Casamenti F, Bracco L, Bartolini L, Pepeu G. Effects of ganglioside treatment in rats with a lesion of the cholinergic forebrain nuclei. Brain Research 1985; 338(1) 45-52.

[162] Wenk G, Sweenay J, Hughey D, Carson J, Olton D. Cholinergic function and memory: extensive inhibition of choline acetyltransferase fails to impair radial maze performance in rats. Pharmacology, Biochemistry and Behavior 1986; 25(3) 521-526.

[163] Wisman L A, Sahin G, Maingay M, Leanz G, Kirik D. Functional convergence of dopaminergic and cholinergic input is critical for hippocampus-dependent working memory. Journal of Neuroscience 2008; 28(31) 7797-7807.

[164] Lee B, Shim I, Lee H, Hahm D H. Effect of Bupleurum falcatum on the stress-induced impairment of spatial working memory in rats. Biological and Pharmaceutical Bulletin 2009; 32(8) 1392-1398.

[165] Barros D M, Pereira P, Medina J, Izquierdo I. Modulation of working memory and of long- but not short-term memory by cholinergic mechanisms in the basolateral amygdala. Behavioural Pharmacology 2002; 13(2) 163-167.

[166] Vuckovich J A, Semel M E, Baxter M G. Extensive lesions of cholinergic basal forebrain neurons do not impair spatial working memory. Learning & Memory (2004); 11(1) 87-94.

[167] Lee B, Choi E J, Lee E J, Han S M, Hahm D H, Lee H J, Shim I. The Neuroprotective Effect of Methanol Extract of Gagamjungjihwan and Fructus Euodiae on Ischemia-Induced Neuronal and Cognitive Impairment in the Rat. Evidence-Based Complementary and Alternative Medicine 2011; 2011:685254. doi: 10.1093/ecam/nep028. http://www.ncbi.nlm.nih.gov/pmc/articles/PMC3137009/ (accessed 2011 March 10).

[168] Izquierdo I, Izquierdo L A, Barros D M, Mello e Souza T, De Souza M M, Quevedo J, Rodrigues C, Sant'Anna M K, Madruga M, Medina J H. Differential involvement of cortical receptor mechanisms in working, short-term and long-term memory. Behavioural Pharmacology 1998; 9(5-6) 421-427.

[169] Izquierdo I, Medina J H, Izquierdo L A, Barros D M, De Souza M M.; Mello e Souza T. Short- and long-term memory are differentially regulated by monoaminergic systems in the rat brain. Neurobiology of Learning and Memory 1998; 69(3) 219-224.

[170] Brown R W, Beale K S, Jay Frye G D. Mecamylamine blocks enhancement of reference memory but not working memory produced by post-training injection of nicotine in rats tested on the radial arm maze. Behavioural Brain Research 2002; 134(1-2) 259-265.

[171] Schweigler H, Lipp H P. Hereditary covariations of neuronal circuity and behavior: Correlation between the proportions of hippocampal synaptic fields in the region inferior and two-way avoidance in mice and rats. Behavioural Brain Research 1983; 7(1) 1-38.

3

The Blood Brain Barrier — Regulation of Fatty Acid and Drug Transport

Siddhartha Dalvi, Ngoc On, Hieu Nguyen,
Michael Pogorzelec, Donald W. Miller and
Grant M. Hatch

1. Introduction

1.1. The blood brain barrier

The blood brain barrier (BBB) is a selectively permeable cellular boundary between the brain and the peripheral circulation. The principal component of the BBB is the capillary or microvessel endothelial cell (Figure 1). The endothelial cells in the brain capillaries differ from those in the peripheral vasculature in several key features:

1. Presence of tight junctions (TJ) that limit the paracellular passage of macromolecules.
2. Restricted rate of fluid-phase endocytosis that limits the transcellular passage of macromolecules [1]
3. Presence of specific transporter and carrier molecules [2]
4. Lack of fenestrations [3]
5. Increased mitochondrial content [3]

Thus, the endothelial cells of the BBB are less "leaky" than those of the peripheral vessels. However, it has been shown that if the endothelial cells of the brain capillaries are removed from their natural environment and allowed to vascularize the peripheral tissue, they become more leaky [1]. In contrast, the endothelial cells from the periphery form tight junctions when allowed to vascularize the brain parenchyma. Morphologically, the tight junctions of the BBB

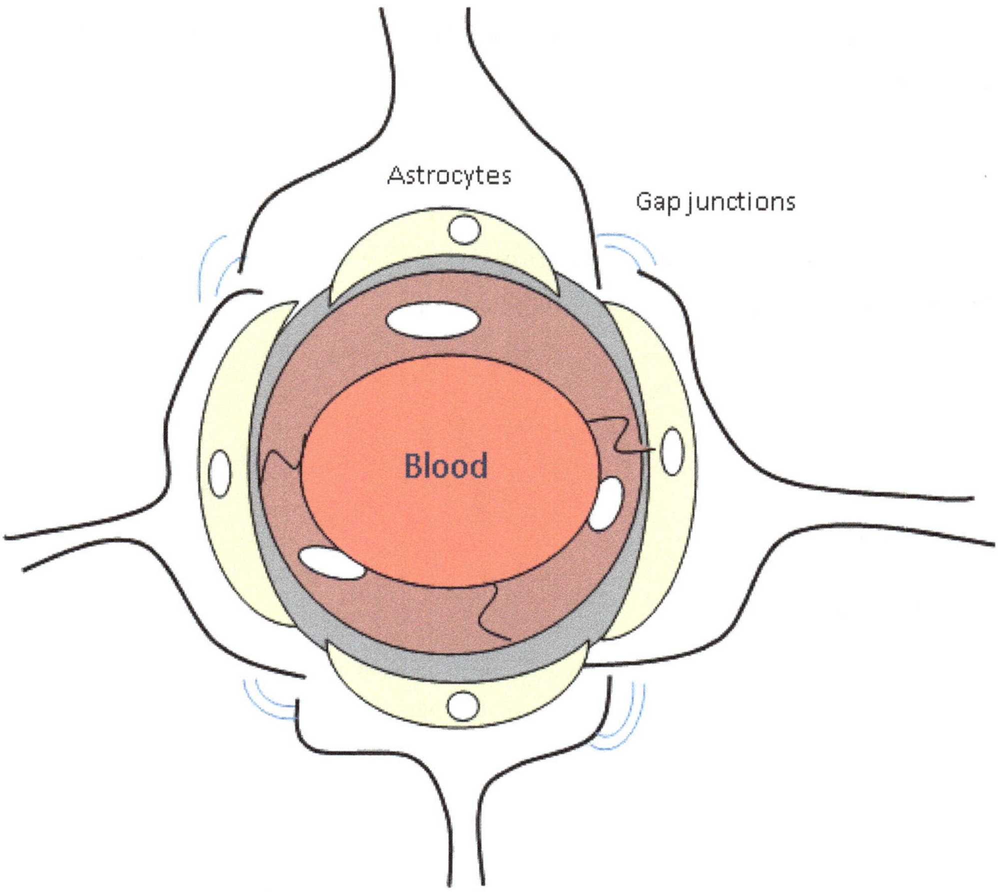

Figure 1. Neurovascular Unit of the blood brain barrier consists of the endothelial cells (pink) surrounded by basement membrane (gray), pericytes (yellow) and astrocyte foot processes. The tight junctions (black lines) formed between two endothelial cells restrict the paracellular diffusion of compounds.

resemble the tight junctions between epithelial cells rather than those between peripheral vascular endothelial cells [4].

The unique tight junctions of the BBB are responsible for producing very high transendothelial electrical resistance (TEER) of 1500 – 2000 Ωcm^2 [2,5,6]. Though the microvessel endothelial cells play a primary role in the formation of the BBB, several other cells are equally important in maintaining the integrity of the BBB. These cells, namely, the astrocytes, pericytes, neurons and other glial cells are said to form a "neurovascular unit" [7]. Integrity of the BBB is of utmost importance in maintaining the homeostasis of the brain microenvironment. Disruption of the BBB is seen in various states of inflammation (multiple sclerosis), neoplasia, infections (meningitis, encephalitis), trauma and Alzheimer disease [8,9]. It would be highly desirable to develop therapeutic strategies to reverse this disruption and tighten the BBB. At the same time, a transient opening of the BBB would be advantageous for delivery of drugs into the brain in conditions like epilepsy or Parkinson disease [2].

1.2. Functions of the BBB

The BBB is responsible for maintaining the appropriate ionic composition of the interstitial fluid of the brain that is required for optimum functioning of the neurons. To achieve this, the BBB functions as a *transport barrier* by facilitating the uptake of the required nutrients, while preventing the uptake of, or actively effluxing certain other molecules or toxic by-products of metabolism [10] The BBB also functions as a *metabolic barrier* by virtue of possessing intracellular and extracellular enzymes. For example, extracellular enzymes such as peptidases and nucleotidases break down peptides and ATP, respectively. Intracellular enzymes like cytochrome P450 (CYP450), primarily CYP1A and CYP2B degrade noxious substances and prevent their entry into the brain parenchyma [10].

1.3. Role of astrocytes in the BBB

It is now known that the astrocytes play a key role in the conditioning and development of the brain microvessel endothelial cells (BMEC). Astrocytes are one of the glial cells of the central nervous system (CNS) that play several important roles in the structure and function of the CNS. They are intimately associated with the BMEC such that their foot processes ensheath 99% of the external surface of the BMEC [11]. Astrocytes have been shown to alter the properties of cocultured brain endothelial cells in the following ways [11,12].

1. Increase in barrier-related marker enzyme activities, such as that of γ-glutamyl transpeptidase (GGT) and alkaline phosphatase.
2. Enhanced expression of a glucose transporter.
3. Elevation of trans-endothelial electrical resistance (TEER).
4. Tightening of the BBB as seen by decreased paracellular permeability of sucrose.
5. Increase in tight junction number, length and complexity.

It has also been shown that BMEC monolayers are less leaky if grown in the presence of astrocyte-conditioned medium (ACM) [1,11]. The precise molecular nature of the astrocyte-derived factors that is responsible for the tightness of the BBB have yet to be unequivocally elucidated. However, several factors have been postulated to play a role including glial cell-derived neurotrophic factor (GDNF), transforming growth factor-beta (TGF-β), and src-suppressed C-kinase substrate (SSeCKS) that leads to increased angiopoietin-1 secretion. The BMEC themselves are known to secrete factors that help in the maintenance of astrocyte health. One such putative factor is the leukemia-inhibitory factor (LIF), a cytokine known to be involved in astrocyte differentiation [11].

1.4. Role of pericytes in the BBB

The pericytes are specialized cells of mesenchymal lineage that have multiple organ-specific roles. For example, they are present in the kidney as mesangial cells, in the liver as perisinusoidal stellate cells and in the bone as osteoblasts [13,14]. The pericytes in the central nervous system are closely associated with the BMEC and play an important role in the maintenance of the BBB. Their functions include [14].

1. Cerebrovascular autoregulation and blood flow distribution
2. Differentiation of the BBB
3. Formation and maintenance of the tight junctions of the BBB.
4. Initiation of the extrinsic (tissue factor) pathway of blood coagulation following cerebrovascular injury
5. Brain angiogenesis via secretion of angiopoietin-1
6. Phagocytic and scavenging (macrophage-like) functions
7. Production of immunoregulatory cytokines like IL-1β, IL-6 and GM-CSF
8. Regulation of leukocyte transmigration, antigen presentation and T-cell activation.

2. Molecular components of the tight junctions

The tight junctions consist of both membrane proteins as well as cytoplasmic proteins [15] (Figure 2). The integral membrane proteins are Claudins, Occludin and Junctional adhesion molecules (JAM). There are also several cytoplasmic accessory proteins that form a plaque and function as adapter proteins to link the membrane proteins to the actin cytoskeleton of the cell [16,17]. These include Zonula occludens proteins (ZO-1, ZO-2, ZO-3), Cingulin, AF-6, 7H6 antigen and Symplekin. These tight junctional complexes are not static structures but rather very dynamic entities that can "bend without breaking", thereby maintaining structural integrity [8].

2.1. Claudins

The claudins are a large family of transmembrane phosphoproteins [15]. Twenty-four members have been characterized so far, claudins 1-24 [18,19]. Of these, claudins 1, 3, 5 and 12 have been shown to form the tight junctions of the BBB [9,17,20,21]. Claudin-5 appears to be specific to the tight junctions of the endothelial cells and is called the "endothelial claudin" [17]. Each claudin molecule has 4 transmembrane domains. The claudin on one cell binds homotypically to the claudin on the adjacent cell to form the seal of the tight junction. The claudins, along with occludin and the JAMs, form the tight Junctional strands that keep the cells together and prevent paracellular flux of macromolecules from the apical to the basolateral side of polarized cells like BMEC [18]. The cytoplasmic carboxy terminal of the claudins binds to the cytoplasmic ZO proteins [20]. Claudin-1 is an integral component of the tight junctions and its loss is associated with certain pathologic conditions like tumours, strokes and inflammatory diseases [21].

2.2. Occludin

Occludin is a 65-kDa transmembrane phosphoprotein and is distinct from the claudins. However, its subcellular localization parallels that of claudins and, like the claudins, it has

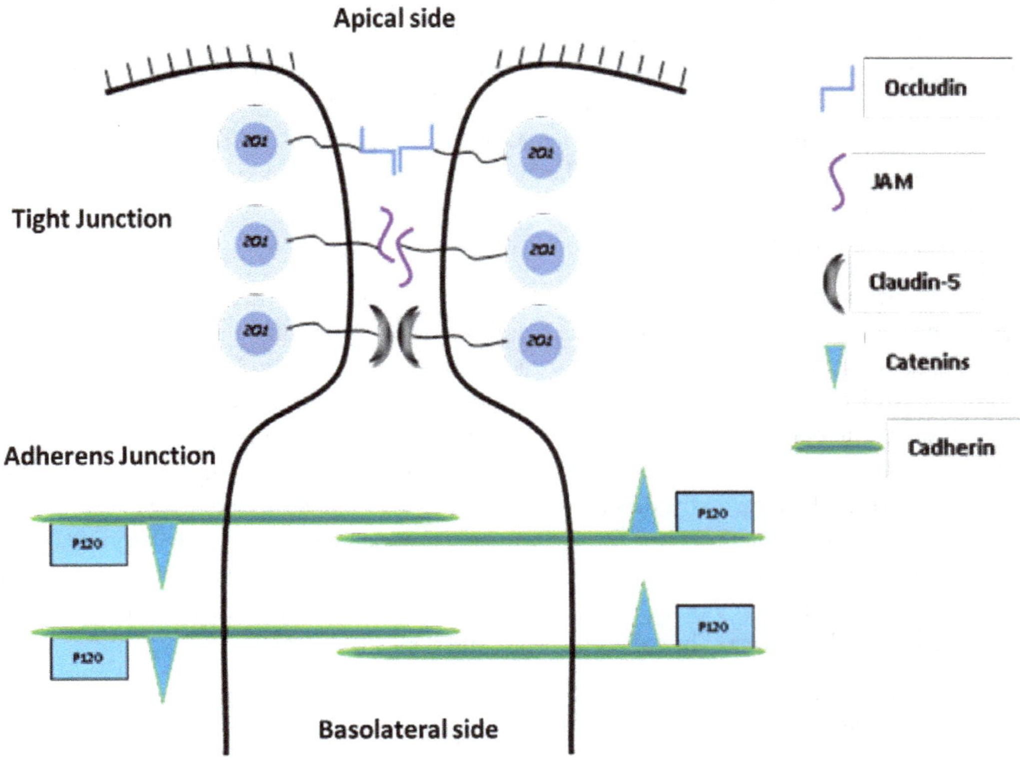

Figure 2. Schematic representation of proteins that are involved in the formation of the tight junction and adherens junctions in brain microvessel endothelial cells.

four transmembrane domains. The expression of occludin is higher in the adult BMEC compared to the peripheral endothelial cells. However, it is not expressed in the fetal or newborn human brain. Occludin plays an important structural, as well as a functional, role in the regulation of BBB permeability. As is the case with several other tight junction-associated proteins, phosphorylation or dephosphorylation of serine, threonine or tyrosine residues on the occludin molecule is crucial for its proper functioning [17,18,22,23]. For example, phosphorylation of occludin at serine and tyrosine residues correlates with tight junction assembly or tightening [8].

Occludin and the claudins interact intricately on the BMEC membrane. Together, they form channels that tightly regulate the paracellular flow of ions and other hydrophilic molecules. Thus, they are both essential in the formation, maintenance and regulation of the BBB [16,18].

2.3. Junctional Adhesion Molecules (JAM)

These molecules play an important role in the regulation of tight junction permeability in endothelial and epithelial cells [24]. These glycoproteins are members of the immunoglobulin superfamily of proteins. Three different JAMs have been characterized in humans, JAM-1,

JAM-2 and JAM-3, also referred to as JAM-A, JAM-B and JAM-C, respectively. Besides endothelial and epithelial cells, these molecules are also found on the surface of erythrocytes, leukocytes and platelets and are thought to contribute to various processes like leukocyte migration, platelet activation, angiogenesis and binding of reovirus [25]. The JAMs have short cytoplasmic tails that interact with cytoplasmic accessory proteins like ZO-1 and may require activation by phosphorylation, mediated by certain atypical protein kinases.

2.4. Cytoplasmic accessory proteins

Several cytoplasmic proteins appear to be essential components of the tight junctions. Among them, the zonula occludens proteins (ZO-1, ZO-2, ZO-3) play an important role. These 3 proteins have a molecular mass of 220, 160 and 130 kDa, respectively. They belong to a family of proteins called MAGUK (membrane-associated guanylate kinase-like protein) and form the submembranous plaque of the tight junction [2,15]. They are structurally complex proteins with several domains that make direct contact with claudins, occludin and JAM on one side and the actin cytoskeleton on the other [15]. Cingulin is a double-stranded myosin-like protein that serves as scaffolding and links the TJ accessory proteins with the cytoskeleton [8]. Actin, the cytoskeletal protein, plays a central role in the maintenance of the TJ. Actin-degrading macromolecules, such as cytochalasin-D, phalloidin and certain cytokines lead to disruption of the actin cytoskeleton and hence, of the tight junctions [8].

The tight junctional proteins can be modulated by several intracellular processes that involve calcium-signaling, phosphorylation, G-proteins, proteases and by TNF-α [4,8]. The tight junctional complexes also help localize the proteins and lipids of the apical and basolateral cell membranes in their respective compartments and prevent free mixing of these cell membrane macromolecules between the two domains. Thus, the BMEC owe much of their polarity to the TJ complexes [2,26].

3. Regulation of BBB permeability

Various factors play a role in regulating the permeability of the BBB as follows [2]:

1. Post-translational modifications of the TJ proteins. For example, phosphorylation and dephosphorylation mediated by protein kinases and phosphatases, respectively.
2. Alteration of the actin cytoskeleton.
3. Proteolytic degradation of certain TJ components like occludin, mediated by metalloproteinases.

4. *In vitro* models to study the BBB

In vitro models of the BBB have proven very effective to study the transport of endogenous macromolecules like fatty acids across the BMEC. They have also been used extensively in pharmaceutical research to study the passage of therapeutic molecules across the BMEC [5-7]. Several studies have shown that the BMEC lose many of their special properties when removed from their natural environment and show "dedifferentiation" behaviour. Thus, one potential limitation of in vitro BBB models is that the BMEC may not behave as site-specific specialized endothelial cells in vitro, but rather as common peripheral endothelial cells [7]. In spite of this shortcoming, several successful in vitro models of the BBB have been described [27]. Many of these have used human, bovine, and porcine or rat endothelial cells:

1. Alone [5,6,28-30], or
2. in combination with astrocyte conditioned medium supplemented with agents that elevate intracellular cAMP [1], or
3. Co-culture of endothelial cells on one side of a filter, with astrocytes on the other [31].

5. FA transport across the BBB and effects of FA on BBB permeability

Fatty acids (FA) are key components of membranes and exhibit many biological functions in a variety of tissues, including the key energy source for mitochondrial β-oxidation [32,33]. Cells acquire fatty acids through *de novo* synthesis, hydrolysis of triglycerides (TG) or uptake from exogenous sources [33]. Minimal amount of FA are derived from TG hydrolysis and most cells are dependent upon fatty acid uptake from the peripheral blood [32,34]. FA from the diet are absorbed by enterocytes in the small intestine and packaged into chylomicrons as TG. The liver also produces very low density lipoprotein (VLDL), a rich source of endogenously generated TG. Circulating chylomicrons and VLDL particles are hydrolyzed by lipoprotein lipase in the capillary lumen of tissues and the released FA from these lipoproteins may be taken up by tissues in the body [35]. FA that enter into cells are then esterified and stored as TG or transported to the mitochondria for β-oxidation. The importance of FA for the developing and adult brain has been recently reviewed [6]. FA transport from blood into parenchymal neurons is much more difficult than other cells since the tight junctions of the BBB severely restrict passage into the brain. FA must first move via transcellular transport across both the luminal (apical) and abluminal (basolateral) membranes of the endothelial cells and then across the plasma membrane of the neural cells [36-38].

The mechanism of FA transport into the brain remains controversial. Several studies support the notion that FA can move across membranes by diffusion [39,40]. Alternatively, others studies indicate that FA may enter into cells via specific protein-mediated transport [32,41,42]. In the diffusion model, once bound to the outer membrane leaflet, they quickly reach ionization equilibrium and the non-ionized form of fatty acids move across the membrane more rapidly than the ionized form [43]. The main problem with the FA diffusion model has always been whether diffusion is rapid enough to supply cells, which have a high long-chain FA metabolic requirement with sufficient amount of FA for β-oxidation [44]. In the protein-mediated transport model selective transport of FA occurs via specific protein transporters found on the cell membrane [33,41,45-47]. The mechanism of FA transport into the brain and the involvement of FA protein transporters has been reviewed [6]. We recently showed that the transport of various FA across confluent layers of HBMEC was, in part, mediated by fatty acid transport proteins (FATPs) [5,6]. Knock down of FATP-1 and CD36 resulted in reduced FA transport. In addition, transport appeared to be dependent upon fatty acyl chain length and degree of unsaturation.

The role of FA, such as arachidonic acid (AA), on BBB permeability is well documented and controversial. Studies have indicated that a rapid influx of AA into the brain occurs upon plasma infusion with AA [48,49]. In addition, a permeability-enhancing and neurotoxic effect of AA has been observed [50-52]. AA is a precursor for the formation of various bioactive molecules including prostaglandins, such as PGE_2, and leukotrienes. Several studies have indicated that the increase in BBB permeability is correlated with the formation of PGE_2 [29,30, 53-56]. The prostaglandin EP2 receptor was shown to be responsible for mediating the neuroinflammatory and neurodegenerative effects of PGE_2 in a mouse model of status epilepticus [57]. The permeability increase caused by AA in pial microvessels of rats was effectively blocked by a combination of indomethacin (COX inhibitor) and nordihyroguaria-retic acid (LOX inhibitor) but not singly by either agent [58]. In that same study, AA-mediated permeability increase was blocked by superoxide dismutase and catalase. These authors concluded that free radicals generated by either COX or LOX pathways were responsible for the permeability response to AA. In a mouse model of diabetic retinopathy 12-HETE and 15-HETE, products of the lipoxygenase pathway, were shown to be responsible for increasing the permeability of retinal endothelial cell barrier via an NADPH oxidase-dependent mechanism [59]. Interestingly, AA inhibited the cytokine-induced up-regulation of several genes involved in endothelial cell inflammation [60].

However, other studies have suggested that AA metabolites, such as PGE_2, have a protective role in the microvessels of the CNS and that PGE_2 prevents permeability increases. For example, the permeability increase caused by bradykinin was prevented or attenuated by exogenously added PGE_2 and iloprost, a prostacyclin analog [61]. In that study, COX-inhibitor drugs potentiated the permeability increases caused by bradykinin, thus suggesting an inhibitory role of PGE_2 in increasing endothelial cell permeability. In addition, PGE_2, acting via EP4 receptors, inhibited the increase in BBB permeability in a mouse model of experimental autoimmune encephalomyelitis [62]. Moreover, PGE_2, acting via EP2 receptors, has neuropro-tective properties and limits ischemic damage in mice stroke models [63]. It has been postulated in these studies [61,62] that engagement of EP2 and EP4 receptors by PGE_2 leads to an increase in cAMP levels. This cAMP accumulation has been shown to potentiate cadherin-mediated cell-cell contact and enhance endothelial barrier function. Thus, PGE_2 may promote BBB integrity via direct action on endothelial cells [62].

Several studies have demonstrated that microvessel endothelial cells from various organs have the capacity to produce a range of eicosanoids, notably, PGE_2, PGI_2 and $PGF_{2\alpha}$. In most of these studies the endothelial cells were stimulated with the calcium ionophore A23187 in addition to exogenously added AA [64-66]. However, in one study endothelial cells exposed to plasma from preeclamptic women showed increased production of prostaglandins [67]. In addition, bovine brain microvessel endothelial cells (BBMEC) exposed to TNF-αreleased large amounts of PGE_2 over a 12-hour period [29].

Previous work has shown that docosahexanoic acid (DHA) is converted to its vasodilator metabolite, 17S-HDoHE in endothelial cells [68]. DHA is a precursor in the formation of several bioactive molecules in human blood cells and in glial cells [69]. However, in those experiments, the cells were exposed to stimulants like zymosan A or the calcium ionophore, A23187 to facilitate the release of DHA metabolites. These metabolites have been shown to have several biological effects like inhibition of inflammation and platelet aggregation, mediation of vasodilation, anti-arrhythmic effects and lowering of triglyceride levels [70].

6. Drug transport across the BBB

The tight junction complex that connects brain microvascular endothelial cells in the BBB as well as the epithelial cells of the choroid plexus that form the blood-cerebral spinal fluid barrier (BCSFB) serve as a physical barrier preventing the paracellular diffusion of endogenous and exogenous compounds. The presence of these tight junctions is essential for maintaining the proper environment required for neuronal transmission. However, paracellular diffusion of nutrients and metabolites between the blood and the extracellular compartment of the brain is also highly restricted. Consequently, the uptake of essential molecules, such as glucose and amino acids, to meet the metabolic requirements of the brain occurs through specific transporter proteins located on the plasma membrane of the endothelial cells. In addition to transporters that facilitate the entry of various solutes into the brain, the brain endothelial cells also express numerous efflux transporters [71]. These transporters are members of the ATP-binding cassette (ABC) protein family and utilize energy from adenosine triphosphate (ATP) hydrolysis to actively remove compounds from the cells against a concentration gradient.

From a drug transport perspective, there are several transporters that are critically involved in the movements of drugs across the BBB. These include organic anion-transporting polypeptide 1A2 (OATP1A2/SLO1A2), organic anion transporter 3 (OAT3/SLC22A8), monocarboxylate transporter 1 (MCT1/SLC16A1), from the solute transporter family, and P-glycoprotein (P-gp; MDR1/ABCB1), breast-cancer-resistance protein (BCRP/ABCG2) and multidrug-resistance-associated proteins 1-9(MRP1-9/ABCC1-9) from the ABC transporter family [72]. The localization of these transporters in both the BBB and BCSF barrier are shown in Figure 3 with each individual transporter is being discussed in greater detail below.

6.1. Organic Anion Transporting Polypeptide (OATP)

Organic anion transporting polypeptides (OATPs) are members of the solute carrier organic anion transporter family (SLCO) [73]. The OATPs accommodate the transport of a wide variety of amphipathic solutes, including bile salts, anionic peptides, steroid conjugates, thyroid hormones and an increasing number of pharmaceutical drugs and xenobiotics [74]. Members of the OATP family, of which there are currently 11 known to be expressed in humans

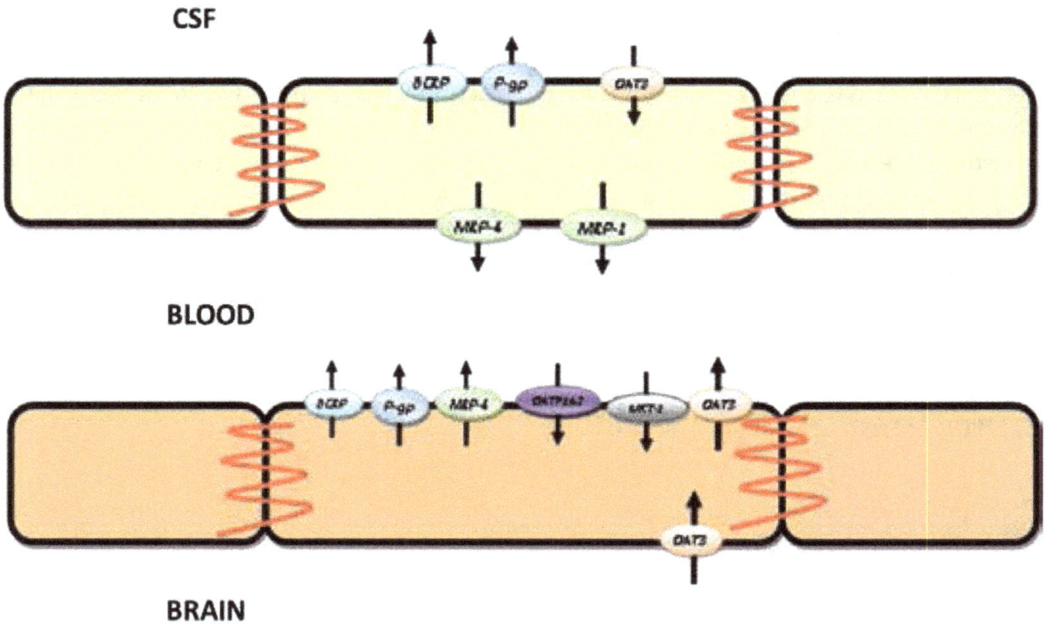

Figure 3. The localization of transporters in the blood brain barrier (BBB) and blood cerebral spinal fluid barrier (BCSFB) of CNS.

(OATP1A2, 1B1, 1B3, 1C1, 2A1, 2B1, 3A1, 4A1, 4C1, 5A1, and 6A1), share a great deal of amino acid sequence identity and transport solutes in a sodium independent manner [75].

Of the various OATPs, both OATP1A2 and OATP1A4 are expressed in the BBB. Organic anion transport protein 1A2 was the first member of the OATP family to be reported in humans, while OATP1A4 is a more recently discovered homolog of hepatic [76]. At the protein level, OATP1A2 (previously designated OATP-A) is expressed in many organs including the liver, intestine, kidney, lung, testes, and the brain. Within the brain, this transporter is localized in the frontal cortex and specifically confined to the endothelial cells of the BBB [74]. Its localization on the luminal side of brain microvessel endothelial cells suggests that OATP1A2 aids in the entry of various solutes and therapeutic agents into the brain [74]. While OATP1A4 is mainly concentrated in the liver, the transporter has also been detected within the brain microvessel endothelial cells [74]. In contrast to OATP1A2, immunohistochemical localization studies indicate that OATP1A4 is expressed on both the apical and basolateral side of the endothelial cells of the BBB and thus, mediates the uptake of compounds from both the brain and the blood compartments [77].

6.2. Organic Anion Transporter (OAT)

Organic anion transporters (OATs) belong to the SLC22A gene family. Similarly to OATPs, the OATs transport a broad range of chemically unrelated endogenous and exogenous compounds. There are at least 10 families of OATs designated by Arabic numbers (eg. OAT1).

OAT1 is predominantly expressed in the kidney although a very small amount is also found in the brain particularly concentrated in regions such as cortex, hypothalamus, hippocampus and cerebellum [78]. This transporter is known to interact with a broad range of drugs including antibiotics (penicillins, benzylpenicillin and carbenicillin), antineoplastics (methotrexate) and even cholesterol lowering drugs including the statins and fibrates such as fluvastatin, pravastatin, and bezafibrate, respectively [78]. OAT2, on the other hand, is predominantly expressed in the liver and very little is found in the kidney and brain. The expression level of this transporter in a particular tissue can be influenced by a variety of factors; including gender and species differences [79]. For example, in the adult male rat, the mRNA for OAT2 expression is greater in the liver than the kidney, and the opposite is true for the adult female rat where the mRNA level in the kidney is greater than in the liver [79]. However, this phenomenon has not been observed in humans. Furthermore, the expression level of OAT2 is also influenced by hepatocyte nuclear factors and endogenous gas molecules including nitric oxide [80,81]. Given the similar molecular structure to OAT1, OAT2 also mediates the transport of a broad range of solutes including cholesterol lowering drugs (i.e. statins), antibiotics such as cephalosporins, and antineoplastic drugs like 5-fluorouracil [78].

From a CNS perspective, OAT3 appears to have the greatest expression levels in the brain [78]. Within the CNS, OAT3 is primarily localized in the brain capillaries and in epithelial cells of the choroid plexus, specifically on the basolateral side of the plasma membrane of the cells [82]. The predominantly basolateral localization of OAT3 in the BBB and BCSFB implies that the primary function of OAT3 is to aid in the removal of compounds from the brain. Endogenous products of neurotransmitter and hormone metabolism are potential candidates for OAT3-mediated removal. Potential therapeutic agents that may be transported out of the brain through OAT3-dependent processes at the BBB and BCSFB include the various statins, diuretics, antibiotics and antivirals [78]. As OAT3 interacts with a large number of therapeutic agents, drug-drug interactions may be of potential concern in the BBB, although specific examples are at present not known.

6.3. Glucose Transporters (GLUT)

Glucose is the major source of energy for most mammalian cells, particularly in the brain. Despite the high dependence of the brain on glycolysis, the source of glucose comes entirely from the blood and is dependent on passage through the BBB. The entry of glucose into the brain is mediated by facilitative glucose transporter proteins. There are currently seven known isoforms, with the designation of GLUT1-7 [83]. The main isoforms found within the CNS are GLUT1 and GLUT3 that bring glucose into the cell through sodium independent transport mechanisms. A summary of the various GLUTs and their distribution within the CNS is shown in Figure 4. GLUT1 within the CNS exists as two distinct forms, which differ only by the extent of glycosylation [84]. A glycosylated, 55 KDa GLUT1 is found primarily in the endothelial cells of the BBB while the non-vascular, non-glycosylated 45 KDa form is mainly found in neural cells as well as the basolateral plasma of epithelial cells isolated from the choroid plexus [83]. Aside from the prominent expression found in the microvessels and choroid plexus, GLUT1 has also been detected in small cells with dark stained nuclei characteristic of glia cells [85].

Immunohistochemistry staining also showed a positive detection of GLUT1 in astrocytes that are in direct contact with the cerebral microvessels of rat brain slices. Electron microscopy also revealed dense distribution of GLUT1 within the astrocyte foot processes surrounding the microvessels of the gray matter and synaptic contacts [86].

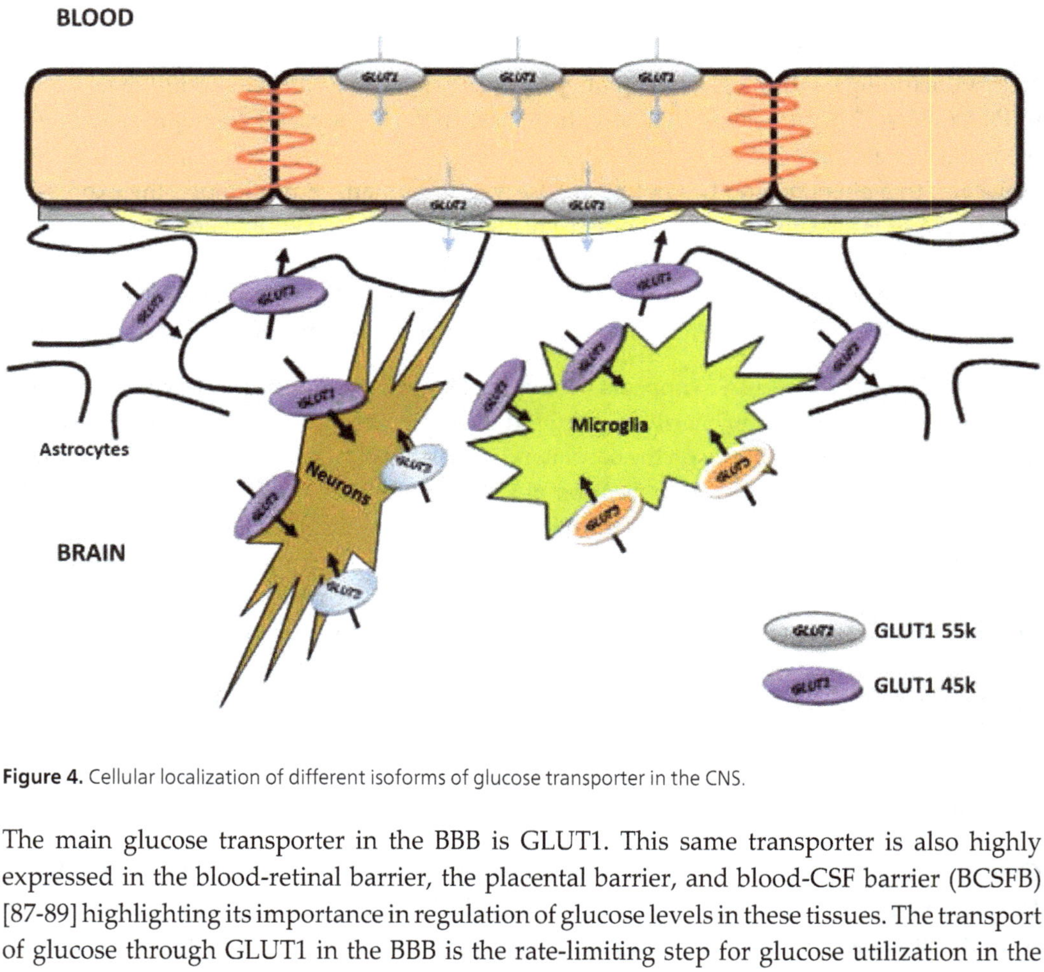

Figure 4. Cellular localization of different isoforms of glucose transporter in the CNS.

The main glucose transporter in the BBB is GLUT1. This same transporter is also highly expressed in the blood-retinal barrier, the placental barrier, and blood-CSF barrier (BCSFB) [87-89] highlighting its importance in regulation of glucose levels in these tissues. The transport of glucose through GLUT1 in the BBB is the rate-limiting step for glucose utilization in the brain and is highly responsive to metabolic changes within the brain. For example, GLUT1 expression in the BBB at both the mRNA and protein level can increase or decrease depending on the ambient concentration of hexose. High concentration of hexose decreases the expression of GLUT1 while low hexose concentration causes an up-regulation of both GLUT1 mRNA and protein levels [90]. Following brain injury such as a stroke and brain tumors, both mRNA and protein levels of GLUT1 are significantly increased [83,85,91].

The endothelial cells forming the BBB also express sodium glucose cotransporter (SGLT) [92]. Unlike GLUT1, glucose transport through SGLT is sodium-dependent. A functional role for SGLT in glucose homeostasis in the brain has not been established; however, it has been speculated that SGLT may help maintain intracellular glucose levels in the brain under stressful conditions such as hypoglycemia [92].

6.4. Monocarboxylate Transporter (MCT)

Monocarboxylic acids, including lactate, pyruvate, and ketones play an important role in energy metabolism within the body. Monocarboxylates such as pyruvate, lactate, and ketone bodies (i.e acetoacetate and β-hydroxybutyarate) can be utilized by neurons, in the absence of glucose, to generate a substantial amount of energy for the brain [93]. Under pathological and physiological conditions including diabetes, prolonged starvation, hypoglycemia, or even intense exercise, the build-up of lactate provides an energy source, which can be utilized by the brain [3,94,95]. In addition, monocarboxylates including lactic acid are a metabolic by-product produced and released within the CNS by neurons [96,97], astrocytes [96] and oligodendrocytes [98]. As monocarboxylates are hydrophilic compounds that cannot readily diffuse cross the BBB, specific transporter systems are required to maintain proper levels of these endogenous metabolic products in the brain [93].

Sequence homology indicates that the monocarboxylate transporter family (previous known as SLC16 gene family) consists of 14 members identified as MCT1-9, MCT11-14 and T-type amino acid transporter 1 (TAT1) [99]. MCT1-4 is a symporter mediating the co-transport of monocarboxylate and proton in a one to one stoichiometry ratio. MCT1-4 is present in almost all tissues including the muscles, liver, kidney, heart, testes, and brain [93,99]. While MCT1 and MCT2 are found in the muscles, liver, kidney, heart and CNS, [93], MCT3 is exclusively expressed on the basolateral side of the retinal pigment epithelium and MCT4 is highly expressed in the skeletal muscles and also in the brain. Within the BBB, MCT1 was the first monocarboxylic acid transporter identified in the brain microvessel endothelial cells and in the ependycytes lining the ventricles [100]. Both electron microscopy and immunohistochemistry revealed a small amount of MCT1 in astrocytic end-feet surrounding the capillaries [100,101]. The presence of MCT1 was found in the cytoplasm of astrocyte and also associated with the plasma membrane [93]. In contrast, MCT2 is found in endothelial cells forming the BBB, but absent in astrocytes [93,100]. MCT4, on the other hand, was exclusively expressed in the astrocytes and glial cells of rodent brain. Furthermore, when the hippocampus and the corpus callosum were labeled, the expression of MCT4 was restricted to astrocytes [93]. MCT8 was recently recognized as thyroid hormone transporter as opposed to monocarboxylate [102].

6.5. ATP-Binding Cassette Transporters (ABC)

The ATP-binding cassette (ABC) superfamily of transporter proteins are responsible for the active transport of a wide variety of compounds including phospholipids, ions, peptides, steroids, polysaccharides, amino acids, organic anions, bile acids, drugs and other xenobiotic compounds across cellular membranes. There are roughly 48 genes encoding the various human ABC transporters, each is organized into seven subfamilies designated ABCA to ABCG [103]. Over-expression of ABC transporters are major contributors to the development of multidrug resistance (MDR) in cancer cells. For instance, when the MDR gene that codes for an efflux transporter is being transfected into drug sensitive cells, the transfectant cells become resistant to the drugs that are substrates for the transporters resulting in a decrease in the intracellular concentration of the drugs, thereby conferring multidrug resistance [104]. MDR in tumor cell lines is often linked to an ATP-dependent decrease in cellular accumulation of drugs namely through p-glycoprotein (p-gp encoded by ABCB1), multidrug resistance proteins (MRP encoded by ABCC), and breast cancer resistance protein (BCRP encoded by ABCG2) drug efflux transporters [105]. In addition to their function as multidrug resistance proteins, these transporters are also expressed in normal tissue such as intestines, liver, kidney and the BBB and BCSFB, suggesting that they also have a protective function in limiting accumulation and distribution and speeding the elimination of xenobiotic compounds which could result in tissue toxicity [106].

6.6. Multidrug Resistance Protein (MRP)

The multidrug resistance-associated proteins (MRPs) are a subfamily of ABC transporters. There are currently 12 members of this subfamily designated as ABCC1-12. Of the 12, 9 have demonstrated drug efflux transporter function and play an important role in absorption, distribution and elimination of various drugs and metabolites. While all MRPs have the capability to transport amphiphatic organic anions, transport substrates are not limited to anionic species. Examples of this include the transport of nucleotide based analogs by MRP4 and MRP5, efflux of prostaglandins by MRP1, co-transport of neutral or cationic solutes as well as glucoronide drug conjugates by MRP1 and MRP2 [107]. Within the MRPs and other ABC transport proteins there tends to be substantial substrate affinity overlap. This is a fascinating feature considering most members are structurally and functionally distinct from other ABC binding cassette transporters. For example, there is only approximately 15% amino acid sequence homology between MRPs and P-gp [108]. In addition, when comparing amino acid sequence between different members within the MRP subfamily to MRP1, amino acid sequence homology ranges between 33% for MRP8 and 58% for MRP3 [109].

The brain endothelial cells that form the BBB express several different MRP. Collectively the MRP efflux transporters function to restrict the uptake and aid in the elimination of drugs, xenobiotics and endogenous compounds from the brain. Currently, members of the MRP family that have been reported in the BBB include MRP1, 2,4-9. The evidence for the localization and function of each of the MRPs within the BBB are discussed below.

6.6.1. MRP1

MRP1 is expressed in primary cultured bovine, murine [110], rat [111] and porcine [112] brain microvessel endothelial cells. While studies by Seetharaman and coworkers [113] suggested up-regulation of MRP1 expression in human culture brain microvessel endothelial cells compared to freshly isolated human brain capillaries, more recent studies support robust expression of MRP1 within the brain capillaries isolated from human brain tissue [114]. Two independent studies reported that MRP1 is localized primarily to the apical (luminal) plasma membrane in brain microvessel endothelial cells [114,115]. This is in contrast to studies by Roberts et al. [116] suggesting MRP1 has a basolateral (abluminal) plasma membrane localization in rat brain microvessels. As MRP1 shows high transporter activity for conjugated compounds such as estradiol 17β glucuronides [117], it is interesting to note that Sugiyama and colleagues [118] demonstrated a reduction in elimination of estradiol 17β glucuronide from the brain of *Mrp1* knockout mice compared to that observed in the wild-type controls with functional MRP1. These functional studies support the luminal expression of MRP1 and suggest a role in limiting brain exposure to drugs and endogenous solutes.

6.6.2. MRP2

The expression and localization of MRP2 within the BBB is the subject of much debate. Studies by Miller et al. [119] indicated MRP2 was expressed in the luminal plasma membrane of isolated rat brain capillaries. These initial findings were supported by reports of MRP2 expression in both human brain capillaries as well as zebrafish [120,121]. In contrast, no detectable expression of MRP2 was found, at either the mRNA or protein level, in bovine brain microvessel endothelial cells [122,123] or mouse brain microvessel endothelial cells [110,118]. Furthermore, studies examining MRP2 protein expression in isolated human brain capillaries were below detection limits [114,124]. Interestingly, expression of MRP2 in rat brain endothelial cells was inducible by activation of either pregnane X receptor (PXR) or constitutive androstane receptor (CAR) pathways [125,126].

Functionally, MRP2 mediates the transport of glucuronide and GSH conjugates to a lesser extent than MRP1 [127]. It also actively transports chemotherapeutics such as methotrexate, vinca alkaloids, anthracyclins, antiepileptics such as phenytoin and endogenous agents like leukotriene C4 [107,109,128,129]. Thus if MRP2 is expressed in the BBB, it could have a profound effect on the brain distribution of many therapeutic agents. However, there are few studies showing a significant impact of MRP2 on the BBB permeability. One such study demonstrated an increased accumulation of phenytoin in the brain of Mrp2 deficient rats compared to controls [129]. There is also evidence for MRP2-mediated changes in brain penetration of drugs in epileptic animals. Based on available information, most evidence indicates that MRP2 expression in the BBB is low or below detectable limits and as such has negligible effects on solute and macromolecule distribution into the brain. However, as MRP2 expression appears highly inducible, there is a possibility that MRP2 activity in the BBB could be of importance during pathological events within the CNS.

6.6.3. MRP3

Studies by Zhang et al. [122] identified low and variable expression of MRP3 in bovine brain microvessel endothelial cells. Subsequent proteomics based studies of both mouse [130] and human [131] BBB indicated that MRP3 expression was below detection limits.

6.6.4. MRP4

Evidence supporting a significant functional role for MRP4 in the BBB is perhaps the strongest of all the MRPs. The first evidence of MRP4 expression in the BBB was the studies by Zhang et al. [122] in bovine brain microvessel endothelial cells. Follow-up studies examining the localization of MRP4 suggested both luminal and abluminal presence of the transporter [115]. The expression of MRP4 has since been reported in human, mouse and rat BBB [114,116,132]. Comparison of MRP4 expression in the brains of wild-type and *Mrp4* knockout mice confirmed BBB localization as well as expression in the choroid plexus epithelial cells forming the BCSFB [132].

Functionally, MRP4 can transport a wide variety of substrates and is important in the efflux of many nucleotide analog based chemotherapeutics. As with MRP1 and MRP2, MRP4 transports the endogenous substrate leukotriene C4 [133,134]. However, in addition, MRP4 can also transport endogenous nucleotides such as cAMP and cGMP [135]. Common chemotherapeutic purine nucleotide anion analogs that are effluxed by this transporter include bis(pivaloyloxymethyl)-9-[2-(phosphonomethoxy)ethyl]-adenine (PMEA), and active metabolites of 6-mercaptopurine and 6-thioguanine [72,107,136]. Using *Mrp4 -/-* knockout mice significant increases in topotecan [132] and PMEA [137] accumulation in the brain was observed.

6.6.5. MRP5 and MRP6

Within the BBB, MRP5 is highly expressed, whereas MRP6 is expressed to a lesser extent [122]. Presently their locations within the BBB remain unclear. Previous studies by Zhang et al. [115] found MRP5 protein expression to be primarily in the apical membrane fraction of brain microvessel endothelial cells. These findings were supported by Nies et al. [114]. In contrast, Roberts et al. [116] found low levels of abluminal MRP5 expression when staining in rat brain microvessel endothelial cells. Currently, the location of MRP6 remains to be seen because no specific MRP6 antibody is available at this time [115].

MRP5 can transport purine nucleotide analogs [127] and is the primary active transporter of cGMP and cAMP [138]. Therefore MRP5 and -4 may work in concert to regulate cGMP and cAMP levels [127] in the brain. MRP6 can transport anionic organic ions but cannot transport glucuronide or GSH [127] and has been shown to transport leukotrinene C4 [139].

6.6.6. MRP7, -8 and -9

Currently, little is known about these transporters with regards to the BBB. MRP7, -8 and -9 have been found to be expressed in brain [140]. MRP7 can transport glucuronide E2 17betaG and exhibits high levels of resistance to taxane docetaxel, approximately 9 to 13 fold [140]. MRP8 is able to transport nucleotide analogues such as PMEA, glutathione conjugates and methotrexate [140]. No substrates for MRP9 have been identified at this time [109].

When looking at drug resistant efflux transport in the literature, major focus has been put on P-gp and BCRP and limited research has been focused on members within the MRP subfamily as it relates to the BBB. As has been demonstrated here, many of these MRP transporters can transport substrates that are important both physiologically and in the clinic. Particularly within the CNS, it is important to decipher any discrepancies in location and expression of MRP members within the BBB because they can have relevant impact on CNS drug concentrations reaching therapeutic levels within the brain and thus can affect our ability to treat important brain pathologies.

6.7. Breast Cancer Resistance Protein (BCRP)

BCRP was originally discovered in the MCF-7 AdrVp breast cancer cell line after observing that the cells are resistant to chemotherapeutic drugs including mitoxantrone, doxorubicin, and daunorubicin [141]. The gene sequence of the protein was isolated shortly after and was classified as the group G subfamily of ABC transporters. There are at least 5 members of ABCG subfamily identified in humans (ABCG1, ABCG2, ABCG4, ABCG5, and ABCG8). However, the primary form that plays a crucial role in the transport of substances between the blood and the CNS is ABCG2 [141]. At the protein level, ABCG2 is approximately 72-kDa with 665 amino acids and is considered as a half-transporter as shown in Figure 5. Other ABC transporters have two sets of membrane spanning regions (6 transmembrane α-helices) and two nucleotide binding domains (NBD); the G subfamily of protein consists of only one set of membrane spanning domain 6 transmembrane α-helices and only one NBD [141]. In order to function, it is believed that these half-transporters form homodimers [142].

The specific localization of ABCG2 within the CNS is primarily confined to the luminal plasma membrane of the brain microvessel endothelial cells. Given the localization within the BBB and the compounds that are transported by ABCG2, it has been suggested that ABCG2 most likely protects the brain from xenobiotics and toxins similar to other ABC transporters [141]. Furthermore, ABCG2 also plays a role in the accumulation and disposition of various endogenous substrates including sulfate and glucuronide conjugates of estrone and dehydroepiandrosterone [143,144]. In addition to endogenous substrates, ABCG2 also binds and recognizes a broad range of structurally-unrelated drugs and xenobiotics [141]. Many of these transport substrates also interact with other ABC transporters including ABCB1 and the ABCC subfamily; thus, the accumulation and distribution of drugs can be significantly altered.

6.8. P-glycoprotein (P-gp)

P-glycoprotein (P-gp) was the first ABC transporter to be characterized. First identified by Juliano and Ling [145] in 1976 using Chinese hamster ovary cells with selected resistance to colchicine, they discovered that the drug resistance properties of the mutated cells were consistently correlated with a high molecular weight component found in the plasma membrane with an approximate weight of 170,000 Da [145]. They also observed that the component was likely a glycoprotein associated with the plasma membrane of the mutated cells and was consistently absent or expressed at a lower level in the wild-type cells. Furthermore, they also noticed that the mutant cells with high levels of glycoprotein displayed an alter drug permeability; thus, they designated it as "P-glycoprotein" [145]. P-gp is also expressed in numerous tissues, including adrenal glands, kidneys, liver, colon, small intestine, heart, testes, peripheral nerves, and the brain. At the BBB, it is the most extensively studied ABC transporter being expressed in the luminal plasma membrane of brain endothelial cells [104]. Under normal conditions, the presence of P-gp in the BBB limits a broad range of substances from penetrating the brain tissue. Some notable drug classes with reduced brain penetration due to P-gp efflux at the BBB include anti-epileptics, anti-cancer drugs, anti-histamines and HIV protease inhibitors [103]. Numerous studies using drugs such as cyclosporine, digoxin, domperidone, etoposide, loperamide, ondansetron, taxol and vinblastine have shown the important role of

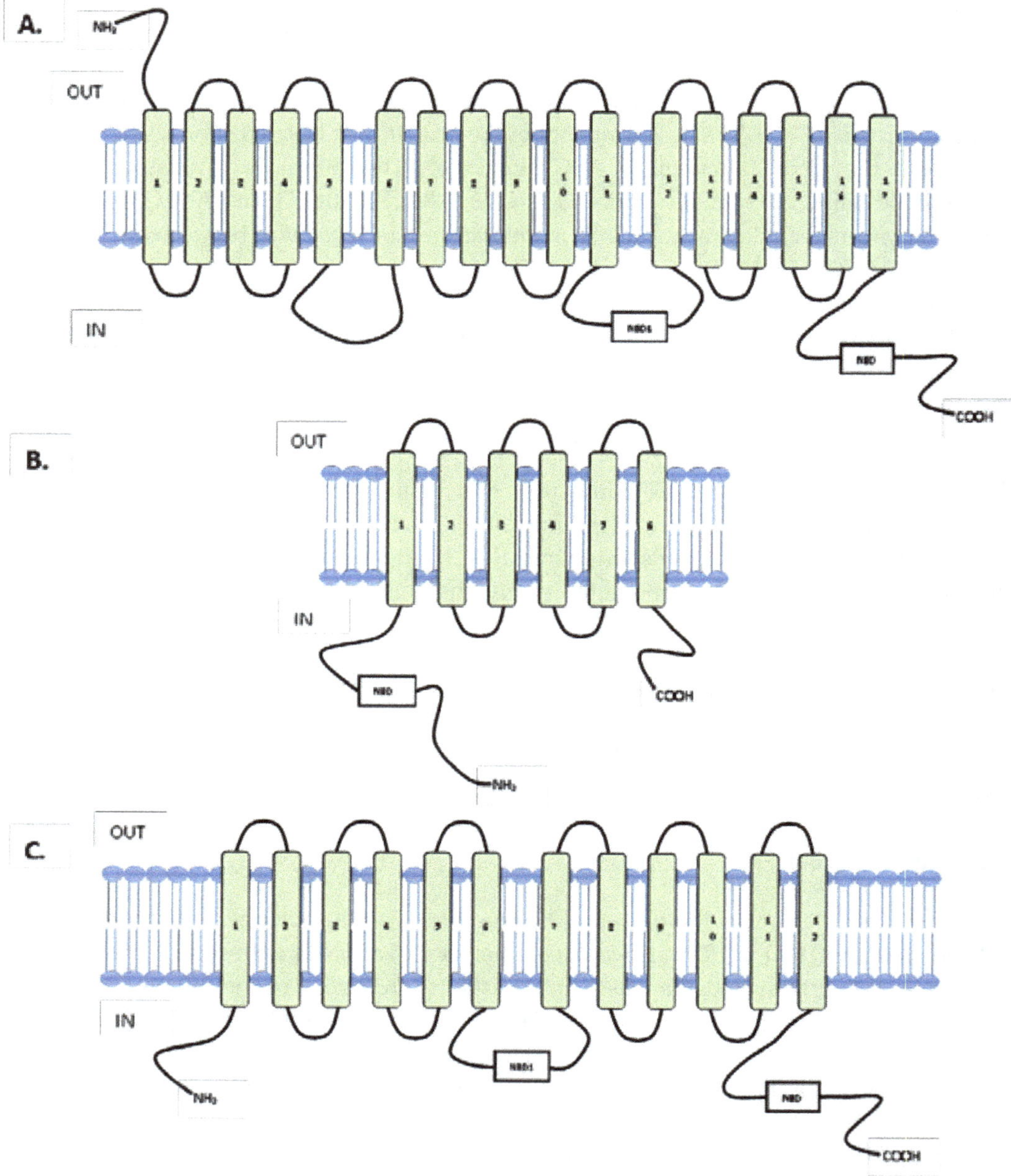

Figure 5. Structures of (A) MRP transporter, (B) BCRP transporter, and (C) P-glycoprotein transporter.

P-gp in the pharmacokinetics of P-gp substrates in multiple parts of the body. Table 1 shows some of the drugs that are known substrates for P-gp.

Similar to other ABC transporters, P-gp is a transmembrane protein with a molecular weight of 170 KDa formed by two homologous subunits that function as an efflux pump in an ATP-dependent manner (shown in Figure 5). The protein is assembled in two halves connected by a 75 amino acid linker region. Each half contains 6 transmembrane segments, an intracellular nucleotide binding domain, and both intracellular N and C terminal regions. The exact localization of P-gp had been a subject of some debate with evidence supporting both luminal and abluminal expression of the protein. Luminal P-gp expression had been observed in rat and mouse brain capillaries [115,146,147]. Furthermore, the luminal expression of P-gp has also been isolated in human brain microvessels [113,148]. In contrast, electron microscope techniques have shown an enhanced expression of P-gp on the abluminal side of the rat brain endothelial cells [149]. Nevertheless, recent studies using immunoreactivity support the localization of P-gp on the luminal side of the endothelial cells [116].

Cancer Drugs	Immuno-suppressive Drugs	Lipid Lowering Agent	Steroids	HIV Protease Inhibitors	Cardiac Drugs	Anti-Diarrheal Drugs	Anti-Gout Agent	Anti-Bacterial Agents	Anti-Helminthic Agent
Doxorubicin	Cyclosporin A	Lovastatin	Aldosterone	Amprenavir	Digoxin	Loperamide	Colchicine	Erythromyccin	Ivermectin
Daunourbicin	FK506		Cortisol	Indinavir	Quinidine	Antiemetics		Rifampin	Abamectin
Vinblastine	Tacrolimus		Corticosterone	Nelfinavir		Domperidone		Valinomycin	
Vincristine			Hydrocortisone	Ritonavir		Ondansetron		Gramicidin	
Vindesine			Dexamethasone	Saquinavir				Grepafloxacin	
Vinorelbine			Triamcinolone	Lopinavir					
Paclitaxel									
Etoposide									
Teniposide									
Epirubicin									
Irinotecan									
Tamoxifen									
Methotrexate									
Amsacrine									
Imatinib									

Table 1 Representative compounds that are known to be P-glycoprotein substrates. (Adapted from [156])

Numerous studies have attempted to identify and characterize P-gp substrates. Unlike conventional transporters, which recognize specific substrates, P-gp recognizes a broad range of compounds and has the capacity to extract its substrates directly from the plasma membrane [150]. Some of the most common features of P-gp substrates include their lipophilic nature that enables them to cross the lipid bilayer of the cell membrane. Furthermore, many P-gp substrates commonly consist of two aromatic rings and a basic nitrogen atom. These molecules can be uncharged or basic in nature, although some acidic compounds including methotrexate and phenytoin can also bind to P-gp but at a lower rate. Molecules with molecular weight ranges from 300 to 2000 Da are capable of binding to the protein and being transported [151]. Peptide substrates consisting of 3 to 15 amino acids with molecular weight ranges from 380 to

1880 Da can also interact with P-gp [151]. Most recently, beta amyloid protein, the component found in amyloid plaques in Alzheimer's disease was reported to be a transport substrate of both P-gp but not BCRP [152,153].

One method for overcoming the limited permeability of P-gp transport substrates is to pharmacologically inhibit Pgp. P-glycoprotein inhibitors are themselves non-cytotoxic agents that can be used in combination with P-gp substrates to maintain the intracellular drug concentration. An inhibitor binds to P-gp and prevents the transport of P-gp substrates. There are at least three generations of P-gp inhibitors. The first generation compounds are less potent and non-selective with undesirable side effects at inhibitory concentrations. Examples of first generation inhibitors include the calcium channel blocker, verapamil, and the immunosuppressive agent cyclosporin A. First generation P-gp inhibitors act as competitive inhibitors of P-gp transport [154].

The second-generation compounds including dexverapamil or dexniguldipine were developed to reduce the toxicity associated with P-gp inhibition. They eliminate the undesirable side effects while retaining the ability to inhibit P-gp. The third generation inhibitors including tariquidar and elacridar are much more specific and more potent than earlier compounds. Unlike the first and second generation of P-gp inhibitors, the third generation of drugs acts as non-competitive inhibitors of P-gp, and the compounds themselves are not transported by P-gp [155]. Table 2 summarizes representative P-gp inhibitors [104].

Cyclopropylibenzosuberane	Immunosupp-ressant	Calcuim channel blocker	Progesterone antagonist	Antiarrhythmic agent	Antifungal agent	Acridonecarboxamide derivative	Topoisomerase
LY335979	Cyclosporin A Valspodar (PSC833)	Verapamil	Mefiprostone (RU486)	Quinidine	Ketoconazole	GG918 (GF120918)	Xenova (XR 5944)

Table 2 Representative compounds that are known to be P-glycoprotein inhibitors. (Adapted from [156])

The ability of P-gp to extrude xenobiotics provides protection and detoxification of cells under normal conditions. For example, knockout mice (MDR1a$^{-/-}$) have been shown to be more sensitive to ivermectin and are susceptible to serious neurotoxicity compared to wild type control mice [156]. Considering the broad range of P-gp substrates and the expression of P-gp in tissues responsible for absorption, distribution and elimination of drugs, it is no surprise that this particular drug efflux transporter can significantly affect the absorption and distribution of drugs. This is especially true for cancer therapies used in the treatment of brain tumors. The tight junctions of the BBB restrict paracellular diffusion of chemotherapeutic agents into the CNS, while the presence of the various drug efflux transporters, such as P-gp, within the endothelial cells of the BBB reduces transcellular passage of chemotherapeutic agents into the brain and tumor sites.

7. Conclusion

The brain capillaries are structurally and functionally different from capillaries formed in the other organs. The selectiveness and permissiveness of the endothelial cell monolayer within the CNS is dependent on the tight junctions as wells as the numerous transporter systems located on the luminal and the abluminal surface of the endothelial cells forming the BBB. The restrictive nature of the tight junctions along with transporter systems expressed in the BBB can significantly altered the accumulation and distribution of fatty acids and drugs in the CNS under pathological conditions. Improved delivery to the brain can be achieved by reversibly disrupting the physical tight junctions and/or inhibiting the activity of efflux transporter systems.

Author details

Siddhartha Dalvi[1], Ngoc On[1], Hieu Nguyen[1], Michael Pogorzelec[1], Donald W. Miller[1] and Grant M. Hatch[1,2]

*Address all correspondence to: ghatch@mich.ca

1 Departments of Pharmacology & Therapeutics, Center for Research and Treatment of Atherosclerosis, University of Manitoba, DREAM Manitoba Institute of Child Health, Canada

2 Biochemistry and Medical Genetics, Center for Research and Treatment of Atherosclerosis, University of Manitoba, DREAM Manitoba Institute of Child Health, Canada

References

[1] Rubin LL, Hall DE, Porter S, Barbu K, Cannon C, Horner HC, et al. A cell culture model of the blood-brain barrier. J Cell Biol 1991 Dec;115(6):1725-1735.

[2] Gloor SM, Wachtel M, Bolliger MF, Ishihara H, Landmann R, Frei K. Molecular and cellular permeability control at the blood-brain barrier. Brain Res Brain Res Rev 2001 Oct;36(2-3):258-264.

[3] Hawkins BT, Davis TP. The blood-brain barrier/neurovascular unit in health and disease. Pharmacol Rev 2005 Jun;57(2):173-185.

[4] Kniesel U, Wolburg H. Tight junctions of the blood-brain barrier. Cell Mol Neurobiol 2000 Feb;20(1):57-76.

[5] Mitchell RW, Edmundson CL, Miller DW, Hatch GM. On the mechanism of oleate transport across human brain microvessel endothelial cells. J Neurochem 2009 Aug; 110(3):1049-1057.

[6] Mitchell RW, On NH, Del Bigio MR, Miller DW, Hatch GM. Fatty acid transport protein expression in human brain and potential role in fatty acid transport across human brain microvessel endothelial cells. J Neurochem 2011 May;117(4):735-746.

[7] Urich E, Lazic SE, Molnos J, Wells I, Freskgård P. Transcriptional Profiling of Human Brain Endothelial Cells Reveals Key Properties Crucial for Predictive In Vitro Blood-Brain Barrier Models. PloS one 2012;7(5).

[8] Huber JD, Egleton RD, Davis TP. Molecular physiology and pathophysiology of tight junctions in the blood-brain barrier. Trends Neurosci 2001 Dec;24(12):719-725.

[9] Zlokovic BV. The blood-brain barrier in health and chronic neurodegenerative disorders. Neuron 2008 Jan 24;57(2):178-201.

[10] Abbott NJ, Ronnback L, Hansson E. Astrocyte-endothelial interactions at the blood-brain barrier. Nat Rev Neurosci 2006 Jan;7(1):41-53.

[11] Haseloff RF, Blasig IE, Bauer HC, Bauer H. In search of the astrocytic factor(s) modulating blood-brain barrier functions in brain capillary endothelial cells in vitro. Cell Mol Neurobiol 2005 Feb;25(1):25-39.

[12] Janzer RC, Raff MC. Astrocytes induce blood-brain barrier properties in endothelial cells. Nature 1987 Jan 15-21;325(6101):253-257.

[13] Balabanov R, Dore-Duffy P. Role of the CNS microvascular pericyte in the blood-brain barrier. J Neurosci Res 1998 Sep 15;53(6):637-644.

[14] Lai CH, Kuo KH. The critical component to establish in vitro BBB model: Pericyte. Brain Res Brain Res Rev 2005 Dec 15;50(2):258-265.

[15] Ballabh P, Braun A, Nedergaard M. The blood-brain barrier: an overview: structure, regulation, and clinical implications. Neurobiol Dis 2004 Jun;16(1):1-13.

[16] Matter K, Balda MS. Signalling to and from tight junctions. Nat Rev Mol Cell Biol 2003 Mar;4(3):225-236.

[17] Morita K, Sasaki H, Furuse M, Tsukita S. Endothelial claudin: claudin-5/TMVCF constitutes tight junction strands in endothelial cells. J Cell Biol 1999 Oct 4;147(1): 185-194.

[18] Sonoda N, Furuse M, Sasaki H, Yonemura S, Katahira J, Horiguchi Y, et al. Clostridium perfringens enterotoxin fragment removes specific claudins from tight junction strands: Evidence for direct involvement of claudins in tight junction barrier. J Cell Biol 1999 Oct 4;147(1):195-204.

[19] Krause G, Winkler L, Mueller SL, Haseloff RF, Piontek J, Blasig IE. Structure and function of claudins. Biochim Biophys Acta 2008 Mar;1778(3):631-645.

[20] Furuse M, Fujita K, Hiiragi T, Fujimoto K, Tsukita S. Claudin-1 and -2: novel integral membrane proteins localizing at tight junctions with no sequence similarity to occludin. J Cell Biol 1998 Jun 29;141(7):1539-1550.

[21] Liebner S, Fischmann A, Rascher G, Duffner F, Grote EH, Kalbacher H, et al. Claudin-1 and claudin-5 expression and tight junction morphology are altered in blood vessels of human glioblastoma multiforme. Acta Neuropathol 2000 Sep;100(3): 323-331.

[22] Hirase T, Staddon JM, Saitou M, Ando-Akatsuka Y, Itoh M, Furuse M, et al. Occludin as a possible determinant of tight junction permeability in endothelial cells. J Cell Sci 1997 Jul;110 (Pt 14)(Pt 14):1603-1613.

[23] Feldman GJ, Mullin JM, Ryan MP. Occludin: structure, function and regulation. Adv Drug Deliv Rev 2005 Apr 25;57(6):883-917.

[24] Aurrand-Lions M, Johnson-Leger C, Wong C, Du Pasquier L, Imhof BA. Heterogeneity of endothelial junctions is reflected by differential expression and specific subcellular localization of the three JAM family members. Blood 2001 Dec 15;98(13): 3699-3707.

[25] Mandell KJ, Parkos CA. The JAM family of proteins. Adv Drug Deliv Rev 2005 Apr 25;57(6):857-867.

[26] Lippoldt A, Kniesel U, Liebner S, Kalbacher H, Kirsch T, Wolburg H, et al. Structural alterations of tight junctions are associated with loss of polarity in stroke-prone spontaneously hypertensive rat blood-brain barrier endothelial cells. Brain Res 2000 Dec 8;885(2):251-261.

[27] Gumbleton M, Audus KL. Progress and limitations in the use of in vitro cell cultures to serve as a permeability screen for the blood-brain barrier. J Pharm Sci 2001 Nov; 90(11):1681-1698.

[28] Miller D.W., Audus K.L. and Borchardt R.T. Application of cultured endothelial cells of the brain microvasculature in the study of the blood-brain barrier. J. Tiss. Cult. Meth 1992;14:217-224.

[29] Trickler WJ, Mayhan WG, Miller DW. Brain microvessel endothelial cell responses to tumor necrosis factor-alpha involve a nuclear factor kappa B (NF-kappaB) signal transduction pathway. Brain Res 2005 Jun 28;1048(1-2):24-31.

[30] de Vries HE, Blom-Roosemalen MC, de Boer AG, van Berkel TJ, Breimer DD, Kuiper J. Effect of endotoxin on permeability of bovine cerebral endothelial cell layers in vitro. J Pharmacol Exp Ther 1996 Jun;277(3):1418-1423.

[31] Cecchelli R, Dehouck B, Descamps L, Fenart L, Buee-Scherrer VV, Duhem C, et al. In vitro model for evaluating drug transport across the blood-brain barrier. Adv Drug Deliv Rev 1999 Apr 5;36(2-3):165-178.

[32] Abumrad N, Coburn C, Ibrahimi A. Membrane proteins implicated in long-chain fatty acid uptake by mammalian cells: CD36, FATP and FABPm. Biochim Biophys Acta 1999 Oct 18;1441(1):4-13.

[33] Schaffer JE. Fatty acid transport: the roads taken. Am J Physiol Endocrinol Metab 2002 Feb;282(2):E239-46.

[34] Brouns F, van der Vusse GJ. Utilization of lipids during exercise in human subjects: metabolic and dietary constraints. Br J Nutr 1998 Feb;79(2):117-128.

[35] Pohl J, Ring A, Ehehalt R, Schulze-Bergkamen H, Schad A, Verkade P, et al. Long-chain fatty acid uptake into adipocytes depends on lipid raft function. Biochemistry 2004 Apr 13;43(14):4179-4187.

[36] Drewes LR. What is the blood-brain barrier? A molecular perspective. Cerebral vascular biology. Adv Exp Med Biol 1999;474:111-122.

[37] Kamp F, Hamilton JA, Kamp F, Westerhoff HV, Hamilton JA. Movement of fatty acids, fatty acid analogues, and bile acids across phospholipid bilayers. Biochemistry 1993 Oct 19;32(41):11074-11086.

[38] Watkins PA, Hamilton JA, Leaf A, Spector AA, Moore SA, Anderson RE, et al. Brain uptake and utilization of fatty acids: applications to peroxisomal biogenesis diseases. J Mol Neurosci 2001 Apr-Jun;16(2-3):87-92; discussion 151-7.

[39] Hamilton JA, Johnson RA, Corkey B, Kamp F. Fatty acid transport: the diffusion mechanism in model and biological membranes. J Mol Neurosci 2001 Apr-Jun; 16(2-3):99-108; discussion 151-7.

[40] Hamilton JA, Guo W, Kamp F. Mechanism of cellular uptake of long-chain fatty acids: Do we need cellular proteins? Mol Cell Biochem 2002 Oct;239(1-2):17-23.

[41] Abumrad N, Harmon C, Ibrahimi A. Membrane transport of long-chain fatty acids: evidence for a facilitated process. J Lipid Res 1998 Dec;39(12):2309-2318.

[42] Schwenk RW, Holloway GP, Luiken JJ, Bonen A, Glatz JF. Fatty acid transport across the cell membrane: regulation by fatty acid transporters. Prostaglandins Leukot Essent Fatty Acids 2010 Apr-Jun;82(4-6):149-154.

[43] Hamilton JA. Transport of fatty acids across membranes by the diffusion mechanism. Prostaglandins Leukot Essent Fatty Acids 1999 May-Jun;60(5-6):291-297.

[44] Hamilton JA. Fatty acid transport: difficult or easy? J Lipid Res 1998 Mar;39(3): 467-481.

[45] Frohnert BI, Bernlohr DA. Regulation of fatty acid transporters in mammalian cells. Prog Lipid Res 2000 Jan;39(1):83-107.

[46] Hui TY, Bernlohr DA. Fatty acid transporters in animal cells. Front Biosci 1997 May 15;2:d222-31.

[47] Storch J, Corsico B. The emerging functions and mechanisms of mammalian fatty acid-binding proteins. Annu Rev Nutr 2008;28:73-95.

[48] Rapoport SI, Chang MC, Spector AA. Delivery and turnover of plasma-derived essential PUFAs in mammalian brain. J Lipid Res 2001 May;42(5):678-685.

[49] Duncan RE, Bazinet RP. Brain arachidonic acid uptake and turnover: implications for signaling and bipolar disorder. Curr Opin Clin Nutr Metab Care 2010 Mar;13(2): 130-138.

[50] Katsuki H, Okuda S. Arachidonic acid as a neurotoxic and neurotrophic substance. Prog Neurobiol 1995 Aug;46(6):607-636.

[51] Chan PH, Fishman RA, Caronna J, Schmidley JW, Prioleau G, Lee J. Induction of brain edema following intracerebral injection of arachidonic acid. Ann Neurol 1983 Jun;13(6):625-632.

[52] Chan PH, Fishman RA, Longar S, Chen S, Yu A. Cellular and molecular effects of polyunsaturated fatty acids in brain ischemia and injury. Prog Brain Res 1985;63:227-235.

[53] Jaworowicz DJ,Jr, Korytko PJ, Singh Lakhman S, Boje KM. Nitric oxide and prostaglandin E2 formation parallels blood-brain barrier disruption in an experimental rat model of bacterial meningitis. Brain Res Bull 1998 Aug;46(6):541-546.

[54] Stanimirovic D, Satoh K. Inflammatory mediators of cerebral endothelium: a role in ischemic brain inflammation. Brain Pathol 2000 Jan;10(1):113-126.

[55] Deli MA, Abraham CS, Kataoka Y, Niwa M. Permeability studies on in vitro blood-brain barrier models: physiology, pathology, and pharmacology. Cell Mol Neurobiol 2005 Feb;25(1):59-127.

[56] Mark KS, Trickler WJ, Miller DW. Tumor necrosis factor-alpha induces cyclooxygenase-2 expression and prostaglandin release in brain microvessel endothelial cells. J Pharmacol Exp Ther 2001 Jun;297(3):1051-1058.

[57] Jiang J, Quan Y, Ganesh T, Pouliot WA, Dudek FE, Dingledine R. Inhibition of the prostaglandin receptor EP2 following status epilepticus reduces delayed mortality and brain inflammation. Proc Natl Acad Sci U S A 2013 Feb 26;110(9):3591-3596.

[58] Easton AS, Fraser PA. Arachidonic acid increases cerebral microvascular permeability by free radicals in single pial microvessels of the anaesthetized rat. J Physiol 1998 Mar 1;507 (Pt 2)(Pt 2):541-547.

[59] Othman A, Ahmad S, Megyerdi S, Mussell R, Choksi K, Maddipati KR, et al. 12/15-Lipoxygenase-derived lipid metabolites induce retinal endothelial cell barrier dysfunction: contribution of NADPH oxidase. PLoS One 2013;8(2):e57254.

[60] Stuhlmeier KM, Tarn C, Csizmadia V, Bach FH. Selective suppression of endothelial cell activation by arachidonic acid. Eur J Immunol 1996 Jul;26(7):1417-1423.

[61] Farmer PJ, Bernier SG, Lepage A, Guillemette G, Regoli D, Sirois P. Permeability of endothelial monolayers to albumin is increased by bradykinin and inhibited by prostaglandins. Am J Physiol Lung Cell Mol Physiol 2001 Apr;280(4):L732-8.

[62] Esaki Y, Li Y, Sakata D, Yao C, Segi-Nishida E, Matsuoka T, et al. Dual roles of PGE2-EP4 signaling in mouse experimental autoimmune encephalomyelitis. Proc Natl Acad Sci U S A 2010 Jul 6;107(27):12233-12238.

[63] Ahmad M, Saleem S, Shah Z, Maruyama T, Narumiya S, Dore S. The PGE2 EP2 receptor and its selective activation are beneficial against ischemic stroke. Exp Transl Stroke Med 2010 Jul 8;2(1):12-7378-2-12.

[64] Denning GM, Figard PH, Spector AA. Effect of fatty acid modification on prostaglandin production by cultured 3T3 cells. J Lipid Res 1982 May;23(4):584-596.

[65] Eldor A, Vlodavsky I, Hy-Am E, Atzmon R, Weksler BB, Raz A, et al. Cultured endothelial cells increase their capacity to synthesize prostacyclin following the formation of a contact inhibited cell monolayer. J Cell Physiol 1983 Feb;114(2):179-183.

[66] Gerritsen ME, Nganele DM, Rodrigues AM. Calcium ionophore (A23187)- and arachidonic acid-stimulated prostaglandin release from microvascular endothelial cells: effects of calcium antagonists and calmodulin inhibitors. J Pharmacol Exp Ther 1987 Mar;240(3):837-846.

[67] Baker PN, Davidge ST, Barankiewicz J, Roberts JM. Plasma of preeclamptic women stimulates and then inhibits endothelial prostacyclin. Hypertension 1996 Jan;27(1):56-61.

[68] Li X, Hong S, Li PL, Zhang Y. Docosahexanoic acid-induced coronary arterial dilation: actions of 17S-hydroxy docosahexanoic acid on K+ channel activity. J Pharmacol Exp Ther 2011 Mar;336(3):891-899.

[69] Hong S, Gronert K, Devchand PR, Moussignac RL, Serhan CN. Novel docosatrienes and 17S-resolvins generated from docosahexaenoic acid in murine brain, human blood, and glial cells. Autacoids in anti-inflammation. J Biol Chem 2003 Apr 25;278(17):14677-14687.

[70] Adkins Y, Kelley DS. Mechanisms underlying the cardioprotective effects of omega-3 polyunsaturated fatty acids. J Nutr Biochem 2010 Sep;21(9):781-792.

[71] Hermann DM, Bassetti CL. Implications of ATP-binding cassette transporters for brain pharmacotherapies. Trends Pharmacol Sci 2007 Mar;28(3):128-134.

[72] Urquhart BL, Kim RB. Blood-brain barrier transporters and response to CNS-active drugs. Eur J Clin Pharmacol 2009 Nov;65(11):1063-1070.

[73] Meier-Abt F, Mokrab Y, Mizuguchi K. Organic anion transporting polypeptides of the OATP/SLCO superfamily: identification of new members in nonmammalian species, comparative modeling and a potential transport mode. J Membr Biol 2005 Dec; 208(3):213-227.

[74] Gao B, Stieger B, Noe B, Fritschy JM, Meier PJ. Localization of the organic anion transporting polypeptide 2 (Oatp2) in capillary endothelium and choroid plexus epithelium of rat brain. J Histochem Cytochem 1999 Oct;47(10):1255-1264.

[75] Hagenbuch B, Meier PJ. Organic anion transporting polypeptides of the OATP/ SLC21 family: phylogenetic classification as OATP/ SLCO superfamily, new nomenclature and molecular/functional properties. Pflugers Arch 2004 Feb;447(5):653-665.

[76] Kalliokoski A, Niemi M. Impact of OATP transporters on pharmacokinetics. Br J Pharmacol 2009 Oct;158(3):693-705.

[77] Ose A, Kusuhara H, Endo C, Tohyama K, Miyajima M, Kitamura S, et al. Functional characterization of mouse organic anion transporting peptide 1a4 in the uptake and efflux of drugs across the blood-brain barrier. Drug Metab Dispos 2010 Jan;38(1): 168-176.

[78] Burckhardt G, Burckhardt BC. In vitro and in vivo evidence of the importance of organic anion transporters (OATs) in drug therapy. Handb Exp Pharmacol 2011;(201): 29-104. doi(201):29-104.

[79] Buist SC, Cherrington NJ, Choudhuri S, Hartley DP, Klaassen CD. Gender-specific and developmental influences on the expression of rat organic anion transporters. J Pharmacol Exp Ther 2002 Apr;301(1):145-151.

[80] Aoki K, Saso N, Kato S, Sugiyama Y, Sato H. Nitric oxide and peroxynitrite regulate transporter transcription in rat liver slices. Biol Pharm Bull 2008 Oct;31(10):1882-1887.

[81] Popowski K, Eloranta JJ, Saborowski M, Fried M, Meier PJ, Kullak-Ublick GA. The human organic anion transporter 2 gene is transactivated by hepatocyte nuclear factor-4 alpha and suppressed by bile acids. Mol Pharmacol 2005 May;67(5):1629-1638.

[82] Kikuchi R, Kusuhara H, Sugiyama D, Sugiyama Y. Contribution of organic anion transporter 3 (Slc22a8) to the elimination of p-aminohippuric acid and benzylpenicillin across the blood-brain barrier. J Pharmacol Exp Ther 2003 Jul;306(1):51-58.

[83] Vannucci SJ, Maher F, Simpson IA. Glucose transporter proteins in brain: delivery of glucose to neurons and glia. Glia 1997 Sep;21(1):2-21.

[84] Birnbaum MJ, Haspel HC, Rosen OM. Cloning and characterization of a cDNA encoding the rat brain glucose-transporter protein. Proc Natl Acad Sci U S A 1986 Aug; 83(16):5784-5788.

[85] Bondy CA, Lee WH, Zhou J. Ontogeny and cellular distribution of brain glucose transporter gene expression. Mol Cell Neurosci 1992 Aug;3(4):305-314.

[86] Morgello S, Uson RR, Schwartz EJ, Haber RS. The human blood-brain barrier glucose transporter (GLUT1) is a glucose transporter of gray matter astrocytes. Glia 1995 May;14(1):43-54.

[87] Pardridge WM. Blood-brain barrier biology and methodology. J Neurovirol 1999 Dec;5(6):556-569.

[88] Pardridge WM, Boado RJ, Farrell CR. Brain-type glucose transporter (GLUT-1) is selectively localized to the blood-brain barrier. Studies with quantitative western blotting and in situ hybridization. J Biol Chem 1990 Oct 15;265(29):18035-18040.

[89] Farrell CL, Yang J, Pardridge WM. GLUT-1 glucose transporter is present within apical and basolateral membranes of brain epithelial interfaces and in microvascular endothelia with and without tight junctions. J Histochem Cytochem 1992 Feb;40(2): 193-199.

[90] Klip A, Tsakiridis T, Marette A, Ortiz PA. Regulation of expression of glucose transporters by glucose: a review of studies in vivo and in cell cultures. FASEB J 1994 Jan; 8(1):43-53.

[91] Au KK, Liong E, Li JY, Li PS, Liew CC, Kwok TT, et al. Increases in mRNA levels of glucose transporters types 1 and 3 in Ehrlich ascites tumor cells during tumor development. J Cell Biochem 1997 Oct 1;67(1):131-135.

[92] Vemula S, Roder KE, Yang T, Bhat GJ, Thekkumkara TJ, Abbruscato TJ. A functional role for sodium-dependent glucose transport across the blood-brain barrier during oxygen glucose deprivation. J Pharmacol Exp Ther 2009 Feb;328(2):487-495.

[93] Pierre K, Pellerin L. Monocarboxylate transporters in the central nervous system: distribution, regulation and function. J Neurochem 2005 Jul;94(1):1-14.

[94] Nybo L, Secher NH. Cerebral perturbations provoked by prolonged exercise. Prog Neurobiol 2004 Mar;72(4):223-261.

[95] Gjedde A, Crone C. Induction processes in blood-brain transfer of ketone bodies during starvation. Am J Physiol 1975 Nov;229(5):1165-1169.

[96] Bouzier-Sore AK, Merle M, Magistretti PJ, Pellerin L. Feeding active neurons: (re)emergence of a nursing role for astrocytes. J Physiol Paris 2002 Apr-Jun;96(3-4): 273-282.

[97] Pellerin L. Lactate as a pivotal element in neuron-glia metabolic cooperation. Neurochem Int 2003 Sep-Oct;43(4-5):331-338.

[98] Waniewski RA, Martin DL. Astrocytes and synaptosomes transport and metabolize lactate and acetate differently. Neurochem Res 2004 Jan;29(1):209-217.

[99] Simpson IA, Carruthers A, Vannucci SJ. Supply and demand in cerebral energy metabolism: the role of nutrient transporters. J Cereb Blood Flow Metab 2007 Nov; 27(11):1766-1791.

[100] Pierre K, Pellerin L, Debernardi R, Riederer BM, Magistretti PJ. Cell-specific localization of monocarboxylate transporters, MCT1 and MCT2, in the adult mouse brain revealed by double immunohistochemical labeling and confocal microscopy. Neuroscience 2000;100(3):617-627.

[101] Leino RL, Gerhart DZ, Drewes LR. Monocarboxylate transporter (MCT1) abundance in brains of suckling and adult rats: a quantitative electron microscopic immunogold study. Brain Res Dev Brain Res 1999 Mar 12;113(1-2):47-54.

[102] Friesema EC, Ganguly S, Abdalla A, Manning Fox JE, Halestrap AP, Visser TJ. Identification of monocarboxylate transporter 8 as a specific thyroid hormone transporter. J Biol Chem 2003 Oct 10;278(41):40128-40135.

[103] Tai LM, Reddy PS, Lopez-Ramirez MA, Davies HA, Male DK, Loughlin AJ, et al. Polarized P-glycoprotein expression by the immortalised human brain endothelial cell line, hCMEC/D3, restricts apical-to-basolateral permeability to rhodamine 123. Brain Res 2009 Oct 6;1292:14-24.

[104] Dantzig AH, de Alwis DP, Burgess M. Considerations in the design and development of transport inhibitors as adjuncts to drug therapy. Adv Drug Deliv Rev 2003 Jan 21;55(1):133-150.

[105] Potschka H. Targeting regulation of ABC efflux transporters in brain diseases: a novel therapeutic approach. Pharmacol Ther 2010 Jan;125(1):118-127.

[106] Loscher W, Potschka H. Role of drug efflux transporters in the brain for drug disposition and treatment of brain diseases. Prog Neurobiol 2005 May;76(1):22-76.

[107] Kruh GD, Belinsky MG. The MRP family of drug efflux pumps. Oncogene 2003 Oct 20;22(47):7537-7552.

[108] Su W, Pasternak GW. The role of multidrug resistance-associated protein in the blood-brain barrier and opioid analgesia. Synapse 2013 Sep;67(9):609-619.

[109] Keppler D. Multidrug resistance proteins (MRPs, ABCCs): importance for pathophysiology and drug therapy. Handb Exp Pharmacol 2011;(201):299-323. doi(201): 299-323.

[110] Kusuhara H, Suzuki H, Naito M, Tsuruo T, Sugiyama Y. Characterization of efflux transport of organic anions in a mouse brain capillary endothelial cell line. J Pharmacol Exp Ther 1998 Jun;285(3):1260-1265.

[111] Regina A, Koman A, Piciotti M, El Hafny B, Center MS, Bergmann R, et al. Mrp1 multidrug resistance-associated protein and P-glycoprotein expression in rat brain microvessel endothelial cells. J Neurochem 1998 Aug;71(2):705-715.

[112] Gutmann H, Torok M, Fricker G, Huwyler J, Beglinger C, Drewe J. Modulation of multidrug resistance protein expression in porcine brain capillary endothelial cells in vitro. Drug Metab Dispos 1999 Aug;27(8):937-941.

[113] Seetharaman S, Barrand MA, Maskell L, Scheper RJ. Multidrug resistance-related transport proteins in isolated human brain microvessels and in cells cultured from these isolates. J Neurochem 1998 Mar;70(3):1151-1159.

[114] Nies AT, Jedlitschky G, Konig J, Herold-Mende C, Steiner HH, Schmitt HP, et al. Expression and immunolocalization of the multidrug resistance proteins, MRP1-MRP6 (ABCC1-ABCC6), in human brain. Neuroscience 2004;129(2):349-360.

[115] Zhang Y, Schuetz JD, Elmquist WF, Miller DW. Plasma membrane localization of multidrug resistance-associated protein homologs in brain capillary endothelial cells. J Pharmacol Exp Ther 2004 Nov;311(2):449-455.

[116] Roberts LM, Black DS, Raman C, Woodford K, Zhou M, Haggerty JE, et al. Subcellular localization of transporters along the rat blood-brain barrier and blood-cerebral-spinal fluid barrier by in vivo biotinylation. Neuroscience 2008 Aug 13;155(2): 423-438.

[117] Stanley LA, Horsburgh BC, Ross J, Scheer N, Wolf CR. Drug transporters: gatekeepers controlling access of xenobiotics to the cellular interior. Drug Metab Rev 2009;41(1):27-65.

[118] Sugiyama D, Kusuhara H, Lee YJ, Sugiyama Y. Involvement of multidrug resistance associated protein 1 (Mrp1) in the efflux transport of 17beta estradiol-D-17beta-glucuronide (E217betaG) across the blood-brain barrier. Pharm Res 2003 Sep;20(9): 1394-1400.

[119] Miller DS, Nobmann SN, Gutmann H, Toeroek M, Drewe J, Fricker G. Xenobiotic transport across isolated brain microvessels studied by confocal microscopy. Mol Pharmacol 2000 Dec;58(6):1357-1367.

[120] Dombrowski SM, Desai SY, Marroni M, Cucullo L, Goodrich K, Bingaman W, et al. Overexpression of multiple drug resistance genes in endothelial cells from patients with refractory epilepsy. Epilepsia 2001 Dec;42(12):1501-1506.

[121] Miller DS, Graeff C, Droulle L, Fricker S, Fricker G. Xenobiotic efflux pumps in isolated fish brain capillaries. Am J Physiol Regul Integr Comp Physiol 2002 Jan; 282(1):R191-8.

[122] Zhang Y, Han H, Elmquist WF, Miller DW. Expression of various multidrug resistance-associated protein (MRP) homologues in brain microvessel endothelial cells. Brain Res 2000 Sep 8;876(1-2):148-153.

[123] Berezowski V, Landry C, Dehouck MP, Cecchelli R, Fenart L. Contribution of glial cells and pericytes to the mRNA profiles of P-glycoprotein and multidrug resistance-

associated proteins in an in vitro model of the blood-brain barrier. Brain Res 2004 Aug 20;1018(1):1-9.

[124] Ma JJ, Chen BL, Xin XY. Inhibition of multi-drug resistance of ovarian carcinoma by small interfering RNA targeting to MRP2 gene. Arch Gynecol Obstet 2009 Feb;279(2): 149-157.

[125] Bauer B, Hartz AM, Lucking JR, Yang X, Pollack GM, Miller DS. Coordinated nuclear receptor regulation of the efflux transporter, Mrp2, and the phase-II metabolizing enzyme, GSTpi, at the blood-brain barrier. J Cereb Blood Flow Metab 2008 Jun;28(6): 1222-1234.

[126] Lombardo L, Pellitteri R, Balazy M, Cardile V. Induction of nuclear receptors and drug resistance in the brain microvascular endothelial cells treated with antiepileptic drugs. Curr Neurovasc Res 2008 May;5(2):82-92.

[127] Kruh GD, Zeng H, Rea PA, Liu G, Chen ZS, Lee K, et al. MRP subfamily transporters and resistance to anticancer agents. J Bioenerg Biomembr 2001 Dec;33(6):493-501.

[128] Bakos E, Evers R, Sinko E, Varadi A, Borst P, Sarkadi B. Interactions of the human multidrug resistance proteins MRP1 and MRP2 with organic anions. Mol Pharmacol 2000 Apr;57(4):760-768.

[129] Potschka H, Fedrowitz M, Loscher W. Multidrug resistance protein MRP2 contributes to blood-brain barrier function and restricts antiepileptic drug activity. J Pharmacol Exp Ther 2003 Jul;306(1):124-131.

[130] Agarwal S, Elmquist WF. Insight into the cooperation of P-glycoprotein (ABCB1) and breast cancer resistance protein (ABCG2) at the blood-brain barrier: a case study examining sorafenib efflux clearance. Mol Pharm 2012 Mar 5;9(3):678-684.

[131] Uchida Y, Ohtsuki S, Katsukura Y, Ikeda C, Suzuki T, Kamiie J, et al. Quantitative targeted absolute proteomics of human blood-brain barrier transporters and receptors. J Neurochem 2011 Apr;117(2):333-345.

[132] Leggas M, Adachi M, Scheffer GL, Sun D, Wielinga P, Du G, et al. Mrp4 confers resistance to topotecan and protects the brain from chemotherapy. Mol Cell Biol 2004 Sep;24(17):7612-7621.

[133] Chen ZS, Lee K, Kruh GD. Transport of cyclic nucleotides and estradiol 17-beta-D-glucuronide by multidrug resistance protein 4. Resistance to 6-mercaptopurine and 6-thioguanine. J Biol Chem 2001 Sep 7;276(36):33747-33754.

[134] Lai L, Tan TM. Role of glutathione in the multidrug resistance protein 4 (MRP4/ABCC4)-mediated efflux of cAMP and resistance to purine analogues. Biochem J 2002 Feb 1;361(Pt 3):497-503.

[135] van Aubel RA, Smeets PH, Peters JG, Bindels RJ, Russel FG. The MRP4/ABCC4 gene encodes a novel apical organic anion transporter in human kidney proximal tubules:

putative efflux pump for urinary cAMP and cGMP. J Am Soc Nephrol 2002 Mar; 13(3):595-603.

[136] Sampath J, Adachi M, Hatse S, Naesens L, Balzarini J, Flatley RM, et al. Role of MRP4 and MRP5 in biology and chemotherapy. AAPS PharmSci 2002;4(3):E14.

[137] Belinsky MG, Guo P, Lee K, Zhou F, Kotova E, Grinberg A, et al. Multidrug resistance protein 4 protects bone marrow, thymus, spleen, and intestine from nucleotide analogue-induced damage. Cancer Res 2007 Jan 1;67(1):262-268.

[138] Jedlitschky G, Burchell B, Keppler D. The multidrug resistance protein 5 functions as an ATP-dependent export pump for cyclic nucleotides. J Biol Chem 2000 Sep 29;275(39):30069-30074.

[139] Belinsky MG, Chen ZS, Shchaveleva I, Zeng H, Kruh GD. Characterization of the drug resistance and transport properties of multidrug resistance protein 6 (MRP6, ABCC6). Cancer Res 2002 Nov 1;62(21):6172-6177.

[140] Kruh GD, Guo Y, Hopper-Borge E, Belinsky MG, Chen ZS. ABCC10, ABCC11, and ABCC12. Pflugers Arch 2007 Feb;453(5):675-684.

[141] Nicolazzo JA, Katneni K. Drug transport across the blood-brain barrier and the impact of breast cancer resistance protein (ABCG2). Curr Top Med Chem 2009;9(2): 130-147.

[142] Ozvegy C, Litman T, Szakacs G, Nagy Z, Bates S, Varadi A, et al. Functional characterization of the human multidrug transporter, ABCG2, expressed in insect cells. Biochem Biophys Res Commun 2001 Jul 6;285(1):111-117.

[143] Imai Y, Asada S, Tsukahara S, Ishikawa E, Tsuruo T, Sugimoto Y. Breast cancer resistance protein exports sulfated estrogens but not free estrogens. Mol Pharmacol 2003 Sep;64(3):610-618.

[144] Suzuki M, Suzuki H, Sugimoto Y, Sugiyama Y. ABCG2 transports sulfated conjugates of steroids and xenobiotics. J Biol Chem 2003 Jun 20;278(25):22644-22649.

[145] Juliano RL, Ling V. A surface glycoprotein modulating drug permeability in Chinese hamster ovary cell mutants. Biochim Biophys Acta 1976 Nov 11;455(1):152-162.

[146] Beaulieu E, Demeule M, Ghitescu L, Beliveau R. P-glycoprotein is strongly expressed in the luminal membranes of the endothelium of blood vessels in the brain. Biochem J 1997 Sep 1;326 (Pt 2)(Pt 2):539-544.

[147] Tatsuta T, Naito M, Oh-hara T, Sugawara I, Tsuruo T. Functional involvement of P-glycoprotein in blood-brain barrier. J Biol Chem 1992 Oct 5;267(28):20383-20391.

[148] Virgintino D, Robertson D, Errede M, Benagiano V, Girolamo F, Maiorano E, et al. Expression of P-glycoprotein in human cerebral cortex microvessels. J Histochem Cytochem 2002 Dec;50(12):1671-1676.

[149] Bendayan R, Ronaldson PT, Gingras D, Bendayan M. In situ localization of P-glycoprotein (ABCB1) in human and rat brain. J Histochem Cytochem 2006 Oct;54(10): 1159-1167.

[150] Seelig A, Landwojtowicz E. Structure-activity relationship of P-glycoprotein substrates and modifiers. Eur J Pharm Sci 2000 Nov;12(1):31-40.

[151] Ueda K, Taguchi Y, Morishima M. How does P-glycoprotein recognize its substrates? Semin Cancer Biol 1997 Jun;8(3):151-159.

[152] Wijesuriya HC, Bullock JY, Faull RL, Hladky SB, Barrand MA. ABC efflux transporters in brain vasculature of Alzheimer's subjects. Brain Res 2010 Oct 28;1358:228-238.

[153] Kania KD, Wijesuriya HC, Hladky SB, Barrand MA. Beta amyloid effects on expression of multidrug efflux transporters in brain endothelial cells. Brain Res 2011 Oct 18;1418:1-11.

[154] Hollo Z, Homolya L, Hegedus T, Sarkadi B. Transport properties of the multidrug resistance-associated protein (MRP) in human tumour cells. FEBS Lett 1996 Mar 25;383(1-2):99-104.

[155] Bauer F, Kuntner C, Bankstahl JP, Wanek T, Bankstahl M, Stanek J, et al. Synthesis and in vivo evaluation of [11C]tariquidar, a positron emission tomography radiotracer based on a third-generation P-glycoprotein inhibitor. Bioorg Med Chem 2010 Aug 1;18(15):5489-5497.

[156] Balayssac D, Authier N, Cayre A, Coudore F. Does inhibition of P-glycoprotein lead to drug-drug interactions? Toxicol Lett 2005 Apr 28;156(3):319-329.

4

High Temporal Resolution Brain Microdialysis as a Tool to Investigate the Dynamics of Interactions Between Olfactory Cortex and Amygdala in Odor Fear Conditioning

Chloé Hegoburu, Luc Denoroy,
Anne-Marie Mouly and Sandrine Parrot

1. Introduction

Fear conditioning is one of the most widely used paradigms for studying the neurobiology of emotional learning. In this paradigm, an emotionally neutral stimulus (the conditioned stimulus or CS) is paired with an aversive unconditioned stimulus (US), generally a mild foot shock. After a few trials, re-exposure to the CS alone elicits a fear response, proceeding through the necessary connecting structures, and ending with the autonomic and motoric effector outputs. This fear response is part of an anticipatory response to danger [1], initiating a range of defensive reactions that counter threats to survival [2]. The most universal response is a postural immobility, called freezing [3, 4]. Moreover, the threatening stimulus also triggers the activation of the hypothalamic subnuclei to induce an increase in blood pressure, ultrasonic vocalizations emission, or the release of stress hormones.

The vast majority of studies devoted to investigate the neural basis of fear conditioning have used auditory cues as conditioned stimuli and the neural pathways involved in auditory fear conditioning have been well characterized [5-8]. The information carried by the auditory CS can take one of two pathways: either directly from the thalamus to quickly reach the amygdala or the CS can travel from the auditory thalamus to the auditory cortex before reaching the amygdala. These thalamic and cortical areas send projections to the lateral nucleus of the amygdala, which is a site of CS-US convergence. The lateral nucleus, in turn, projects to the central amygdala, which controls the expression of fear responses by way of projections to brainstem areas. The major conclusion of these studies is that the amygdala plays a critical role in linking external stimuli to defense responses through synaptic plasticity. However, although the amygdala seems to be essential to the formation and storage of fear memories, it might not store all aspects of the aversive event. Indeed, plasticity also occurs in cortical areas during fear conditioning, which could support declarative memories of the learning episode mainly through interactions with the medial temporal lobe memory system [9-13]. Thus, the amygdala may store some aspects of fear memory and facilitate the storage of other, more sensory-related, aspects of fear memory in cortical areas [14]. Yet few studies have investigated this question [15].

Intriguingly, whereas olfaction plays a dominant role in rat behavior from birth throughout adulthood, very few studies have used odor cues as CS in fear conditioning paradigms. Yet, odors have a rather unique status for eliciting emotional memories.[16]. This particularity might be linked to the uniqueness of the anatomy of the olfactory system. Indeed, in contrast to the other sensory pathways, olfactory information has a direct access to the amygdala and olfactory (piriform) cortex with no obligatory thalamic relay [17-19]. The literature suggests that, similarly to what is observed in auditory fear conditioning, the amygdala is a key brain structure involved in the acquisition, consolidation and expression of odor fear conditioning [20-26]. Recently, some studies also suggest that the posterior piriform cortex (PPC) may play a critical role in this associative learning [23, 26, 27]. Therefore, the olfactory system constitutes a particularly relevant model for studying the relative contribution of sensory cortices and amygdalar nuclei to odor fear learning.

For several years now, the glutamatergic transmission in the amygdala is known to play a critical role in the acquisition of fear conditioning [28, 29]. Indeed, pharmacological studies show that NMDA and AMPA subclasses of glutamate receptors are crucial for synaptic plasticity and long-term potentiation to occur in the amygdala, sustaining the formation of the CS-US association [25, 30-35]. In addition, the GABAergic transmission seems to be also involved in the acquisition of fear learning. Intra-amygdala infusion of the $GABA_A$ receptor agonist muscimol before training impairs learning [36, 37]. Therefore, glutamate and GABA neurotransmission are thought to play a critical role in the acquisition and expression of fear memories (for review, see [38]).

Beside these neuropharmacological studies, a few neurochemical studies have directly measured glutamate or GABA levels in the amygdala during auditory fear conditioning, using a 10-min sampling rate [39, 40]. However, this sampling rate is too long as compared to the rapid neurobiological events underlying fear conditioning. An approach allowing rapid, sub-minute sampling is required to better characterize the dynamics of neurotransmitter changes evoked by the stimuli involved in fear conditioning experiments [41]. Until now, the precise time course of the differential involvement of the amygdala and sensory cortices in fear conditioning has received little investigation. The aim of this chapter is to show that intra-cerebral in vivo microdialysis with high temporal resolution is an interesting tool to investigate the time course of activation of amygdala and sensory cortices in this learning.

2. Monitoring neurotransmitters using microdialysis

2.1. Principle of the technique and analytical considerations

Microdialysis has become a conventional technique for sampling low molecular weight molecules present in the extracellular medium of many organs from animals or humans [42]. In the brain, it has been used *in vivo* or *ex vivo* to monitor amino acids neurotransmitters as excitatory or inhibitory amino acids as glutamate and GABA, monoamines as dopamine, noradrenaline, serotonin and/or neuropeptides for instance. The microdialysis relies on a semi-permeable membrane that allows free diffusion of solutes between the extracellular space and an artificial fluid. A microdialysis probe consists of two concentric tubes with the distal part (1–5 mm) covered by a dialysis hollow fibre whose cut-off ranges between 6,000 and 100,000 Da. Such a probe is inserted into a living brain tissue and is perfused by an isotonic physiological fluid. Molecules diffuse down their concentration gradient across the dialysis membrane in a bidirectional way ("dialysis" for collecting endogenous molecules or "reverse dialysis" for applying exogenous compounds) (Figure 1). In the case of collection, the relative recovery across the probe membrane, defined as the ratio between the extracellular concentration and the concentration of a compound in the dialysate collected at the outlet of the probe, depends on several factors: it increases with the surface of the membrane, it decreases with higher flow rate of the perfusion fluid, and it varies with the chemical and physical characteristics of the membrane [43]. The choice of the dialysis membrane can be crucial for compounds present at trace concentration or when the limit of detection of the analytical method is relatively moderate. For instance, a short length (i.e. 1-2 mm) of the membrane chosen to sample a very small brain area in rats, such as the periaqueductal grey matter, the locus coeruleus, the amygdala and hypothalamic nuclei leads to a low recovery of sampling, making difficult the monitoring of low concentrated compounds as monoamines or neuropeptides. Depending on the methodological parameters, recovery values usually reported in literature are between 5 and 25 % for amino acids or monoamines and can reach < 1 % for neuropeptides. Another point to take into account is the choice of the geometry of the probe tubings when considering the sampling rate, especially when designing in vivo microdialysis on awake animals. These latter peculiar points will be explained and detailed in the next section part of the manuscript.

As the microdialysis probe is continuously perfused at a constant flow rate, continuous sampling of neurotransmitters is possible with no loss. Indeed, neurotransmitters present in the microdialysate can be directly analyzed without clean-up procedures as high molecular weight proteins cannot cross the dialysis membrane thanks to the cut-off of the membrane used. However, manipulation of microdialysis samples requires precaution in case of amino acids: use of sterile tubes, filtered aCSF and wear of gloves avoiding contamination due to the ubiquitous presence of free amino acids on labware and skin. Eventually, samples may be usually analyzed by a separative method like high performance liquid chromatography (HPLC) or capillary electrophoresis (CE) [44, 45]. Microdialysates can be analyzed on-line, i.e., at the outlet of the probe, through an analytical interface, or off-line i.e., after sample collection in micro-tubes, in combination with a separative method [44, 46, 47]. Thus, the determination

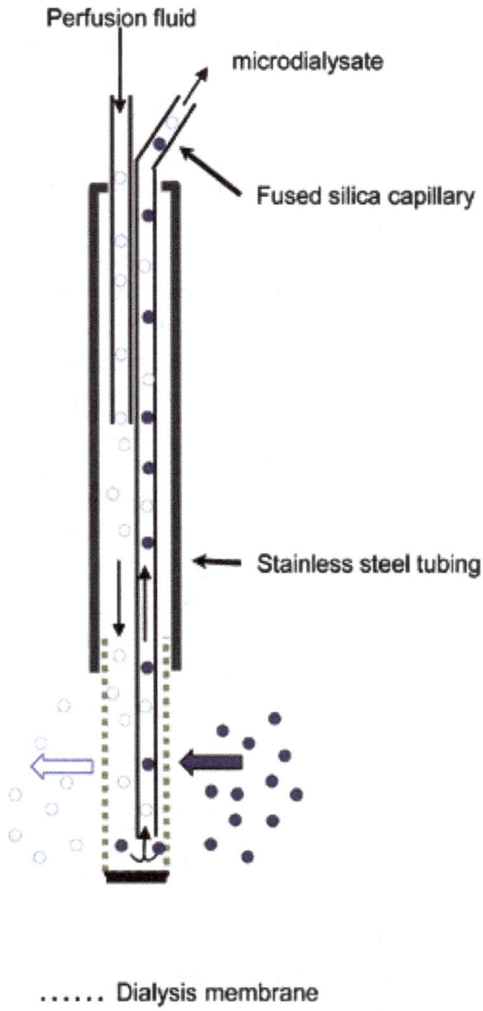

Figure 1. Schematic representation of a microdialysis probe. The probe is continuously perfused by an isotonic physiological fluid. Endogenous compounds (filled circles) diffuse through the dialysis membrane (filled arrow) and are sampled in the microdialysate collected at the outlet of the probe. Drugs (open circles) can be added to the perfusion medium and can diffuse out of the probe into the extracellular medium (open arrow) providing a means of local administration. From [109], with permission from John Wiley and Sons.

of concentrations in each sample reflects the average concentration over the defined sampling duration. Data are classically expressed as % of the average of the first samples collected, corresponding to baseline. As a consequence, microdialysis (except in very peculiar methodological contexts not explained in this chapter) is considered as a semi-quantitative method as it permits to monitor precisely relative variations of neurotransmitters.

Analysis of microdialysates has commonly used HPLC with electrochemical [48, 49] or fluorometric detection [50, 51], and also enzymatic methods [52]. However, these analytical techniques exhibit poor mass sensitivity and require large volume samples to determine neurotransmitter contents. As a consequence, despite constant improvements in HPLC [50, 51, 53], the required sample volume may still be too large, leading to lengthy dialysis sampling times and poor temporal resolution. Consequently, most microdialysis experiments were severely limited by the temporal resolution of microdialysis (5–30 min) compared to rapid changes occurring in the extracellular concentrations of neurotransmitters. In contrast, microdialysis coupled to CE, a more recent technique, allows the monitoring of rapid changes in the extracellular concentration of neurotransmitters by analysing nanovolume dialysates with low limits of detection. At present, it appears to be suitable for microdialysis with high sampling rate. Often coupled to laser-induced fluorescence (LIF) detection or mass spectrometry (MS), capillary electrophoresis has become one of the most powerful analytical tools for the routine determination of neurotransmitters because it offers the advantage of rapidity, high resolution and sensitivity, while requiring very small sample sizes [44, 54, 55]. In brain microdialysates, glutamate and GABA [56-64] were often analysed using CE with LIF detection. However, as amino acid neurotransmitters are not fluorescent at wavelengths of most commercially available lasers, derivatization prior to the separation is needed. Fluorescent reagents, as naphthalene-2,3-dicarboxaldehyde (NDA), orthophtaldehyde (OPA) or fluorescein isothiocyanate, reacting with the primary amine function of neurotransmitters, allow their detection following laser excitation at 442, 325, or 488 nm, respectively [63-65]. Several groups, including our own, have developed methodologies for the CE–LIF analysis of brain microdialysates after a derivatization of samples with fluorogenic agents, even on sub-microliter dialysates obtained with high temporal resolution microdialysis (5s – 1 min, [44] for mini-review).

2.2. Set-up for high temporal microdialysis on behaving animal

According to the neurophysiological question asked, the experimental set-up for microdialysis experiments has to be carefully designed: the choice of microdialysis probe according to the targeted brain area, the choice of the analytical method to quantify dialysate neurotransmitters and the coupling of the experimental set-ups or approaches are all crucial to succeed in neurochemical studies. The aim of the study described here [66] was to monitor amino acid neurotransmitters as glutamate and GABA in brain areas involved in emotional learning and memory using odor fear conditioning. Indeed, while a few studies have investigated the time course of events separately in the auditory cortex and the amygdala during auditory fear conditioning [11, 12], no study up to date has been conducted to investigate simultaneously the changes in amygdala and sensory cortical areas in the same animal during fear conditioning.

Our group previously reported lasting changes in electrophysiological field potential signals in both posterior piriform cortex (PPC) and amygdala (basolateral nucleus, BLA) after a session of odor fear conditioning [23]. As a consequence, we conducted an experiment using a dual-microdialysis probe implantation, in order to compare the time courses of changes in GABA and glutamate concentrations, monitored simultaneously in BLA and PPC during odor fear conditioning. Very few groups have developed dual (or triple) implantation of microdialysis probes on the same animal [67, 68]. Indeed in most studies using brain microdialysis, dialysates collection is usually performed in one brain structure at a time, sometimes on different days. Literature on microdialysis experiments in BLA is rather abundant, mainly for monoamines.

There are only a few papers in the literature reporting microdialysis studies in the piriform cortex in an epileptic model [69] or during a feeding/diet procedure [70]. Two other studies were devoted to glutamate monitoring at 20 or 30-min sampling rate in anesthetized [71] or awake rats [72]. In order to target the centre of each brain structure and avoid excluding rats with inaccurate implantation on one hand, and in order to optimize the amount of collected glutamate and GABA in the microdialysates for analytical quantification on the other hand, 1.5-mm microdialysis probes were used for both BLA and PPC. However, due to the size of the probes and the vicinity of amygdala and olfactory cortex, we implanted one probe per hemisphere, BLA probe on one side, PPC probe contralaterally (Figure 2). As the acquisition session of odor fear conditioning was short-lasting (30 min), we monitored glutamate and GABA at high sampling rate using CE-LIFD as analytical technique. When performing high sampling rate, it is crucial to optimize the geometry of the probe tubings.

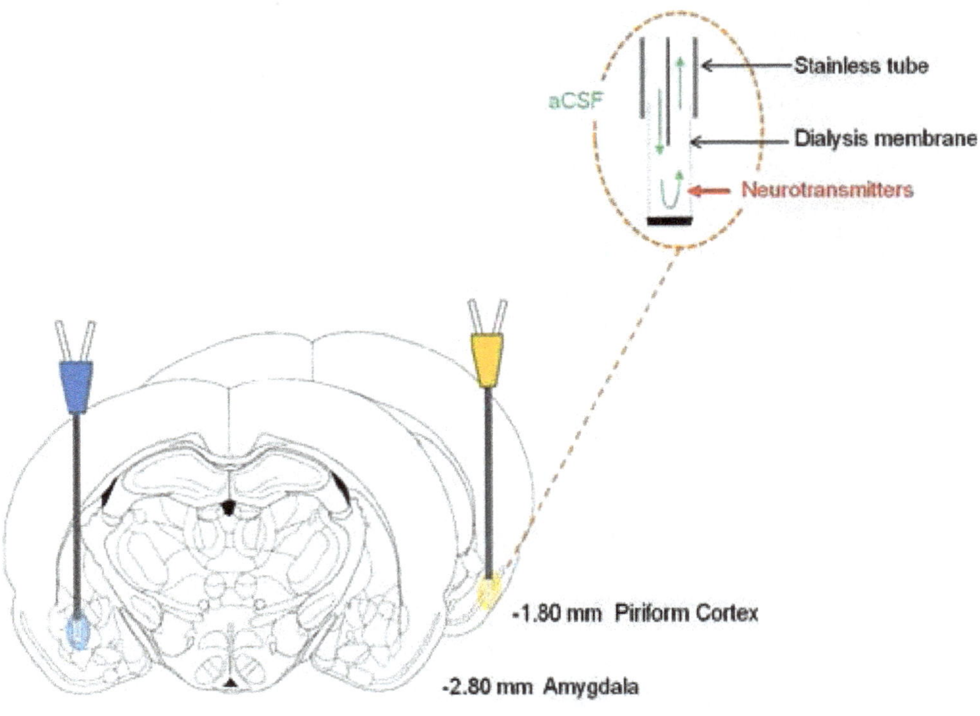

Figure 2. Brain sections from Paxinos & Watson's atlas with a schematic probe implanted in the left basolateral amygdala and the other implanted in the right posterior piriform cortex of the same freely-moving rat for simultaneous glutamate and GABA monitoring.

Indeed, a high sampling rate requires appropriate probe tubings since solutes could undergo more longitudinal diffusion in the outlet probe tubing if the interval of time between dialysis and collection, also called 'dead time, is superior to the sampling time [56]. As a consequence, to avoid mixing of analytes between successive samples, the dead volume of these tubings has to be minimized. This is particularly relevant when microdialysis experiments are carried out on awake animals because the setting requires long inlet and outlet probe tubings in order to let the animals move freely. In our odor fear conditioning, the set-up includes specific characteristics: an experimental chamber with a grid for electrical stimulation which is a mild footshock (Unconditioned Stimulus, US) and with an ventilation system bringing and removing the odor (Conditioned Stimulus, CS); besides, this experimental chamber has to be placed in a soundproof box in which we can position cameras to record the behavior of the animal. Material for microdialysis (perfusion pump) and collection have to be placed outside the box for not disturbing the animal in learning. In our set-up, the height of the box reaches almost one meter (Figure 3). The dead volume can be greatly minimized by using capillary tubings with sub-50 µm inner diameters, as previously demonstrated by our group [56]. By using a 40-µm inner diameter, we have optimized the microdialysis set-up for odor conditioning by adapting methods that our group previously used for an accurate monitoring of 30-s pharmacologically-induced increases [73] or 20-s behaviourally-induced variations [56] in extracellular levels of amino acids neurotransmitters. We showed that the experimental determination of the dead time is necessary in order to adapt each set-up to the sampling rate required (Figure 4). The final length of the outlet tubing is 120 cm with a dead time of 1 min 30 at 2µL/min as sampling rate and the final sampling resolution is 1 min. The time scale in the figures corresponds to the real time of collection of the fractions. Administration of odor was timed to take into account the outlet dead time of the dialysate system.

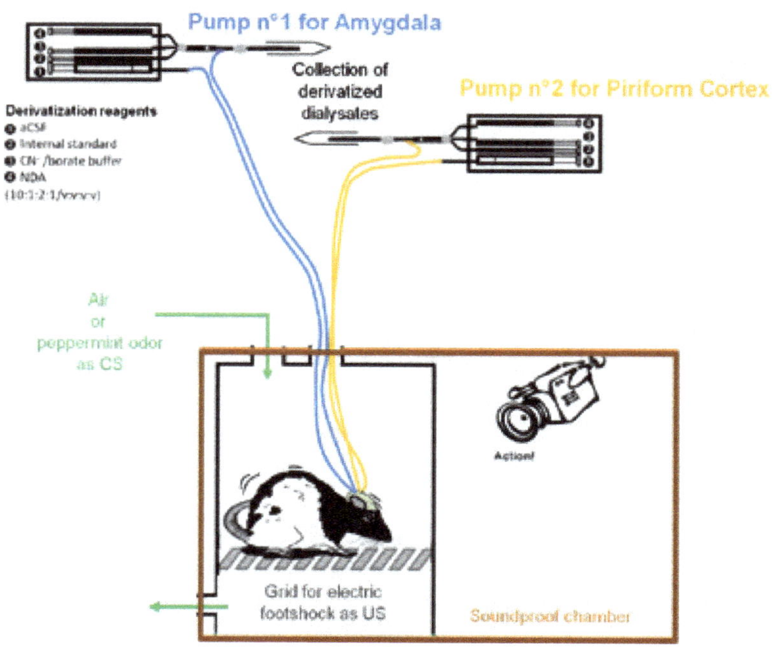

Figure 3. Experimental set-up for both microdialysis sampling and dialysates derivatization during the acquisition of odor fear conditioning. The dual probe-implanted animal is placed in an experimental chamber for odor (conditional stimulus) and shock (unconditional stimulus) deliveries, required in the learning procedure. This chamber is soundproof in order to prevent external noise to interfere with the animal's behaviour. Microdialysis and derivatization are performed simultaneously using one pump per brain area and four syringes delivering artificial cerebrospinal fluid (aCSF) in the inlet of the probe or reagents (NDA as derivatization agent in presence of cyanide ions at pH 8.7 and internal standard for better quantification by capillary electrophoresis with laser-induced fluorescence detection) to tag the neurotransmitters at the outlet of the probe.

Another analytical constraint is to tag the sample in order to detect the amino acids collected during the dialysis experiment. As glutamate and GABA are not fluorescent, we employed a validated home-made on-line system able to deliver the derivatization reagents directly in the collection tube [56], allowing to derivatize the dialysate while dialyzing, without sample loss, noticeable dilution or contamination and without increasing the dead volume of the probe. Thus, the collection tube is not only the micro-reactor of derivatization, but also the injection tube for capillary electrophoresis analysis (Figure 3).

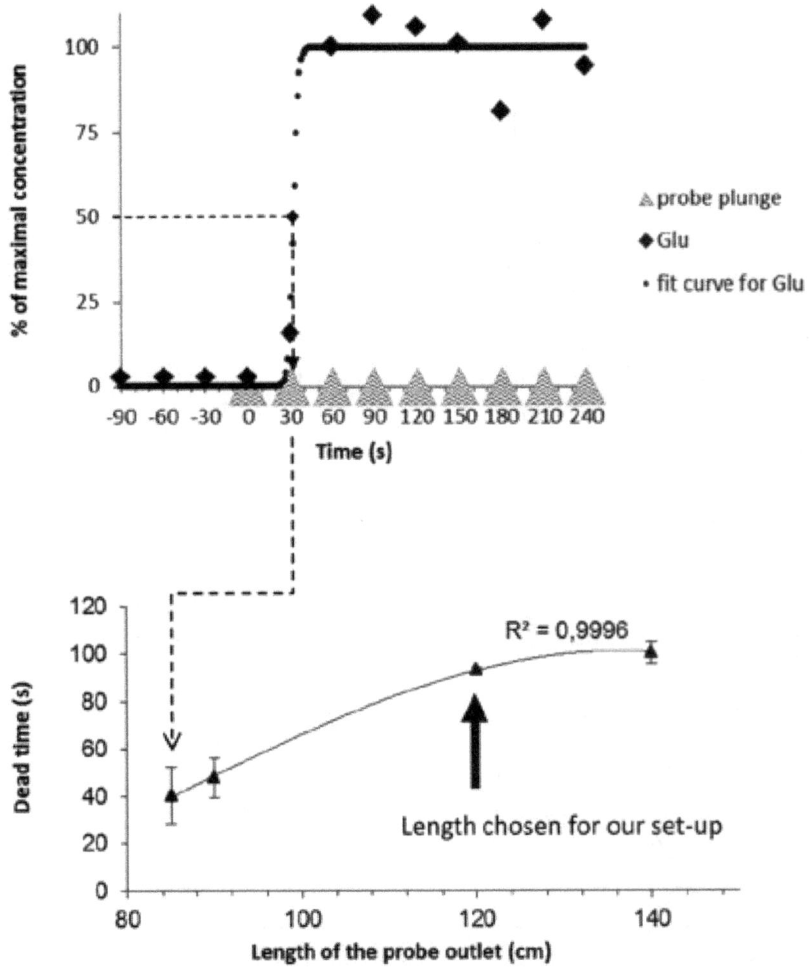

Figure 4. Example of determination of the dead time of an 85-cm outlet home-made probe perfused at 2µL/min by plunging the probe into a known concentration of glutamate at t=0s. The dead time is determined as the time when 50% of the maximal response is reached using a sigmoid curve fitting the 30-s glutamate monitoring (up). By varying the length of the outlet tubing of customized probes (n=3), the dead time of probes can be interpolated and the final length of outlet tubing (here, 120 cm for a dead time of 1 min 30 s) can be chosen according to the height of our experimental set-up and the 1-min sampling rate (bottom). As a consequence, administration of odor was timed to take into account the outlet dead volume of the dialysate system.

Figure 5 presents an example of typical electropherogramm obtained from 1 minute sampling rate of brain microdialysate in freely-moving rat during the acquisition of fear conditioning. Note that the concentrations for GABA and glutamate are similar in PPC or in BLA.

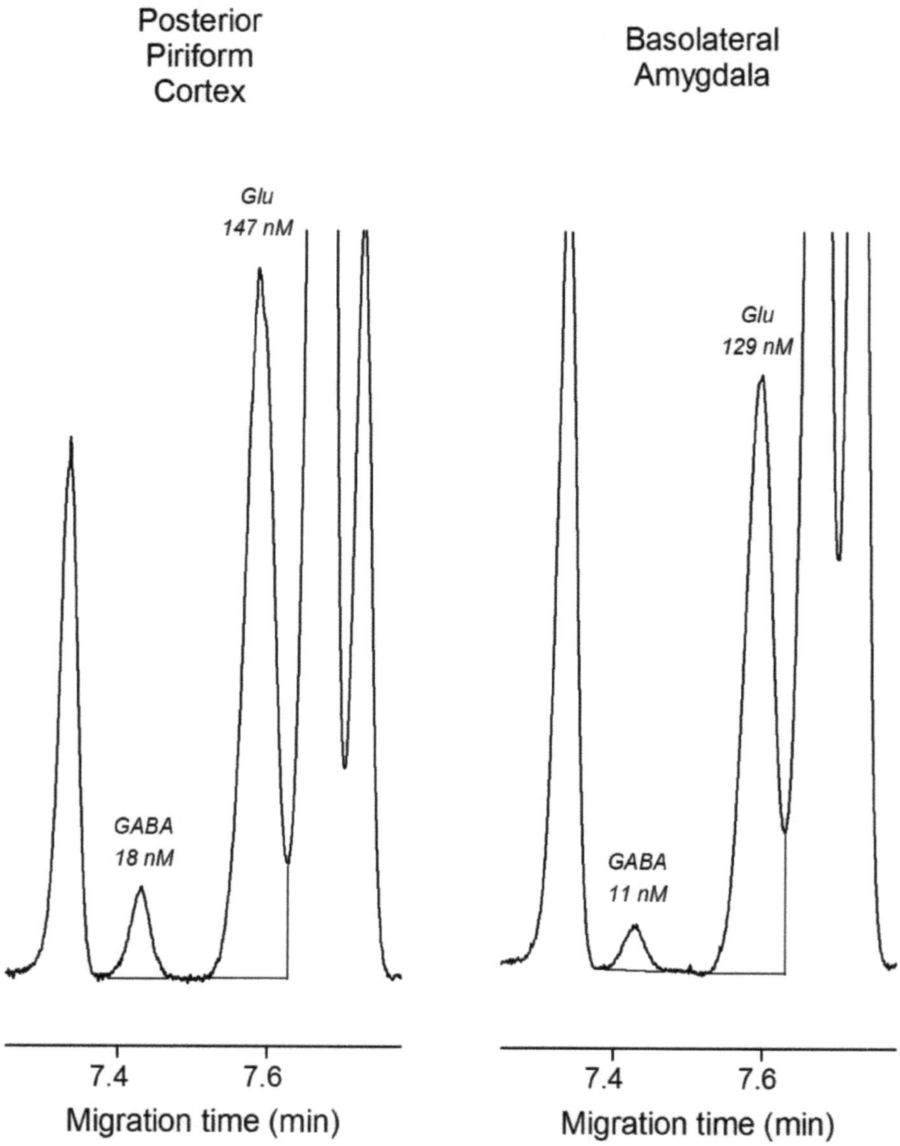

Figure 5. Typical electropherograms from microdialysates obtained in posterior piriform cortex and basolateral amygdala on the same freely-moving Long-Evans rat. Samples were collected every minute at 2μL/min and derivatized online as described in Figure 3 of this chapter. Adapted from [110].

3. Neurochemistry of odor fear conditioning

3.1. Interactions between amygdala and piriform cortex in odor fear conditioning

The odor fear conditioning paradigm consisted of six 20-s odor/ 2-s shock associations presented with an interval of 4 minutes between each pairing. In the amygdala, the first odor-shock association is accompanied by a significant but transient +40%-increase of glutamate release. During the next trials, the concentrations returned to the baseline levels or slightly below. In contrast, in piriform cortex, each odor-shock association is followed by a transient +25%-increase in glutamate release. The comparison of the pattern of release observed in the two structures has also shown that the increase in the amygdala during the first association occurred 1-2 min before the first response in the piriform cortex (Figure 6).

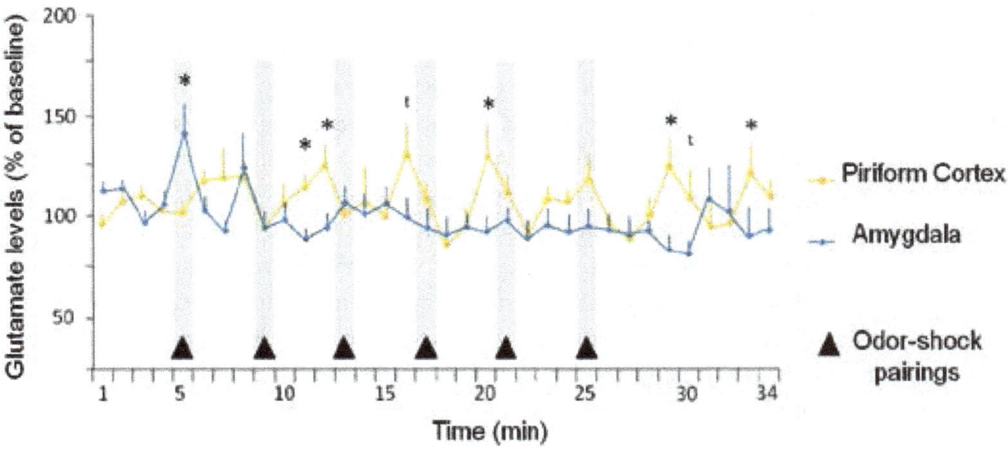

Figure 6. Comparison of glutamate concentration fluctuations in the amygdala and the piriform cortex during odor fear acquisition session. Glutamate concentrations were measured throughout the session and expressed as a percentage of baseline calculated as the mean of concentration for the four points preceding the first pairing. Black arrowheads above the x-axis symbolize trial occurrence. Light gray vertical bars indicate the timing of the 4-min intertrial intervals. (*) Significant difference between the two structures ($p < 0.05$); (#) tendency toward significant difference ($p < 0.09$). Adapted from [66].

The profile of GABA variations during odor fear conditioning was similar in duration and amplitude to that obtained for glutamate presented in Figure 6, i.e. with an enhancement of GABA levels in the amygdala during the first pairing and increases of GABA concentrations in piriform cortex 1-2 min after each pairing. As glutamate and GABA fluctuations were not overall significantly different throughout the experiment, it can be suggested that GABA increases could be induced by glutamate increases, as shown by [74, 75] in the prefrontal cortex.

The high temporal resolution microdialysis allowed us to highlight a differential dynamics of neurotransmitters release in the piriform cortex and amygdala during odor fear acquisition. Taken together, these results suggest that there is a temporal sequence of neurochemical events in the amygdala and piriform cortex, a very precise dynamics of neurotransmitters during the early stages of the acquisition session, which could be involved in the initiation of plastic changes supporting the formation of the memory.

3.2. Functional significance of neurochemical data

Glutamate collected from the BLA and PPC may have originated from both extrinsic and intrinsic sources. Indeed, the BLA receives afferences from primary olfactory cortex [76-78] and from other associative areas [19, 79], providing an extrinsic source of glutamate. Similarly, PPC receives a strong glutamatergic input from the olfactory bulb as well as inputs from the BLA, prefrontal cortex, and hippocampus [80-82]. In addition, both the BLA and PPC contain glutamatergic pyramidal cells that send axon collaterals to neighboring cells, thus providing an intrinsic source of glutamate [79, 83, 84]. Concerning GABA origin, in both BLA and PPC, GABA is released by local inhibitory interneurons [79, 85].

While *in vivo* microdialysis is a useful method for monitoring the neurotransmitters present in the brain extracellular fluid [86], many studies have questioned to what extent dialysate glutamate concentration reflects the amount of glutamate released by the presynaptic neuron. Indeed, due to the ubiquitous localization of its metabolism enzymes and transporters in all brain cells and its paramount role in protein synthesis and general metabolism, numerous works attempted to determine the origin of extracellular glutamate. If the proportion of extracellular glutamate taken up by astrocytes is about 80–90% of the whole glutamate pool [87], the part of the neuronal glutamate, i.e. released for the only neurotransmission purpose, is still matter of debate, because glutamate may come from many sources of effluxes as neuronal "classical" release [88], exchange via cysteine/glutamate transporters [89-92], inversion of transporters [93] and glial release via exocytosis or non-exocytosis [94-96]. Former methodological strategies used for monoamine neurotransmitters to impair the vesicular neuronal release by lowering or removing calcium in aCSF or by blocking nerve impulse Na^+-dependent channels with tetrodotoxine (TTX) gave contradictory answers: some studies reported decreases in basal level of glutamate in dialysate, which is in favour of the neuronal origin of basal extracellular glutamate. In contrast, other studies described no change or even increases under such experimental conditions [97]. Consequently, it was suggested that most part of neurotransmitter glutamate released into synaptic cleft in basal conditions may be taken up into surrounding glia and diffuses poorly to the dialysis probe. The same question can be asked for extracellular GABA because its metabolism is tightly linked to glutamate. As for glutamate, unsuccessful conclusions were also reported regarding the origin of dialysate GABA in basal conditions [97]. However, increasing the microdialysis sampling rate had been proposed in order to observe the rapid variations in glutamate extracellular level which are expected to occur in neurophysiological events [73, 98]. Recent studies using high sampling rate microdialysis showed that NMDA application [99] or electrical stimulation of the prefrontal cortex [100] increases dialysate glutamate concentrations in brain regions receiving projections from this area and that the increase is suppressed or partly altered by TTX [99, 100]. These studies strongly suggest that the transient increase in dialysate glutamate detected under these conditions really represents evoked neurotransmitter glutamate release [101].

Extracellular (or dialysate) concentrations of glutamate and GABA may not always provide a reliable index of their synaptic exocytotic release. Indeed, a strict compartment between intra-synaptic and extra-synaptic was evidenced with poor spill-over from synaptic compartment to extra-synaptic part [102, 103], mainly due to a strong glial uptake. So that, the changes in extracellular concentrations of glutamate and GABA under specific pharmacological and behavioural stimuli should not be only interpreted as a consequence of the activation of specific neurochemical circuits, but as an expression of the activity of the neuron-astrocyte unit in specific circuits of the brain. Several authors proposed that dialysate changes in glutamate and GABA could be used as an index of volume transmission mediated actions of these two neurotransmitters. This hypothesis is based firstly on the assumption that the activity of neurons is functionally linked to the activity of astrocytes, which can release glutamate and GABA to the extracellular space [94, 104]; secondly, on the existence of extrasynaptic glutamate and GABA receptors with functional properties different from those of receptors located in the synapse [105, 106]; and thirdly, on the experimental evidence reporting specific electrophysiological and neurochemical effects of glutamate and GABA when their levels are increased in the extracellular space [107]. Thus, glutamate and GABA, once released into the extracellular compartment, can diffuse and have long-lasting effects modulating glutamatergic and/or GABAergic neuron-astrocytic networks and interact with neurons containing other neurotransmitters and located in the same areas of the brain. In conclusion, monitoring of glutamate and GABA concentrations in the extracellular space using microdialysis may provide an indirect index of amino acids synaptic neurotransmission while giving direct indications of amino acids volume neurotransmission [101].

A few studies have specifically measured extracellular glutamate or GABA in brain structures involved in fear conditioning, investigating the neurotransmitters changes in amygdala during auditory fear learning. More precisely, these microdialysis studies have described a long-lasting decrease in GABA during expression of conditioned fear [39] and a small increase in glutamate during auditory fear conditioning [40]. However, these studies suffer from poor (10–20 min) temporal resolution associated with traditional microdialysis. Only one study has used high temporal resolution microdialysis to measured glutamate and GABA into the amygdala during the acquisition of auditory fear conditioning [108] and suggests that the co-variations of glutamate and GABA may be explained as a glutamate-induced increase in GABA. This study also showed an increase in neurotransmitters levels in the amygdala only for the first association after which the concentration returned to baseline levels. This last result is in agreement with our microdialysis data for the amygdala in odor fear conditioning. Unfortunately, microdialysis was not performed in the auditory cortex, thus precluding any comparison with our own data on the piriform cortex. Nevertheless, there are some electrophysiological data which show that the amygdala is activated before the auditory cortex in auditory fear learning [9, 11]. These data are in accordance with our findings and confirm the differential activation of the amygdala and sensory cortices within the acquisition session of fear conditioning.

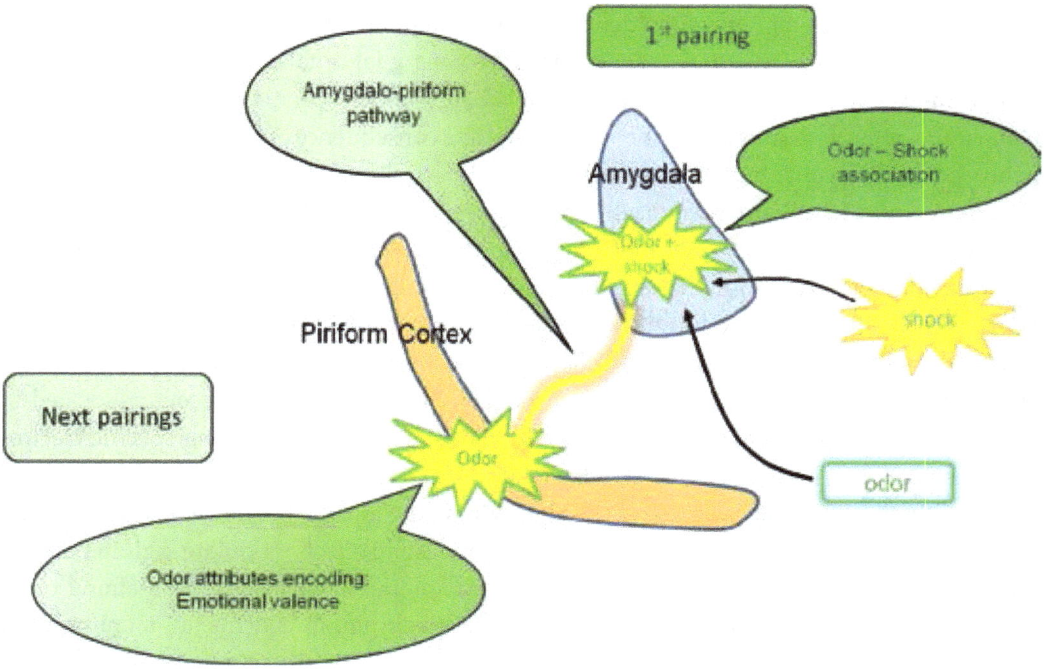

Figure 7. Functional hypotheses on the interactions between the amygdala and the piriform cortex during the acquisition of odor fear learning. An early transient response in the amygdala may allow fast signaling following the first CS-US pairing. Projections from the amygdala to the piriform cortex may provide a pathway through which the amygdala can modulate cortical processing of olfactory information and initiate the storage of the various attributes of the learned odor. The piriform cortex might store certain aspects of the conditioning experience, including the learned hedonic value of the CS odor.

Our microdialysis data led us to formulate the following working hypothesis (Figure 7). During the first pairing, the amygdala glutamatergic transmission would allow the formation of the memory of the CS-US association as it is the case for auditory fear conditioning. The new idea brought by our data is that this could be initiated by a single trial, since no further increase in glutamate was detected in the amygdala for the next pairings. In parallel, the amygdala would trigger the first glutamate increase detected in the olfactory cortex. This would be achieved through the involvement of a direct projection pathway between the amygdala and the piriform cortex [82]. After that, the piriform cortex would progressively build the memory of the different attributes of the learned odor across the next trials.

What are the strengths of our data? This work was aimed at studying the neurochemical interaction between the amygdala and the piriform cortex in odor fear conditioning. We described a differential activation dynamics between the amygdala and the olfactory cortex within the acquisition session. This dynamic reveals an early and transient involvement of the amygdala, restricted to the first odor-shock association followed by the activation of the olfactory cortex during the next associations, which persists until the end of the acquisition session. Until now, most studies questioning the role of the amygdala and sensory areas in fear conditioning have used local lesions or inactivation before or after the acquisition session. Our technical approach is one of the very few allowing online monitoring of neurochemical events occurring in parallel in the amygdala and olfactory cortex, using a temporal resolution compatible with the observation of very transient changes.

4. Conclusion and perspectives

The recent development of high sampling rate microdialysis coupled with high-performance separative microtechniques able to handle sub-microliter sample allows monitoring rapid changes in extracellular levels of amino acid neurotransmitters. Such a platform allows in vivo investigating neurotransmission in freely-moving animals learning fear as in odor fear conditioning. Using two microdialysis probes, we were able to study the neurochemical interactions between two major brain areas involved in the acquisition and consolidation of odor fear conditioning: the amygdala which role is crucial for the formation of fear memory and the piriform cortex which could encode other aspects of the aversive event. Our data suggest that projections from the amygdala to the piriform cortex might provide a pathway via which the amygdala could modulate the cortical processing of olfactory information and initiate the progressive storage of the different attributes of the learned odor in long-term memory.

Author details

Chloé Hegoburu[1,2,4], Luc Denoroy[3,4], Anne-Marie Mouly[2,4] and Sandrine Parrot[4,5]

*Address all correspondence to: sandrine.parrot@univ-lyon1.fr

1 Present address: Center for Psychiatric Neuroscience, Prilly, University of Lausanne, Lausanne, Switzerland

2 CNRS, UMR 5292, Lyon Neuroscience Research Center, Olfaction: From Coding to Memory Team, Lyon, France

3 University Lyon, Lyon Neuroscience Research Center, BioRaN team, Lyon, France

4 University Lyon , Lyon, France

5 INSERM, U1028, Lyon Neuroscience Research Center, NeuroDialyTics, Lyon, France

References

[1] Bevins RA, Ayres JJB. One-trial context fear conditioning as a function of the interstimulus interval. Animal Learning & Behavior. 1995;23 (4):400-10.

[2] Davis M, Shi C. The amygdala. Current biology : CB. 2000;10(4):R131.

[3] Blanchard RJ, Blanchard DC. Crouching as an index of fear. J Comp Physiol Psychol. 1969;67(3):370-5.

[4] Blanchard DC, Blanchard RJ. Innate and conditioned reactions to threat in rats with amygdaloid lesions. J Comp Physiol Psychol. 1972;81(2):281-90. Epub 1972/11/01.

[5] LeDoux JE. Emotion circuits in the brain. Annu Rev Neurosci. 2000;23:155-84. Epub 2000/06/09.

[6] Maren S. Neurobiology of Pavlovian fear conditioning. Annu Rev Neurosci. 2001;24:897-931. Epub 2001/08/25.

[7] Maren S, Quirk GJ. Neuronal signalling of fear memory. Nat Rev Neurosci. 2004;5(11):844-52. Epub 2004/10/22.

[8] Myers KM, Davis M. Mechanisms of fear extinction. Molecular psychiatry. 2007;12(2):120-50. Epub 2006/12/13.

[9] Edeline JM, Pham P, Weinberger NM. Rapid development of learning-induced receptive field plasticity in the auditory cortex. Behav Neurosci. 1993;107(4):539-51. Epub 1993/08/01.

[10] McClelland JL, McNaughton BL, O'Reilly RC. Why there are complementary learning systems in the hippocampus and neocortex: insights from the successes and failures of connectionist models of learning and memory. Psychol Rev. 1995;102(3): 419-57. Epub 1995/07/01.

[11] Quirk GJ, Armony JL, LeDoux JE. Fear conditioning enhances different temporal components of tone-evoked spike trains in auditory cortex and lateral amygdala. Neuron. 1997;19(3):613-24. Epub 1997/10/23.

[12] Armony JL, Quirk GJ, LeDoux JE. Differential effects of amygdala lesions on early and late plastic components of auditory cortex spike trains during fear conditioning. J Neurosci. 1998;18(7):2592-601. Epub 1998/04/16.

[13] Weinberger NM. Specific long-term memory traces in primary auditory cortex. Nat Rev Neurosci. 2004;5(4):279-90. Epub 2004/03/23.

[14] Maren S. Building and burying fear memories in the brain. Neuroscientist. 2005;11(1):89-99. Epub 2005/01/06.

[15] Sacco T, Sacchetti B. Role of secondary sensory cortices in emotional memory storage and retrieval in rats. Science. 2010;329(5992):649-56. Epub 2010/08/07.

[16] Chu S, Downes JJ. Odour-evoked autobiographical memories: psychological investigations of proustian phenomena. Chem Senses. 2000;25(1):111-6. Epub 2000/02/11.

[17] Price JL. An autoradiographic study of complementary laminar patterns of termination of afferent fibers to the olfactory cortex. J Comp Neurol. 1973;150(1):87-108. Epub 1973/07/01.

[18] Savander V, LeDoux JE, Pitkanen A. Topographic projections from the periamygdaloid cortex to select subregions of the lateral nucleus of the amygdala in the rat. Neurosci Lett. 1996;211(3):167-70. Epub 1996/06/28.

[19] McDonald AJ. Cortical pathways to the mammalian amygdala. Prog Neurobiol. 1998;55(3):257-332. Epub 1998/06/27.

[20] Cousens G, Otto T. Both pre- and posttraining excitotoxic lesions of the basolateral amygdala abolish the expression of olfactory and contextual fear conditioning. Behav Neurosci. 1998;112(5):1092-103.

[21] Rosenkranz JA, Grace AA. Dopamine-mediated modulation of odour-evoked amygdala potentials during pavlovian conditioning. Nature. 2002;417(6886):282-7.

[22] Kilpatrick L, Cahill L. Modulation of memory consolidation for olfactory learning by reversible inactivation of the basolateral amygdala. Behav Neurosci. 2003;117(1): 184-8.

[23] Sevelinges Y, Gervais R, Messaoudi B, Granjon L, Mouly AM. Olfactory fear conditioning induces field potential potentiation in rat olfactory cortex and amygdala. Learn Mem. 2004;11(6):761-9. Epub 2004/11/13.

[24] Sevelinges Y, Moriceau S, Holman P, Miner C, Muzny K, Gervais R, et al. Enduring effects of infant memories: infant odor-shock conditioning attenuates amygdala activity and adult fear conditioning. Biol Psychiatry. 2007;62(10):1070-9. Epub 2007/09/11.

[25] Walker DL, Paschall GY, Davis M. Glutamate receptor antagonist infusions into the basolateral and medial amygdala reveal differential contributions to olfactory vs. context fear conditioning and expression. Learn Mem. 2005;12(2):120-9.

[26] Jones SV, Stanek-Rattiner L, Davis M, Ressler KJ. Differential regional expression of brain-derived neurotrophic factor following olfactory fear learning. Learn Mem. 2007;14(12):816-20.

[27] Sevelinges Y, Sullivan RM, Messaoudi B, Mouly AM. Neonatal odor-shock conditioning alters the neural network involved in odor fear learning at adulthood. Learn Mem. 2008;15(9):649-56. Epub 2008/09/06.

[28] Fanselow MS, Kim JJ. Acquisition of contextual Pavlovian fear conditioning is blocked by application of an NMDA receptor antagonist D,L-2-amino-5-phosphono-

valeric acid to the basolateral amygdala. Behav Neurosci. 1994;108(1):210-2. Epub 1994/02/01.

[29] Maren S, Aharonov G, Fanselow MS. Retrograde abolition of conditional fear after excitotoxic lesions in the basolateral amygdala of rats: absence of a temporal gradient. Behav Neurosci. 1996;110(4):718-26.

[30] Miserendino MJ, Sananes CB, Melia KR, Davis M. Blocking of acquisition but not expression of conditioned fear-potentiated startle by NMDA antagonists in the amygdala. Nature. 1990;345(6277):716-8. Epub 1990/06/21.

[31] Campeau S, Miserendino MJ, Davis M. Intra-amygdala infusion of the N-methyl-D-aspartate receptor antagonist AP5 blocks acquisition but not expression of fear-potentiated startle to an auditory conditioned stimulus. Behav Neurosci. 1992;106(3): 569-74. Epub 1992/06/01.

[32] Gewirtz JC, Davis M. Second-order fear conditioning prevented by blocking NMDA receptors in amygdala. Nature. 1997;388(6641):471-4. Epub 1997/07/31.

[33] Kim JJ, Lee HJ, Han JS, Packard MG. Amygdala is critical for stress-induced modulation of hippocampal long-term potentiation and learning. J Neurosci. 2001;21(14): 5222-8.

[34] Walker DL, Davis M. The role of amygdala glutamate receptors in fear learning, fear-potentiated startle, and extinction. Pharmacol Biochem Behav. 2002;71(3):379-92. Epub 2002/02/07.

[35] Goosens KA, Maren S. NMDA receptors are essential for the acquisition, but not expression, of conditional fear and associative spike firing in the lateral amygdala. Eur J Neurosci. 2004;20(2):537-48. Epub 2004/07/06.

[36] Muller J, Corodimas KP, Fridel Z, LeDoux JE. Functional inactivation of the lateral and basal nuclei of the amygdala by muscimol infusion prevents fear conditioning to an explicit conditioned stimulus and to contextual stimuli. Behav Neurosci. 1997;111(4):683-91. Epub 1997/08/01.

[37] Wilensky AE, Schafe GE, LeDoux JE. Functional inactivation of the amygdala before but not after auditory fear conditioning prevents memory formation. J Neurosci. 1999;19(24):RC48. Epub 1999/12/14.

[38] Ehrlich I, Humeau Y, Grenier F, Ciocchi S, Herry C, Luthi A. Amygdala inhibitory circuits and the control of fear memory. Neuron. 2009;62(6):757-71. Epub 2009/06/27.

[39] Stork O, Ji FY, Obata K. Reduction of extracellular GABA in the mouse amygdala during and following confrontation with a conditioned fear stimulus. Neurosci Lett. 2002;327(2):138-42. Epub 2002/07/06.

[40] Yokoyama M, Suzuki E, Sato T, Maruta S, Watanabe S, Miyaoka H. Amygdalic levels of dopamine and serotonin rise upon exposure to conditioned fear stress without elevation of glutamate. Neurosci Lett. 2005;379(1):37-41.

[41] Young AM. Increased extracellular dopamine in nucleus accumbens in response to unconditioned and conditioned aversive stimuli: studies using 1 min microdialysis in rats. J Neurosci Methods. 2004;138(1-2):57-63. Epub 2004/08/25.

[42] Ungerstedt U. Microdialysis--principles and applications for studies in animals and man. J Intern Med. 1991;230(4):365-73. Epub 1991/10/01.

[43] Benveniste H, Huttemeier PC. Microdialysis--theory and application. Prog Neurobiol. 1990;35(3):195-215. Epub 1990/01/01.

[44] Parrot S, Bert L, Mouly-Badina L, Sauvinet V, Colussi-Mas J, Lambas-Senas L, et al. Microdialysis monitoring of catecholamines and excitatory amino acids in the rat and mouse brain: recent developments based on capillary electrophoresis with laser-induced fluorescence detection--a mini-review. Cell Mol Neurobiol. 2003;23(4-5): 793-804. Epub 2003/09/30.

[45] Zapata A, Chefer VI, Parrot S, Denoroy L. Detection and quantification of neurotransmitters in dialysates. Current protocols in neuroscience / editorial board, Jacqueline N Crawley [et al]. 2013;Chapter 7:Unit7 4. Epub 2013/04/06.

[46] Westerink BH. Brain microdialysis and its application for the study of animal behaviour. Behav Brain Res. 1995;70(2):103-24. Epub 1995/10/01.

[47] Watson CJ, Venton BJ, Kennedy RT. In vivo measurements of neurotransmitters by microdialysis sampling. Anal Chem. 2006;78(5):1391-9. Epub 2006/03/31.

[48] Abercrombie ED, Finlay JM. Monitoring extracellular norepinephrine in brain using in vivo microdialysis and HPLC-EC. In: Robinson TE, Justice JBJ, editors. Microdialysis in Neurosciences. Amsterdam: Elsevier; 1991. p. 253–74.

[49] Smolders I, Sarre S, Michotte Y, Ebinger G. The analysis of excitatory, inhibitory and other amino acids in rat brain microdialysates using microbore liquid chromatography. J Neurosci Methods. 1995;57(1):47-53. Epub 1995/03/01.

[50] Kehr J. Determination of gamma-aminobutyric acid in microdialysis samples by microbore column liquid chromatography and fluorescence detection. J Chromatogr B Biomed Sci Appl. 1998;708(1-2):49-54. Epub 1998/07/08.

[51] Kehr J. Determination of glutamate and aspartate in microdialysis samples by reversed-phase column liquid chromatography with fluorescence and electrochemical detection. J Chromatogr B Biomed Sci Appl. 1998;708(1-2):27-38. Epub 1998/07/08.

[52] Obrenovitch TP, Zilkha E. Microdialysis coupled to online enzymatic assays. Methods. 2001;23(1):63-71. Epub 2001/02/13.

[53] McKenzie JA, Watson CJ, Rostand RD, German I, Witowski SR, Kennedy RT. Automated capillary liquid chromatography for simultaneous determination of neuroactive amines and amino acids. J Chromatogr A. 2002;962(1-2):105-15. Epub 2002/08/30.

[54] Lunte SM, Lunte CE. Microdialysis sampling for pharmacological studies: HPLC and CE analysis. Adv Chromatogr. 1996;36:383-432. Epub 1996/01/01.

[55] Kennedy RT, Watson CJ, Haskins WE, Powell DH, Strecker RE. In vivo neurochemical monitoring by microdialysis and capillary separations. Curr Opin Chem Biol. 2002;6(5):659-65. Epub 2002/11/05.

[56] Parrot S, Sauvinet V, Riban V, Depaulis A, Renaud B, Denoroy L. High temporal resolution for in vivo monitoring of neurotransmitters in awake epileptic rats using brain microdialysis and capillary electrophoresis with laser-induced fluorescence detection. J Neurosci Methods. 2004;140(1-2):29-38. Epub 2004/12/14.

[57] Touret M, Parrot S, Denoroy L, Belin MF, Didier-Bazes M. Glutamatergic alterations in the cortex of genetic absence epilepsy rats. BMC Neurosci. 2007;8:69. Epub 2007/08/30.

[58] Bergquist J, Vona MJ, Stiller CO, O'Connor WT, Falkenberg T, Ekman R. Capillary electrophoresis with laser-induced fluorescence detection: a sensitive method for monitoring extracellular concentrations of amino acids in the periaqueductal grey matter. J Neurosci Methods. 1996;65(1):33-42. Epub 1996/03/01.

[59] Dawson LA, Stow JM, Palmer AM. Improved method for the measurement of glutamate and aspartate using capillary electrophoresis with laser induced fluorescence detection and its application to brain microdialysis. J Chromatogr B Biomed Sci Appl. 1997;694(2):455-60. Epub 1997/07/04.

[60] Lada MW, Vickroy TW, Kennedy RT. High temporal resolution monitoring of glutamate and aspartate in vivo using microdialysis on-line with capillary electrophoresis with laser-induced fluorescence detection. Anal Chem. 1997;69(22):4560-5. Epub 1998/01/07.

[61] Li YM, Qu Y, Vandenbussche E, Arckens L, Vandesande F. Analysis of extracellular gamma-aminobutyric acid, glutamate and aspartate in cat visual cortex by in vivo microdialysis and capillary electrophoresis-laser induced fluorescence detection. J Neurosci Methods. 2001;105(2):211-5. Epub 2001/03/29.

[62] Robert F, Bert L, Parrot S, Denoroy L, Stoppini L, Renaud B. Coupling on-line brain microdialysis, precolumn derivatization and capillary electrophoresis for routine minute sampling of O-phosphoethanolamine and excitatory amino acids. J Chromatogr A. 1998;817(1-2):195-203. Epub 1998/10/09.

[63] Tucci S, Rada P, Sepulveda MJ, Hernandez L. Glutamate measured by 6-s resolution brain microdialysis: capillary electrophoretic and laser-induced fluorescence detec-

tion application. J Chromatogr B Biomed Sci Appl. 1997;694(2):343-9. Epub 1997/07/04.

[64] Zhou SY, Zuo H, Stobaugh JF, Lunte CE, Lunte SM. Continuous in vivo monitoring of amino acid neurotransmitters by microdialysis sampling with on-line derivatization and capillary electrophoresis separation. Anal Chem. 1995;67(3):594-9. Epub 1995/02/01.

[65] Hernandez L, Joshi N, Murzi E, Verdeguer P, Mifsud JC, Guzman N. Colinear laser-induced fluorescence detector for capillary electrophoresis. Analysis of glutamic acid in brain dialysates. J Chromatogr A. 1993;652(2):399-405. Epub 1993/10/22.

[66] Hegoburu C, Sevelinges Y, Thevenet M, Gervais R, Parrot S, Mouly AM. Differential dynamics of amino acid release in the amygdala and olfactory cortex during odor fear acquisition as revealed with simultaneous high temporal resolution microdialysis. Learn Mem. 2009;16(11):687-97. Epub 2009/10/30.

[67] Del Arco A, Segovia G, Prieto L, Mora F. Endogenous glutamate-taurine interaction in striatum and nucleus accumbens of the freely moving rat: studies during the normal process of aging. Mechanisms of ageing and development. 2001;122(4):401-14. Epub 2001/03/10.

[68] Hernandez LF, Segovia G, Mora F. Chronic treatment with a dopamine uptake blocker changes dopamine and acetylcholine but not glutamate and GABA concentrations in prefrontal cortex, striatum and nucleus accumbens of the awake rat. Neurochemistry international. 2008;52(3):457-69. Epub 2007/09/21.

[69] Layton ME, Pazdernik TL. Reactive oxidant species in piriform cortex extracellular fluid during seizures induced by systemic kainic acid in rats. Journal of molecular neuroscience : MN. 1999;13(1-2):63-8. Epub 2000/02/26.

[70] Wang CX, Erecius LF, Beverly JL, 3rd, Gietzen DW. Essential amino acids affect interstitial dopamine metabolites in the anterior piriform cortex of rats. The Journal of nutrition. 1999;129(9):1742-5. Epub 1999/08/25.

[71] Tanaka K, Graham SH, Simon RP. The role of excitatory neurotransmitters in seizure-induced neuronal injury in rats. Brain research. 1996;737(1-2):59-63. Epub 1996/10/21.

[72] Wade JV, Samson FE, Nelson SR, Pazdernik TL. Changes in extracellular amino acids during soman- and kainic acid-induced seizures. Journal of neurochemistry. 1987;49(2):645-50. Epub 1987/08/01.

[73] Bert L, Parrot S, Robert F, Desvignes C, Denoroy L, Suaud-Chagny MF, et al. In vivo temporal sequence of rat striatal glutamate, aspartate and dopamine efflux during apomorphine, nomifensine, NMDA and PDC in situ administration. Neuropharmacology. 2002;43(5):825-35. Epub 2002/10/18.

[74] Del Arco A, Mora F. Effects of endogenous glutamate on extracellular concentrations of GABA, dopamine, and dopamine metabolites in the prefrontal cortex of the freely

moving rat: involvement of NMDA and AMPA/KA receptors. Neurochem Res. 1999;24(8):1027-35.

[75] Del Arco A, Mora F. Endogenous dopamine potentiates the effects of glutamate on extracellular GABA in the prefrontal cortex of the freely moving rat. Brain Res Bull. 2000;53(3):339-45. Epub 2000/12/13.

[76] Haberly LB, Price JL. Association and commissural fiber systems of the olfactory cortex of the rat. II. Systems originating in the olfactory peduncle. J Comp Neurol. 1978;181(4):781-807. Epub 1978/10/15.

[77] Ottersen OP. Connections of the amygdala of the rat. IV: Corticoamygdaloid and intraamygdaloid connections as studied with axonal transport of horseradish peroxidase. J Comp Neurol. 1982;205(1):30-48. Epub 1982/02/10.

[78] Luskin MB, Price JL. The laminar distribution of intracortical fibers originating in the olfactory cortex of the rat. J Comp Neurol. 1983;216(3):292-302. Epub 1983/05/20.

[79] Sah P, Faber ES, Lopez De Armentia M, Power J. The amygdaloid complex: anatomy and physiology. Physiol Rev. 2003;83(3):803-34.

[80] Haberly LB, Price JL. The axonal projection patterns of the mitral and tufted cells of the olfactory bulb in the rat. Brain research. 1977;129(1):152-7. Epub 1977/06/24.

[81] Datiche F, Cattarelli M. Reciprocal and topographic connections between the piriform and prefrontal cortices in the rat: a tracing study using the B subunit of the cholera toxin. Brain Res Bull. 1996;41(6):391-8. Epub 1996/01/01.

[82] Majak K, Ronkko S, Kemppainen S, Pitkanen A. Projections from the amygdaloid complex to the piriform cortex: A PHA-L study in the rat. J Comp Neurol. 2004;476(4):414-28.

[83] Luskin MB, Price JL. The topographic organization of associational fibers of the olfactory system in the rat, including centrifugal fibers to the olfactory bulb. J Comp Neurol. 1983;216(3):264-91. Epub 1983/05/20.

[84] Datiche F, Litaudon P, Cattarelli M. Intrinsic association fiber system of the piriform cortex: a quantitative study based on a cholera toxin B subunit tracing in the rat. J Comp Neurol. 1996;376(2):265-77. Epub 1996/12/09.

[85] Suzuki N, Bekkers JM. Inhibitory interneurons in the piriform cortex. Clin Exp Pharmacol Physiol. 2007;34(10):1064-9. Epub 2007/08/24.

[86] Benveniste H. Brain microdialysis. Journal of neurochemistry. 1989;52(6):1667-79. Epub 1989/06/01.

[87] Kanamori K, Ross BD, Kondrat RW. Glial uptake of neurotransmitter glutamate from the extracellular fluid studied in vivo by microdialysis and (13)C NMR. Journal of neurochemistry. 2002;83(3):682-95. Epub 2002/10/23.

[88] Fonnum F. Glutamate: a neurotransmitter in mammalian brain. Journal of neurochemistry. 1984;42(1):1-11. Epub 1984/01/01.

[89] Melendez RI, Vuthiganon J, Kalivas PW. Regulation of extracellular glutamate in the prefrontal cortex: focus on the cystine glutamate exchanger and group I metabotropic glutamate receptors. J Pharmacol Exp Ther. 2005;314(1):139-47. Epub 2005/03/17.

[90] Xi ZX, Shen H, Baker DA, Kalivas PW. Inhibition of non-vesicular glutamate release by group III metabotropic glutamate receptors in the nucleus accumbens. Journal of neurochemistry. 2003;87(5):1204-12. Epub 2003/11/19.

[91] Baker DA, Xi ZX, Shen H, Swanson CJ, Kalivas PW. The origin and neuronal function of in vivo nonsynaptic glutamate. J Neurosci. 2002;22(20):9134-41. Epub 2002/10/22.

[92] Xi ZX, Ramamoorthy S, Baker DA, Shen H, Samuvel DJ, Kalivas PW. Modulation of group II metabotropic glutamate receptor signaling by chronic cocaine. J Pharmacol Exp Ther. 2002;303(2):608-15. Epub 2002/10/22.

[93] Nicholls D, Attwell D. The release and uptake of excitatory amino acids. Trends Pharmacol Sci. 1990;11(11):462-8. Epub 1990/11/01.

[94] Araque A, Li N, Doyle RT, Haydon PG. SNARE protein-dependent glutamate release from astrocytes. J Neurosci. 2000;20(2):666-73. Epub 2000/01/13.

[95] Bezzi P, Gundersen V, Galbete JL, Seifert G, Steinhauser C, Pilati E, et al. Astrocytes contain a vesicular compartment that is competent for regulated exocytosis of glutamate. Nat Neurosci. 2004;7(6):613-20. Epub 2004/05/25.

[96] Malarkey EB, Parpura V. Mechanisms of glutamate release from astrocytes. Neurochemistry international. 2008;52(1-2):142-54. Epub 2007/08/03.

[97] Timmerman W, Westerink BH. Brain microdialysis of GABA and glutamate: what does it signify? Synapse. 1997;27(3):242-61. Epub 1997/11/05.

[98] Drew KL, Pehek EA, Rasley BT, Ma YL, Green TK. Sampling glutamate and GABA with microdialysis: suggestions on how to get the dialysis membrane closer to the synapse. J Neurosci Methods. 2004;140(1-2):127-31. Epub 2004/12/14.

[99] Parrot S, Bert L, Renaud B, Denoroy L. Glutamate and aspartate do not exhibit the same changes in their extracellular concentrations in the rat striatum after N-methyl-D-aspartate local administration. J Neurosci Res. 2003;71(3):445-54. Epub 2003/01/15.

[100] Lada MW, Vickroy TW, Kennedy RT. Evidence for neuronal origin and metabotropic receptor-mediated regulation of extracellular glutamate and aspartate in rat striatum in vivo following electrical stimulation of the prefrontal cortex. Journal of neurochemistry. 1998;70(2):617-25. Epub 1998/02/07.

[101] Parrot S, Renaud B, Zimmer L, Denoroy L. Monitoring Neurotransmitter Amino Acids by Microdialysis: Pharmacodynamic Applications. In: Tsai T-H, editor. Appli-

cations of Microdialysis in Pharmaceutical Science: John Wiley & Sons, Inc.; 2011. p. 151-206.

[102] Obrenovitch TP, Urenjak J, Zilkha E, Jay TM. Excitotoxicity in neurological disorders--the glutamate paradox. Int J Dev Neurosci. 2000;18(2-3):281-7. Epub 2000/03/15.

[103] Rusakov DA, Kullmann DM. Extrasynaptic glutamate diffusion in the hippocampus: ultrastructural constraints, uptake, and receptor activation. J Neurosci. 1998;18(9): 3158-70. Epub 1998/05/09.

[104] Schousboe A, Waagepetersen HS. Glial modulation of GABAergic and glutamat ergic neurotransmission. Curr Top Med Chem. 2006;6(10):929-34. Epub 2006/06/22.

[105] Sierra-Paredes G, Sierra-Marcuno G. Extrasynaptic GABA and glutamate receptors in epilepsy. CNS Neurol Disord Drug Targets. 2007;6(4):288-300. Epub 2007/08/19.

[106] Galvan A, Kuwajima M, Smith Y. Glutamate and GABA receptors and transporters in the basal ganglia: what does their subsynaptic localization reveal about their function? Neuroscience. 2006;143(2):351-75. Epub 2006/10/25.

[107] Del Arco A, Segovia G, Fuxe K, Mora F. Changes in dialysate concentrations of glutamate and GABA in the brain: an index of volume transmission mediated actions? Journal of neurochemistry. 2003;85(1):23-33. Epub 2003/03/19.

[108] Venton BJ, Robinson TE, Kennedy RT, Maren S. Dynamic amino acid increases in the basolateral amygdala during acquisition and expression of conditioned fear. Eur J Neurosci. 2006;23(12):3391-8. Epub 2006/07/06.

[109] Denoroy L, Bert L, Parrot S, Robert F, Renaud B. Assessment of pharmacodynamic and pharmacokinetic characteristics of drugs using microdialysis sampling and capillary electrophoresis. Electrophoresis. 1998;19(16-17):2841-7. Epub 1998/12/31.

[110] Denoroy L, Renaud B, Parrot S. Capillary Electrophoresis Analysis in Neuroscience. In: He Z, editor. Capillary Electrophoresis: Fundamentals, Techniques and Applications: NOVA Science Publishers; 2012. p. 211-51.

5

TRP Channels in Neuronal and Glial Signal Transduction

Christian Harteneck and Kristina Leuner

1. Introduction

Many physiological processes like muscle contraction, hormone secretion and intracellular signalling processes are triggered by calcium as intracellular signalling molecule. The signal transduction capacity of calcium depends on the 10,000-fold gradient across the plasma membrane with 2.5 mM extracellular and resting intracellular calcium ion concentration of approximately 100 nM. Low intracellular calcium concentrations are managed by the extrusion of calcium by ATPases and transporters [1, 2], whereas rapid and distinct increases in intracellular calcium up to micromolar concentrations are mediated by calcium-permeable ion channels of the plasma membrane as well intracellular calcium storage compartments. Calcium mediates its biological functions by protein structures capable to bind calcium. These calcium-binding domains are building blocks of the proteins modulated by calcium directly or part of calcium sensor proteins (calmodulin, calcium binding protein, calcineurin, S100, NCS etc) mediating calcium-dependent modulation by protein-protein interaction [3].

In excitable cells like neurons, heart or skeletal or smooth muscle cells, calcium currents first identified are mediated by voltage-gated calcium channels [4-6]. Later, additional calcium-permeable ion channels have been identified mediating hormone-induced calcium entry also in non-excitable cells like endothelial, epithelial, immune cells. The identity of these channels has been unravelled via analysis of phototransduction in flies [7]. Montell and Rubin cloned Transient Receptor Potential (TRP) from *Drosophila melanogaster* and described TRP as a phospholipase C-modulated, calcium-permeable ion channel [8]. Mammalian TRP-homologous channels have been identified by comparing the *Drosophila* TRP sequences with sequences resulting from the upcoming genome and expression profiling projects at that time. The first channel protein showing the highest degree of sequence similarities with *Drosophila* TRP were named classic TRP family (TRPC1) [9-11]. Additional TRP-homologous proteins establishing the melastatin-like and vanilloid-like TRP subfamilies, TRPM and TRPV, respectively, were identified by other approaches [12-14]. An additional fascinating feature of TRP channels became obvious with the identification of TRPV1 (vanilloid receptor 1, VR1) as molecular target of capsaicin [15]. Capsaicin is the active molecule of chilli peppers and an irritant that is responsible for providing a sensation of burning, e.g., on the tongue. TRPV1 characterization revealed that TRP channels are targets of many secondary plant compounds and are involved in sensory functions [16]. Last but not least, the TRP superfamily comprises the mucolipin [TRPML [17]] and the polycystin [TRPP [18]] calcium-permeable channel proteins sharing a comparable transmembrane topology and features like ion permeability [13, 14, 19]. TRP channels are integrated in many cellular signal transduction pathways and a variety of physiological processes as discussed below.

TRP channels have been identified and characterized by common biochemical, immunochemical and physiological methods. The function of TRP channels can be directly studied by patch clamp electrophysiology as well as imaging techniques. Patch clamp techniques enable to monitor currents across the plasma membrane mediated by TRP channels using small electrodes in small pipettes together with the ground electrode in the bath solution [20]. In this configuration, the electrical activity of ion channels in the plasma membrane can be monitored. Depending on configuration and access of the electrode within the patch pipette, different configurations can be discriminated (cell-attached, whole cell, inside-out or outside-out). On the other hand, a growing number of methods has been developed to monitor changes in ion concentrations in intact cells using small chemical compounds or artificial proteins constructs [21]. Fura-2 is one of the best known calcium dyes, a small chemical compound changing its fluorescence features depending on calcium concentration [22]. In the meantime a variety of new compounds have been developed characterized by changed ion selectivity, changes in Kd values or fluorescence intensities. The intracellular concentration of the indicator dyes depend on the activity and capability of organic solute carrier to export the dyes and thereby lowering intracellular dye concentrations. This disadvantage can be overcome by the use of the new protein-based probes. These artificial proteins are constructs of ion binding domains conjugated with fluorescence protein domains transcribed transiently from transfected plasmids or permanently from genomic localized expression cassettes [23, 24].

The following review will give an introduction in the broad field of TRP channel research related to their expression in the central nervous system (CNS), their physiological function in neurons as well as in glia cells, and their role in neurological and psychiatric CNS disorders. The involvement of TRP channels in the pathophysiology of glioma and the sensing of pain is not discussed here [for comprehensive reviews please refer to [25, 26]].

2. TRP channels in the brain

2.1. TRPC channels

The classic TRP channel family comprises seven different genes with proteins showing the highest sequence similarity to the prototypic *Drosophila* TRP [8, 12, 19]. The mammalian channel proteins are involved in receptor-regulated calcium entry [27]. Receptor activation by hormones, neurotransmitter and in *Drosophila* light results in the phospholipase C-mediated breakdown of phosphatidylinositides leading to the formation of inositol 1,4,5-trisphosphate and diacylglycerol (Figure 1). Inositol 1,4,5-trisphosphate induces calcium release from intracellular stores via the activation of inositol 1,4,5-trisphosphate receptors (IP3 receptor), whereas diacylglycerol directly activates mammalian classic transient receptor potential (TRPC) channels (TRPC2, TRPC3, TRPC6 and TRPC7) in a protein kinase C-independent manner [27, 28]. The prerequisite of phospholipase C stimulation has been shown for TRPC1, TRPC4 and TRPC5 currents, however the molecular mechanism is still unclear [27].

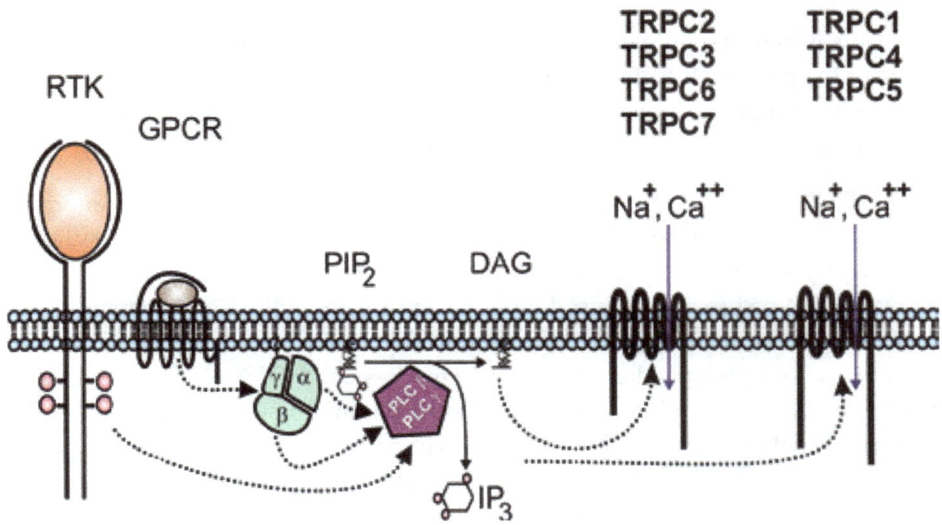

Figure 1. Receptor-induced activation mechanisms of TRP channels in mammals. RTK: receptor tyrosine kinase; GPCR: G protein-coupled receptor; PLC: phospholipase C; PIP2: phosphatidylinositol-4,5-bisphosphate; IP3: inositol-1,4,5-trisphosphate; DAG: diacylglycerol.

In the brain, TRPC1 expression was confirmed using a set of techniques ranging from RT-PCR, western blotting to confocal and electron microscopy. TRPC1 was detected in different brain regions of adult mice including the cerebellum, the hippocampus, the basal ganglia, the amygdala and the forebrain [29-31]. Strübing et al. showed that TRPC1 and TRPC5 channels are expressed in similar brain areas suggesting that they might form heteromers for example in the hippocampus [31]. However, empirical evidence for the existence of these heteromers is still lacking [32]. Only little is known about the distribution of TRPC channels in neurons. TRPC5 channels were suggested to be expressed mainly in distal dendrites and dendritic spines in lateral septal neurons. However, the expression pattern might differ in different brain areas and neurons [33]. Interestingly, TRPC1 protein was not only detected in neurons such as in the hippocampal CA1 or CA3 pyramidal cells [31], but also in astrocytes and oligodendrocyte progenitor cells [34-36]. Furthermore, mRNA for all TRPC channels including TRPC1 was found in the cortex of the mouse developing brain [37]. TRPC1, together with TRPC3 and TRPC5 were the main isoforms detected in this study. This expression pattern might be time dependent and species specific because TRPC4 and TRPC5 were the most prominent isoforms in the adult rat prefrontal cortex [38], whereas TRPC3 and TRPC6 channels are major TRPC mRNAs detected in adult mice [29]. TRPC2 being expressed in the rodent vomeronasal organ is clearly an exception [39]. In humans, TRPC2 is a pseudogene; the transcribed mRNA is functionless due to various stop codons [40]. In rodents, the transcription of the TRPC2 gene results in a functionally active protein involved in sensory responses to pheromones [39]. Genetic inactivation of TRPC2 in mice leads to loss of sex discrimination of male mice [41-43]. TRPC4 mRNA expression was observed in the adult mouse brain in the cortex, the hippocampus, the thalamus, the amygdala, the basal ganglia as well as the prefrontal cortex [29, 30, 38, 44]. TRPC4 protein expression was shown in the hippocampus, the cortex as well as the cerebellum [38, 44]. Using in situ hybridisation or immunocytochemistry, the expression of TRPC4 channels in different brain areas was specified. For example, TRPC4 was detected in cell layers of the prefrontal cortex [38] or in pyramidal CA1 and CA3 neurons of the hippocampus. In lateral septal neurons, TRPC4 channels were found on the cell surface of the soma and primary dendrites [33].

TRPC3 and TRPC6 mRNAs were demonstrated in the basal ganglia, the cerebellum, hippocampus as well as the forebrain [29]. TRPC3 protein expression in the brain especially in the prefrontal cortex and cerebellum was not only shown in rat and mouse tissues but also in human tissue obtained from subjects of different age groups [45]. TRPC3 channel expression was higher in the developing cortex compared to the adult cortex, whereas TRPC3 cerebral expression was not age-dependent. The protein expression of TRPC6 channels in the hippocampus is controversial. While several groups using pharmacological approaches or RT-PCR or western blot analyses describe TRPC6 channels being expressed in all hippocampal regions [46-51], Nagy and co-workers as well as Chung and colleagues show expression of TRPC6 channels selectively in the dentate gyrus and interneurons [52, 53]. Interestingly, in contrast to Tai et al. 2008, who described TRPC6 expression in hippocampal CA1 soma as well as in dendrites, Nagy's data suggest that TRPC6 channels are mainly expressed in dendrites of interneurons and neurons from the dentate gyrus [49, 53]. In the developing brain TRPC6 channels protein expression peaked between postnatal day 7 and 14, a period known to be important for maximal dendritic growth [49]. For TRPC7, only low mRNA expression levels were published [29, 30]. TRPC3 channels are also expressed in astrocytes [54].

2.2. TRPM channels

Melastatin, the founding member of the melastatin-like TRP family, was identified within a screen for proteins differentially regulated in melanocytes and melanoma cells [55]. Analysis of clinical data showed that the presence of melastatin expression in melanoma patients inversely correlates with the severity and survival [56-58]. Although melastatin is the first member of the TRPM family its activation mechanism and physiological role is still unclear. In line with the first description as protein involved in melanocyte physiology several reports confirmed this view. A completely unexpected function, the integration in retinal signal processing, has recently been discovered by the identification of TRPM1 expression in retinal ON bipolar cells [59]. The critical role of TRPM1 in mammalian phototransduction is also highlighted by several reports describing TRPM1 mutations in patients suffering from congenital stationary night blindness [60-63]. Only very little is known about TRPM1 function and expression in the CNS. Rather low mRNA TRPM1 expression was found in three studies in the brain [29, 64, 65].

From sequence similarity, TRPM3 is phylogenetically the closest neighbour to melastatin. TRPM3 is a polymodal ion channel activated by a variety of different stimuli like hypotonicity [66], sphingolipids [67], steroids [68, 69], nifedipine [69], and heat [70]. TRPM3 is activated by hypotonic extracellular solution and represents together with TRPV4, the volume-regulated TRP channels in the kidney [71, 72]. With the help of pharmacological tools, calcium entry induced by the application of hypotonic extracellular solutions can be assigned to TRPV4 and TRPM3 [71, 73-75]. While TRPV4 is activated by 4α-Isomers of phorbolesters and is blocked by ruthenium red, TRPM3 is activated by sphingosine and by pregnenolone-sulphate and blocked by gadolinium ions. TRPM3 is expressed in different areas of the CNS such as the hippocampus, the corpus callosum, the cortex or the hippocampus. These findings were reproduced in different studies using RT-PCR [29], northern blot [66, 76], as well as immunohistochemistry [77, 78]. TRPM3 channels are found in neurons (cerebral Purkinje neurons) as well as in oligodendrocytes [76-78]. Interestingly, neuronal expression of TRPM3 is present throughout development. However, it is almost lost in the adult brain [77]. In contrast, TRPM3 is highly expressed in oligodendrocytes in the adult brain.

The phylogenetically next neighbours to TRPM1 and TRPM3 are TRPM6 and TRPM7 [79]. The latter ones are involved in the body magnesium homeostasis [80]. While TRPM7 is ubiquitously expressed, TRPM6 is expressed in epithelial cells of the gut and the kidney and responsible for magnesium absorption and reabsorption. Loss-of-function mutations in TRPM6 are linked to autosomal-recessive hypomagnesemia with secondary hypocalcemia [81, 82]. TRPM6, TRPM7 and TRPM2 share a common structural feature. All three genes code for chimeric proteins combining a hexahelical transmembrane channel forming domain with a C-terminal enzymatic active domain [83]. In the case of TRPM6 and TRPM7, the pore-forming domains are fused to atypical alpha kinase-like structures. The functional role for the enzymatic domain is still under dispute. TRPM6 and TRPM7 are permeable for magnesium and for other essential divalent cations like Ca^{2+}, Zn^{2+}, Mn^{2+}, Co^{2+} as well as toxic cations like Ba^{2+}, Sr^{2+}, Ni^{2+}, Cd^{2+} [84, 85]. While TRPM6 mRNA was detected at low level in different brain areas [29], nothing is known about its role in the CNS. In contrast to TRPM6 channels, TRPM7 mRNA is highly expressed in the brain [29, 86]. In primary hippocampal neurons as well as in pyramidal hippocampal CA1 neurons in rat brain slices, TRPM7 was detected by different groups using immunocyto- and immunohistochemistry [87-89].

While divalent ions are the preferentially carried ion of TRPM6- and TRPM7-mediated currents, TRPM4 and TRPM5 form ion pores impermeable for divalent ions and allow selectively sodium to pass [90]. As sodium channels, TRPM4 and TRPM5 are paradoxically activated by increased intracellular calcium concentrations and represent calcium-activated sodium channels. TRPM4 is expressed in different brain regions including the thalamus, the hypothalamus, the medulla oblongata, the hippocampus and the spinal cord in mouse, rat as well as human brain (Lein et al., 2007; [29, 91]. In contrast to TRPM4, the expression of TRPM5 is restricted to a few cell types. TRPM5 is expressed in taste buds of the tongue and involved in the sensation of bitter and sweet taste [92, 93].

The remaining two TRPM channels proteins, TRPM2 and TRPM8, can also be discussed in the light of sensory functions. As already mentioned, TRPM2 represents a chimeric protein integrating an ADP-ribose hydrolase domain C-terminal to the pore-forming transmembrane domains [83]. Simultaneously to the ADP-ribose hydrolysing activity of the C-terminal enzymatic domain, TRPM2 is activated by ADP-ribose and it has been shown that the C-terminal part is essential for the function of the pore forming channel protein [94, 95]. Increased intracellular ADP-ribose concentrations are linked to genotoxic and/or oxidative stress of cells leading to the activation of the poly(ADP-ribose) polymerase (PARP) modulating protein stability by the mono and poly ADP-ribosylation of proteins [96]. This process of protein stability regulation is additionally controlled by an enzyme called poly(ADP-ribose) gluco-hydrolase (PARG). PARG reduces the post-translational poly ADP-ribose modifications to mono ADP-ribosylation, thereby increasing the intracellular ADP-ribose concentration leading to the activation of TRPM2. In whole cell calcium imaging experiments, the extracellular application of hydrogen peroxide results in the activation of TRPM2 validating its function as redox sensor. TRPM2 channels are preferentially expressed in microglia cells, the host macrophages of the CNS [97, 98]. In addition, in several brain regions such as the hippocampus, the cortex and the substantia nigra TRPM2 channels were also detected in neurons using RT-PCR, western blotting as well as immunohistochemistry [99, 100]. It was suggested that TRPM2 and TRPM7 channels form heteromers because knock-down of TRPM7 with siRNA is accompanied by down-regulation of TRPM2 channels [101]. TRPM8, the cold sensor, is mainly expressed in sensory neurons. TRPM8 is activated at temperatures between 8 °C to 28 °C as well as the secondary plant compound menthol and synthetic cooling compounds. Together with TRPA1, TRPM8 represent the cold sensors in human. Noxious cold is mediated by TRPA1 [26, 102].

2.3. TRP channels in the brain - TRPV channels

Vanilloid structures, derivates of vanillin comprising eugenol, zingerone and capsaicin, are found in many spice plants and known for their individual characteristic flavour. Beside the use as spice, vanilloid containing plant extracts are used as remedy in the various traditions of folk medicines. Therapeutic and experimental use of capsaicin in pain treatment inspired research resulting in the unravelling of the molecular target of capsaicin. The molecular target, an ion channel related to *Drosophila* TRP, was named capsaicin or vanilloid receptor and became eponym of the subgroup or structurally related ion channels of the TRP channel superfamily [15]. The vanilloid-like TRP channels comprise six members, four proteins (TRPV1 to TRPV4) like TRPV1 are non selective ion channels involved in thermosensation [14, 73, 74, 102, 103], while two ion channels (TRPV5 and TRPV6) represent highly calcium-selective ion channels [75, 104].

The warm and heat sensors (TRPV1 to TRPV4) and the cold sensors (TRPM8 and TRPA1) represent the thermosensors of the human body and cover the complete temperature range necessary for human life. As warning sensors expressed in dorsal root ganglia, the thermo TRPs are also involved in sensation and modulation of pain and therefore interesting as molecular targets for new pain-treating drugs. Most studies dealing with the structural and functional properties of the TRPV channel family in the CNS are focused on TRPV1. However, TRPV2, TRPV3 and TRPV4 are also detected in the CNS. In contrast for TRPV5 and TRPV6, there is no evidence for their expression in the CNS.

Localization	Function	References
Hippocampus (interneurons, dentate gyrus)	involved in anxiety and fear	[132, 151]
	involved in LTD	[152, 153]
	involved in LTP	[152]
	involved in pathogenesis of epilepsy	[126, 127]
hypothalamus	central osmoregulation	[154, 155]
	central regulation of temperature	[108]
Locus coeruleus	potentiation of glutamate,	
	adrenaline or norepinephrine release	[151]
Cortex	involved in cortical excitability	[156]
	involved in pathogenesis of epilepsy	[126]
Striatum	facilitation of glutamatergic	[157]
	postsynaptic neurotransmission	[158]
	glutamate release	[159]

Table 1 Localization and putative function of TRPV1 channels

TRPV1 expression in the CNS was investigated using a variety of methods ranging from pharmacological characterization and immunohistochemistry [105] to RT-PCR [106], western blotting to radio ligand binding [107]. Beside the great variety of methods and studies the expression of TRPV1 in the brain remains controversial. Several studies showed a wide spread TRPV1 expression in the CNS suggesting an expression of TRPV1 in pyramidal neurons of the CA1, CA3 area of the hippocampus, the dentate gyrus, the locus coeruleus, the hypothalamus, the substantia nigra, the cerebellum, the cortex and other limbic structures [108]. Other studies reported TRPV1 expression which was highly restricted to primary sensory ganglia with minimal expression in few brain regions which are adjacent to the caudal hypothalamus [107] (expression profiles and methods are summarized in Table 1). However several groups used TRPV1 agonists or antagonists as well as TRPV1 knock-out mice to define the role of TRPV1 channels in the CNS and reported versatile functions in different brain regions such as the hippocampus, the substantia nigra, the cortex or the hypothalamus. TRPV1 channels are not only activated by capsaicin but also by the CB1 agonist anandamide [109], other endovanilloids such as N-acyldopamines or the endogenous lipoxygenase derivates HPETE which are released for example in the hippocampus after mGluR1 activation [108]. Importantly, colocalization of TRPV1 and CB1 receptors was found in different mouse brain regions including the pyramidal cells of the hippocampus and basal glia [110, 111]. Regarding its cellular localisation, TRPV1 channels were detected in neuronal cell bodies, presynaptic terminals as well as in dendrites on postsynaptic spines [105, 106, 112, 113]. Furthermore, these channels are also present in pericytes and at the feet of astrocytes surrounding small vessels [105, 114].

TRPV2 channels are widely distributed in the brain compromising the colocalisation with TRPV1 in the cortex [19, 112, 115, 116]. TRPV3 mRNA was detected throughout the cortex, hippocampus, thalamus, striatum and cerebellum [117, 118]. TRPV4 mRNA is present in the hypothalamus, the cerebellum, basal ganglia, as well as in pyramidal neurons of the hippocampus [29, 119, 120]. Importantly, TRPV1-4 were also found in astrocytes [121, 122].

3. TRP channels in CNS diseases

3.1. Developmental disorders — Rett syndrome

Rett syndrome (RTT) is severe X-linked neurodevelopmental disorder which is unique among genetic, chromosomal and other developmental disorders because of its extreme female gender bias, early normal development, and subsequent developmental regression with loss of motor and language skills. RTT is caused by heterozygosity for mutations in the X-linked gene *MECP2*, which encodes methyl-CpG binding protein 2. Rett syndrome patients suffer from stereotypic wringing hand movements, social withdrawal, communication dysfunction, cognitive impairment, respiratory dysfunction as well as failing locomotion [123]. MeCP2 regulates expression of multiple genes, including BDNF. BDNF signaling was strongly altered in Mecp2 mutant mice [48].

Importantly, TRPC3 and TRPC6 channel expression and function was significantly lower in the hippocampus and several other brain regions of Mecp2 mutant mice revealing a cellular phenotype certainly contributing to hippocampal dysfunction in Mecp2 mutant mice as well as Rett syndrome etiology. These results suggest that compounds which enhance BDNF release or boost TRPC3/TRPC6 channel function might be an interesting new preclinical concept which needs to be evaluated in Rett mouse models [124, 125].

3.2. Epilepsy

Recent data suggests that TRPV1 channels might contribute to the pathophysiology of epilepsy. In the cortex and hippocampus from patients suffering from mesial temporal lobe epilepsy, the most common form of chronic and intractable epilepsy, TRPV1 mRNA and protein expression was significantly increased compared to healthy controls [126]. In a mouse model of temperal lobe epilepsy, these findings were supported [127]. The expression of TRPV1 in the dentate gyrus was significantly enhanced. Furthermore, capsaicin and anandamide significantly enhanced glutamate release in a TRPV1-dependent manner in mice with temperal lobe epilepsy [128, 129]. In contrast, the TRPV1 antagonist capsazepine reduced 4-aminopyridine-induced seizure-like activity in mice [128].

Beside TRPV1 channels, data from knockout mice point to a role of TRPC1/4/5 as well as for TRPC3/6 channels in the pathophysiology of epilepsy. Phelan et al. described a major role of TRPC1 and TRPC4 channels in the plateau potential of lateral septal neurons which show a high vulnerability to seizure-induced neuronal death as well as direct excitotoxicity by the application of group I mGluR receptor agonists [33]. *In vivo* results using the pilocarpine-induced status epileptics in TRPC1/TRPC4 double knockout animals showed surprising results. Cell death was significantly reduced in the lateral septum but also in the CA1 region of the hippocampus after severe seizures. However, the severity of the seizures *per se* was not altered. The authors concluded that this conundrum might be explained by the hypothesis that TRPC5 channels might be important for epileptiform burst in other limbic brain areas. This hypothesis was recently supported using TRPC5 knockout mice [32]. They exhibit significantly reduced seizures and minimal seizure-induced cell death in the CA1 region of the hippocampus. Importantly, spatial learning was not affected making TRPC5 channels an attractive novel target for the treatment of epilepsy.

TRPC3 channels are also discussed to play a "toxic" role in status epilepticus [46, 130]. After pilocarpine-induced status epilepticus in rats, TRPC3 expression was significantly enhanced in CA1, CA3 pyramidal neurons as well as dentate granule cells, whereas TRPC6 channel expression was reduced in these areas. Using two pharmacological approaches, first the inhibition of TRPC3 with the selective antagonist Pyr3 and second activation of TRPC6 channels with the TRPC6 activator hyperforin protected against neuronal damages following the status epilepticus [46].

3.3. Migraine

TRP channels might be involved in several processes relevant for the pathophysiology of migraine such as altered central calcium homeostasis, multimodal sensory and pain perception, or central or peripheral sensitization. Therefore, a recent study investigated single nucleotide polymorphisms (SNPs) in TRP genes in 1040 patients and 1037 healthy controls in Spain. For TRPV1, a nominal association was found for TRPV1 rs 222741 in the overall migraine group, for TRPV3 a correlation with TRPV3 rs7217270 was detected in the migraine group with aura [131].

3.4. Mood disorders – anxiety, unipolar and bipolar depression

TRPV1 and TRPV3 channels might be involved in fear and anxiety [107, 132]. TRPV1 knockout mice showed decreased anxiety-related behavior in several behavior paradigms such as the elevated plus maze test or the light dark test [107, 132]. Furthermore, fear and stress reaction were also reduced in TRPV1 knockout mice [107]. Therefore, TRPV1 antagonists such as capsazepine were investigated when they were applied directly into the ventral hippocampus or the periaqueductal grey. In both studies capsazepine showed anxiolytic effects. Recent studies investigated if compounds which act on both TRPV1 as well as CB1 receptors might be more effective than selective TRPV1 blocker [133]. N-arachidonoyl-serotonin which blocks TRPV1 channels and indirectly activates CB1 receptors and Arachidonyl-2-chloroethylamide (ACEA) which activates both TRPV1 as well as CB1 receptors were investigated. N-arachidonyl-serotonin was more effective than arachidonyl-2-chloroethylamide in behavioral paradigms for anxiety [134, 135]. The TRPV1/CB1 agonist ACEA showed anxiolytic effects in a bell shaped dose dependency in a mouse model using electrical stimulation of a brain area, the medial dorsal periaqueductal gray, which has an important role in orchestrating anxiety- and panic-related responses [133, 136]. The panicolytic effects are dependent on CB1 receptors. Importantly, in higher concentrations ACEA loses its anxiolytic effect probably via TRPC1 activation. This assumption is supported by the finding that ACEA effects in higher concentrations can be unmasked by the addition of the TRPV1 antagonist capsazepine. TRPV1 blockade per se also showed panicolytic effects suggesting opposite functions for TRPV1 and CB_1 receptors in the modulation of panic-like responses [136].

The evidence for the role of TRPC6 channels in depression comes from the active antidepressant constituent of St. Johns wort, hyperforin. Hyperforin resembles in its effects several classical antidepressants and neurotrophic factors such brain derived neurotrophic factor (BDNF) or nerve growth factor (NGF) [137-140]. Hyperforin inhibits neurotransmitter reuptake and improves synaptic plasticity ranging from increased neuritic outgrowth in PC12 cells to altered spine morphology in CA1 and CA3 neurons of the hippocampus via the activation of TRPC6 channels [137-139]. Recently, we showed that several signal cascades are involved in the alteration of synaptic plasticity such as Ras/MEK/ERK, PI3K/Akt as well as CAMKIV which finally result in CREB phorsphorylation [137]. In addition, enhanced CREB phosphorylation and TRPC6 channel expression was detected in the cortex but not the hippocampus after chronic hyperforin treatment for 4 weeks in adult mice [141]. However, hippocampal neurogenesis remained unchanged. Bouron et al. suggests that not only the hyperforin-mediated calcium influx but also its effects on intracellular zinc might be important for its antidepressant activity [142, 143]

Oxidative stress, mitochondrial dysfunction, and disrupted intracellular Ca^{2+} homeostasis are discussed to play a role in bipolar disorder (BD). TRPM2 channels, as a regulator and connector between reactive oxygen species (ROS) and intracellular Ca^{2+}, seem to be implicated in bipolar disorder. In B-lymphocytes from patients, TRPM2 channel expression is elevated associated with enhanced intracellular Ca^{2+} levels [144]. In addition, several groups reported genetic association between several intronic and extronic single nucleotide polymorphisms in TRPM2 and BD [145-149]. In a recent study using B-lymphocytes from small group of patients (n = 6) suffering from bipolar disorder, no change in TRPM2 expression could be detected. However, they were more susceptible to oxidative stress when stimulated with H_2O_2 [150].

3.5. Multiple sclerosis

Multiple sclerosis is a neurodegenerative disease caused by chronic inflammation of the CNS. Schattling et al. recently demonstrated that TRPM4 channels are involved in the pathogenesis of multiple sclerosis by using TRPM4 knockout mice and inducing an experimental autoimmune encephalomyelitis (EAE) in these animals [91]. TRPM4 channels are located in hippocampal neurons from mice and humans as well as in the spinal cord and cortex. TRPM4 deficiency reduced overall disease severity. Importantly, deficiency or pharmacological inhibition of TRPM4 resulted in reduced axonal and neuronal degeneration without altering

EAE relevant immune function. In addition, axonal TRPM4 expression in axons was significantly elevated in demyelinating white matter brain lesions of patients with multiple sclerosis in comparison to healthy controls. The authors further demonstrate that TRPV4 channels are involved in toxic effects of high glutamate levels which are a major contributor to neurodegeneration in multiple sclerosis.

4. Conclusion

Transient receptor potential (TRP) channels comprise a large family of non selective, calcium-permeable channel proteins which are activated and regulated by different mechanisms. TRP channels respond to secondary plant compounds as well as intracellular stimuli such as calcium, metabolites of the arachidonic acid or phosphatidylinositol signal transduction pathways. TRP channels sense environmental stimuli such as changes in temperature, osmolarity and pH and represent the molecular target of pheromones, taste and secondary plant compounds. The broad function of TRP channels in CNS physiology becomes apparent through their involvement in several psychiatric and neurological CNS disorders. This makes them an interesting topic for further research and drug development. The diversity of the chemical structures and the selectivity of the naturally occurring compounds modulating TRP channels show the possibility for pharmacological modulation of TRP channels and inspire the development of new synthetic structures for TRP channel interference at bench and bedside.

Author details

Christian Harteneck[1] and Kristina Leuner[2]

1 Institute of Pharmacology and Toxicology & Interfaculty Centre for Pharmacogenomics and Drug Research, Eberhard-Karls-University, Tübingen, Germany

2 Molecular und Clinical Pharmacy, Friedrich-Alexander-University Erlangen/Nürnberg, Germany

References

[1] Berridge, M.J., M.D. Bootman, and H.L. Roderick, *Calcium signalling: dynamics, homeostasis and remodelling.* Nat Rev Mol Cell Biol, 2003. 4: p. 517-29.

[2] Berridge, M.J., P. Lipp, and M.D. Bootman, *The versatility and universality of calcium signalling.* Nat Rev Mol Cell Biol, 2000. 1: p. 11-21.

[3] Yanez, M., J. Gil-Longo, and M. Campos-Toimil, *Calcium binding proteins.* Adv Exp Med Biol, 2012. 740: p. 461-82.

[4] Atlas, D., *The voltage-gated calcium channel functions as the molecular switch of synaptic transmission.* Annu Rev Biochem, 2013. 82: p. 607-35.

[5] Catterall, W.A., *Voltage-gated calcium channels.* Cold Spring Harb Perspect Biol, 2011. 3: p. a003947.

[6] Dolphin, A.C., *Calcium channel diversity: multiple roles of calcium channel subunits.* Curr Opin Neurobiol, 2009. 19: p. 237-44.

[7] Montell, C., *Drosophila visual transduction.* Trends Neurosci, 2012. 35: p. 356-63.

[8] Montell, C. and G.M. Rubin, *Molecular characterization of the Drosophila trp locus: a putative integral membrane protein required for phototransduction.* Neuron, 1989. 2: p. 1313-23.

[9] Wes, P.D., et al., *TRPC1, a human homolog of a Drosophila store-operated channel.* Proc Natl Acad Sci U S A, 1995. 92: p. 9652-6.

[10] Zhu, X., et al., *Molecular cloning of a widely expressed human homologue for the Drosophila trp gene.* FEBS Lett, 1995. 373: p. 193-8.

[11] Zitt, C., et al., *Cloning and functional expression of a human Ca^{2+}-permeable cation channel activated by calcium store depletion.* Neuron, 1996. 16: p. 1189-96.

[12] Harteneck, C., T.D. Plant, and G. Schultz, *From worm to man: three subfamilies of TRP channels.* Trends Neurosci, 2000. 23: p. 159-66.

[13] Montell, C., et al., *A unified nomenclature for the superfamily of TRP cation channels.* Mol Cell, 2002. 9: p. 229-31.

[14] Wu, L.J., T.B. Sweet, and D.E. Clapham, *International Union of Basic and Clinical Pharmacology. LXXVI. Current progress in the mammalian TRP ion channel family.* Pharmacol Rev, 2010. 62: p. 381-404.

[15] Caterina, M.J., et al., *The capsaicin receptor: a heat-activated ion channel in the pain pathway.* Nature, 1997. 389: p. 816-24.

[16] Voets, T., et al., *Sensing with TRP channels.* Nat Chem Biol, 2005. 1: p. 85-92.

[17] Puertollano, R. and K. Kiselyov, *TRPMLs: in sickness and in health.* Am J Physiol Renal Physiol, 2009. 296: p. F1245-54.

[18] Hofherr, A. and M. Kottgen, *TRPP channels and polycystins.* Adv Exp Med Biol, 2011. 704: p. 287-313.

[19] Venkatachalam, K. and C. Montell, *TRP channels.* Annu Rev Biochem, 2007. 76: p. 387-417.

[20] Talavera, K. and B. Nilius, *Electrophysiological Methods for the Study of TRP Channels*, in *TRP Channels*, M.X. Zhu, Editor. 2011: Boca Raton (FL).

[21] Yang, F. and J. Zheng, *Fluorescence Microscopy in ThermoTRP Channel Research*, in *TRP Channels*, M.X. Zhu, Editor. 2011: Boca Raton (FL).

[22] Grynkiewicz, G., M. Poenie, and R.Y. Tsien, *A new generation of Ca^{2+} indicators with greatly improved fluorescence properties.* J Biol Chem, 1985. 260: p. 3440-50.

[23] Shaner, N.C., P.A. Steinbach, and R.Y. Tsien, *A guide to choosing fluorescent proteins.* Nat Methods, 2005. 2: p. 905-9.

[24] Wallace, D.J., et al., *Single-spike detection in vitro and in vivo with a genetic Ca^{2+} sensor.* Nat Methods, 2008. 5: p. 797-804.

[25] Chung, M.K., S.J. Jung, and S.B. Oh, *Role of TRP channels in pain sensation.* Adv Exp Med Biol, 2011. 704: p. 615-36.

[26] Vay, L., C. Gu, and P.A. McNaughton, *The thermo-TRP ion channel family: properties and therapeutic implications.* Br J Pharmacol, 2012. 165: p. 787-801.

[27] Birnbaumer, L., *The TRPC class of ion channels: a critical review of their roles in slow, sustained increases in intracellular Ca^{2+} concentrations.* Annu Rev Pharmacol Toxicol, 2009. 49: p. 395-426.

[28] Dietrich, A., et al., *Functional characterization and physiological relevance of the TRPC3/6/7 subfamily of cation channels.* Naunyn Schmiedebergs Arch Pharmacol, 2005. 371: p. 257-65.

[29] Kunert-Keil, C., et al., *Tissue-specific expression of TRP channel genes in the mouse and its variation in three different mouse strains.* BMC Genomics, 2006. 7: p. 159.

[30] Riccio, A., et al., *mRNA distribution analysis of human TRPC family in CNS and peripheral tissues.* Brain Res Mol Brain Res, 2002. 109: p. 95-104.

[31] Strübing, C., et al., *TRPC1 and TRPC5 form a novel cation channel in mammalian brain.* Neuron, 2001. 29: p. 645-55.

[32] Phelan, K.D., et al., *Canonical transient receptor channel 5 (TRPC5) and TRPC1/4 contribute to seizure and excitotoxicity by distinct cellular mechanisms.* Mol Pharmacol, 2013. 83: p. 429-38.

[33] Phelan, K.D., et al., *Heteromeric canonical transient receptor potential 1 and 4 channels play a critical role in epileptiform burst firing and seizure-induced neurodegeneration.* Mol Pharmacol, 2012. 81: p. 384-92.

[34] Li, B., et al., *Effects of chronic treatment with fluoxetine on receptor-stimulated increase of $[Ca^{2+}]_i$ in astrocytes mimic those of acute inhibition of TRPC1 channel activity.* Cell Calcium, 2011. 50: p. 42-53.

[35] Malarkey, E.B., Y. Ni, and V. Parpura, *Ca^{2+} entry through TRPC1 channels contributes to intracellular Ca^{2+} dynamics and consequent glutamate release from rat astrocytes.* Glia, 2008. 56: p. 821-35.

[36] Paez, P.M., et al., *Modulation of canonical transient receptor potential channel 1 in the proliferation of oligodendrocyte precursor cells by the golli products of the myelin basic protein gene.* J Neurosci, 2011. 31: p. 3625-37.

[37] Boisseau, S., et al., *Heterogeneous distribution of TRPC proteins in the embryonic cortex.* Histochem Cell Biol, 2009. 131: p. 355-63.

[38] Fowler, M.A., et al., *Corticolimbic expression of TRPC4 and TRPC5 channels in the rodent brain.* PLoS One, 2007. 2: p. e573.

[39] Liman, E.R., D.P. Corey, and C. Dulac, *TRP2: a candidate transduction channel for mammalian pheromone sensory signaling.* Proc Natl Acad Sci U S A, 1999. 96: p. 5791-6.

[40] Vannier, B., et al., *Mouse trp2, the homologue of the human trpc2 pseudogene, encodes mTrp2, a store depletion-activated capacitative Ca^{2+} entry channel.* Proc Natl Acad Sci U S A, 1999. 96: p. 2060-4.

[41] Leypold, B.G., et al., *Altered sexual and social behaviors in trp2 mutant mice.* Proc Natl Acad Sci U S A, 2002. 99: p. 6376-81.

[42] Lucas, P., et al., *A diacylglycerol-gated cation channel in vomeronasal neuron dendrites is impaired in TRPC2 mutant mice: mechanism of pheromone transduction.* Neuron, 2003. 40: p. 551-61.

[43] Stowers, L., et al., *Loss of sex discrimination and male-male aggression in mice deficient for TRP2.* Science, 2002. 295: p. 1493-500.

[44] Zechel, S., S. Werner, and O. von Bohlen Und Halbach, *Distribution of TRPC4 in developing and adult murine brain.* Cell Tissue Res, 2007. 328: p. 651-6.

[45] Roedding, A.S., et al., *TRPC3 protein is expressed across the lifespan in human prefrontal cortex and cerebellum.* Brain Res, 2009. 1260: p. 1-6.

[46] Kim, D.S., et al., *The reverse roles of transient receptor potential canonical channel-3 and -6 in neuronal death following pilocarpine-induced status epilepticus.* Cell Mol Neurobiol, 2013. 33: p. 99-109.

[47] Li, H., et al., *TRPC6 inhibited NMDA receptor activities and protected neurons from ischemic excitotoxicity.* J Neurochem, 2012. 123: p. 1010-8.

[48] Li, W., et al., *Activity-dependent BDNF release and TRPC signaling is impaired in hippocampal neurons of Mecp2 mutant mice.* Proc Natl Acad Sci U S A, 2012. 109: p. 17087-92.

[49] Tai, Y., et al., *TRPC6 channels promote dendritic growth via the CaMKIV-CREB pathway.* J Cell Sci, 2008. 121: p. 2301-7.

[50] Xu, P., et al., *Expression of TRPC6 in renal cortex and hippocampus of mouse during postnatal development.* PLoS One, 2012. 7: p. e38503.

[51] Zhou, J., et al., *Critical role of TRPC6 channels in the formation of excitatory synapses.* Nat Neurosci, 2008. 11: p. 741-3.

[52] Chung, Y.H., et al., *Immunohistochemical study on the distribution of TRPC channels in the rat hippocampus.* Brain Res, 2006. 1085: p. 132-7.

[53] Nagy, G.A., et al., *DAG-sensitive and Ca^{2+} permeable TRPC6 channels are expressed in dentate granule cells and interneurons in the hippocampal formation.* Hippocampus, 2013. 23: p. 221-32.

[54] Shirakawa, H., et al., *Transient receptor potential canonical 3 (TRPC3) mediates thrombin-induced astrocyte activation and upregulates its own expression in cortical astrocytes.* J Neurosci, 2010. 30: p. 13116-29.

[55] Hunter, J.J., et al., *Chromosomal localization and genomic characterization of the mouse melastatin gene (Mlsn1).* Genomics, 1998. 54: p. 116-23.

[56] Deeds, J., F. Cronin, and L.M. Duncan, *Patterns of melastatin mRNA expression in melanocytic tumors.* Hum Pathol, 2000. 31: p. 1346-56.

[57] Duncan, L.M., et al., *Down-regulation of the novel gene melastatin correlates with potential for melanoma metastasis.* Cancer Res, 1998. 58: p. 1515-20.

[58] Fang, D. and V. Setaluri, *Expression and Up-regulation of alternatively spliced transcripts of melastatin, a melanoma metastasis-related gene, in human melanoma cells.* Biochem Biophys Res Commun, 2000. 279: p. 53-61.

[59] Shen, Y., et al., *A transient receptor potential-like channel mediates synaptic transmission in rod bipolar cells.* J Neurosci, 2009. 29: p. 6088-93.

[60] Audo, I., et al., *TRPM1 is mutated in patients with autosomal-recessive complete congenital stationary night blindness.* Am J Hum Genet, 2009. 85: p. 720-9.

[61] Li, Z., et al., *Recessive mutations of the gene TRPM1 abrogate ON bipolar cell function and cause complete congenital stationary night blindness in humans.* Am J Hum Genet, 2009. 85: p. 711-9.

[62] Nakamura, M., et al., *TRPM1 mutations are associated with the complete form of congenital stationary night blindness.* Mol Vis, 2010. 16: p. 425-37.

[63] van Genderen, M.M., et al., *Mutations in TRPM1 are a common cause of complete congenital stationary night blindness.* Am J Hum Genet, 2009. 85: p. 730-6.

[64] Dong, H.W., et al., *Expression of transient receptor potential (TRP) channel mRNAs in the mouse olfactory bulb.* Neurosci Lett, 2012. 524: p. 49-54.

[65] Yang, J., et al., *Receptor for activated C kinase 1 (RACK1) inhibits function of transient receptor potential (TRP)-type channel Pkd2L1 through physical interaction.* J Biol Chem, 2012. 287: p. 6551-61.

[66] Grimm, C., et al., *Molecular and functional characterization of the melastatin-related cation channel TRPM3.* J Biol Chem, 2003. 278: p. 21493-501.

[67] Grimm, C., et al., *Activation of the melastatin-related cation channel TRPM3 by D-erythro-sphingosine [corrected].* Mol Pharmacol, 2005. 67: p. 798-805.

[68] Majeed, Y., et al., *Cis-isomerism and other chemical requirements of steroidal agonists and partial agonists acting at TRPM3 channels.* Br J Pharmacol, 2010. 161: p. 430-41.

[69] Wagner, T.F., et al., *Transient receptor potential M3 channels are ionotropic steroid receptors in pancreatic beta cells.* Nat Cell Biol, 2008. 10: p. 1421-30.

[70] Vriens, J., et al., *TRPM3 is a nociceptor channel involved in the detection of noxious heat.* Neuron, 2011. 70: p. 482-94.

[71] Harteneck, C. and B. Reiter, *TRP channels activated by extracellular hypo-osmoticity in epithelia.* Biochem Soc Trans, 2007. 35: p. 91-5.

[72] Harteneck, C. and G. Schultz, *TRPV4 and TRPM3 as Volume-Regulated Cation Channels,* in *TRP Ion Channel Function in Sensory Transduction and Cellular Signaling Cascades,* W.B. Liedtke and S. Heller, Editors. 2007: Boca Raton (FL).

[73] Liedtke, W., *Role of TRPV ion channels in sensory transduction of osmotic stimuli in mammals.* Exp Physiol, 2007. 92: p. 507-12.

[74] Vriens, J., G. Appendino, and B. Nilius, *Pharmacology of vanilloid transient receptor potential cation channels.* Mol Pharmacol, 2009. 75: p. 1262-79.

[75] Woudenberg-Vrenken, T.E., R.J. Bindels, and J.G. Hoenderop, *The role of transient receptor potential channels in kidney disease.* Nat Rev Nephrol, 2009. 5: p. 441-9.

[76] Oberwinkler, J., et al., *Alternative splicing switches the divalent cation selectivity of TRPM3 channels.* J Biol Chem, 2005. 280: p. 22540-8.

[77] Hoffmann, A., et al., *TRPM3 is expressed in sphingosine-responsive myelinating oligodendrocytes.* J Neurochem, 2010. 114: p. 654-65.

[78] Zamudio-Bulcock, P.A., et al., *Activation of steroid-sensitive TRPM3 channels potentiates glutamatergic transmission at cerebellar Purkinje neurons from developing rats.* J Neurochem, 2011. 119: p. 474-85.

[79] Runnels, L.W., *TRPM6 and TRPM7: A Mul-TRP-PLIK-cation of channel functions.* Curr Pharm Biotechnol, 2011. 12: p. 42-53.

[80] Ferre, S., J.G. Hoenderop, and R.J. Bindels, *Insight into renal Mg^{2+} transporters.* Curr Opin Nephrol Hypertens, 2011. 20: p. 169-76.

[81] Schlingmann, K.P., et al., *Hypomagnesemia with secondary hypocalcemia is caused by mutations in TRPM6, a new member of the TRPM gene family.* Nat Genet, 2002. 31: p. 166-70.

[82] Walder, R.Y., et al., *Mutation of TRPM6 causes familial hypomagnesemia with secondary hypocalcemia.* Nat Genet, 2002. 31: p. 171-4.

[83] Harteneck, C., *Function and pharmacology of TRPM cation channels.* Naunyn Schmiedebergs Arch Pharmacol, 2005. 371: p. 307-14.

[84] Gwanyanya, A., et al., *Magnesium-inhibited, TRPM6/7-like channel in cardiac myocytes: permeation of divalent cations and pH-mediated regulation.* J Physiol, 2004. 559: p. 761-76.

[85] Kerschbaum, H.H., J.A. Kozak, and M.D. Cahalan, *Polyvalent cations as permeant probes of MIC and TRPM7 pores.* Biophys J, 2003. 84: p. 2293-305.

[86] Fonfria, E., et al., *Tissue distribution profiles of the human TRPM cation channel family.* J Recept Signal Transduct Res, 2006. 26: p. 159-78.

[87] Sun, H.S., et al., *Suppression of hippocampal TRPM7 protein prevents delayed neuronal death in brain ischemia.* Nat Neurosci, 2009. 12: p. 1300-7.

[88] Wei, W.L., et al., *TRPM7 channels in hippocampal neurons detect levels of extracellular divalent cations.* Proc Natl Acad Sci U S A, 2007. 104: p. 16323-8.

[89] Zhang, J., et al., *Hypoxia induces an increase in intracellular magnesium via transient receptor potential melastatin 7 (TRPM7) channels in rat hippocampal neurons in vitro.* J Biol Chem, 2011. 286: p. 20194-207.

[90] Guinamard, R., L. Salle, and C. Simard, *The non-selective monovalent cationic channels TRPM4 and TRPM5.* Adv Exp Med Biol, 2011. 704: p. 147-71.

[91] Schattling, B., et al., *TRPM4 cation channel mediates axonal and neuronal degeneration in experimental autoimmune encephalomyelitis and multiple sclerosis.* Nat Med, 2012. 18: p. 1805-11.

[92] Perez, C.A., et al., *A transient receptor potential channel expressed in taste receptor cells.* Nat Neurosci, 2002. 5: p. 1169-76.

[93] Zhang, Y., et al., *Coding of sweet, bitter, and umami tastes: different receptor cells sharing similar signaling pathways.* Cell, 2003. 112: p. 293-301.

[94] Perraud, A.L., et al., *ADP-ribose gating of the calcium-permeable LTRPC2 channel revealed by Nudix motif homology.* Nature, 2001. 411: p. 595-9.

[95] Sano, Y., et al., *Immunocyte Ca^{2+} influx system mediated by LTRPC2.* Science, 2001. 293: p. 1327-30.

[96] Eisfeld, J. and A. Lückhoff, *Trpm2.* Handb Exp Pharmacol, 2007: p. 237-52.

[97] Kraft, R., et al., *Hydrogen peroxide and ADP-ribose induce TRPM2-mediated calcium influx and cation currents in microglia.* Am J Physiol Cell Physiol, 2004. 286: p. C129-37.

[98] Naziroglu, M., *TRPM2 cation channels, oxidative stress and neurological diseases: where are we now?* Neurochem Res, 2011. 36: p. 355-66.

[99] Jia, J., et al., *Sex differences in neuroprotection provided by inhibition of TRPM2 channels following experimental stroke.* J Cereb Blood Flow Metab, 2011. 31: p. 2160-8.

[100] Roedding, A.S., et al., *Chronic oxidative stress modulates TRPC3 and TRPM2 channel expression and function in rat primary cortical neurons: relevance to the pathophysiology of bipolar disorder.* Brain Res, 2013. 1517: p. 16-27.

[101] Aarts, M., et al., *A key role for TRPM7 channels in anoxic neuronal death.* Cell, 2003. 115: p. 863-77.

[102] Talavera, K., B. Nilius, and T. Voets, *Neuronal TRP channels: thermometers, pathfinders and life-savers.* Trends Neurosci, 2008. 31: p. 287-95.

[103] Basbaum, A.I., et al., *Cellular and molecular mechanisms of pain.* Cell, 2009. 139: p. 267-84.

[104] Hoenderop, J.G. and R.J. Bindels, *Calciotropic and magnesiotropic TRP channels.* Physiology (Bethesda), 2008. 23: p. 32-40.

[105] Toth, A., et al., *Expression and distribution of vanilloid receptor 1 (TRPV1) in the adult rat brain.* Brain Res Mol Brain Res, 2005. 135: p. 162-8.

[106] Mezey, E., et al., *Distribution of mRNA for vanilloid receptor subtype 1 (VR1), and VR1-like immunoreactivity, in the central nervous system of the rat and human.* Proc Natl Acad Sci U S A, 2000. 97: p. 3655-60.

[107] Marsch, R., et al., *Reduced anxiety, conditioned fear, and hippocampal long-term potentiation in transient receptor potential vanilloid type 1 receptor-deficient mice.* J Neurosci, 2007. 27: p. 832-9.

[108] Kauer, J.A. and H.E. Gibson, *Hot flash: TRPV channels in the brain.* Trends Neurosci, 2009. 32: p. 215-24.

[109] Ross, R.A., *Anandamide and vanilloid TRPV1 receptors.* Br J Pharmacol, 2003. 140: p. 790-801.

[110] Hajos, N. and T.F. Freund, *Pharmacological separation of cannabinoid sensitive receptors on hippocampal excitatory and inhibitory fibers.* Neuropharmacology, 2002. 43: p. 503-10.

[111] Rouach, N. and R.A. Nicoll, *Endocannabinoids contribute to short-term but not long-term mGluR-induced depression in the hippocampus.* Eur J Neurosci, 2003. 18: p. 1017-20.

[112] Liapi, A. and J.N. Wood, *Extensive co-localization and heteromultimer formation of the vanilloid receptor-like protein TRPV2 and the capsaicin receptor TRPV1 in the adult rat cerebral cortex.* Eur J Neurosci, 2005. 22: p. 825-34.

[113] Roberts, J.C., J.B. Davis, and C.D. Benham, *$[_3H]$Resiniferatoxin autoradiography in the CNS of wild-type and TRPV1 null mice defines TRPV1 (VR-1) protein distribution.* Brain Res, 2004. 995: p. 176-83.

[114] Mannari, T., et al., *Astrocytic TRPV1 ion channels detect blood-borne signals in the sensory circumventricular organs of adult mouse brains.* Glia, 2013. 61: p. 957-71.

[115] Lewinter, R.D., G. Scherrer, and A.I. Basbaum, *Dense transient receptor potential cation channel, vanilloid family, type 2 (TRPV2) immunoreactivity defines a subset of motoneurons in the dorsal lateral nucleus of the spinal cord, the nucleus ambiguus and the trigeminal motor nucleus in rat.* Neuroscience, 2008. 151: p. 164-73.

[116] Wainwright, A., et al., *Discrete expression of TRPV2 within the hypothalamo-neurohypophysial system: Implications for regulatory activity within the hypothalamic-pituitary-adrenal axis.* J Comp Neurol, 2004. 474: p. 24-42.

[117] Smith, G.D., et al., *TRPV3 is a temperature-sensitive vanilloid receptor-like protein.* Nature, 2002. 418: p. 186-90.

[118] Xu, H., et al., *TRPV3 is a calcium-permeable temperature-sensitive cation channel.* Nature, 2002. 418: p. 181-6.

[119] Mutai, H. and S. Heller, *Vertebrate and invertebrate TRPV-like mechanoreceptors.* Cell Calcium, 2003. 33: p. 471-8.

[120] Vriens, J., et al., *Cell swelling, heat, and chemical agonists use distinct pathways for the activation of the cation channel TRPV4.* Proc Natl Acad Sci U S A, 2004. 101: p. 396-401.

[121] Benfenati, V., et al., *Expression and functional characterization of transient receptor potential vanilloid-related channel 4 (TRPV4) in rat cortical astrocytes.* Neuroscience, 2007. 148: p. 876-92.

[122] Benfenati, V., et al., *An aquaporin-4/transient receptor potential vanilloid 4 (AQP4/TRPV4) complex is essential for cell-volume control in astrocytes.* Proc Natl Acad Sci U S A, 2011. 108: p. 2563-8.

[123] Briggs, A., *Primary care of a child with Rett syndrome.* J Am Assoc Nurse Pract, 2013.

[124] Chapleau, C.A., et al., *Evaluation of current pharmacological treatment options in the management of Rett syndrome: from the present to future therapeutic alternatives.* Curr Clin Pharmacol, 2013. 8: p. 358-69.

[125] Li, W. and L. Pozzo-Miller, *BDNF deregulation in Rett syndrome.* Neuropharmacology, 2014. 76 Pt C: p. 737-46.

[126] Sun, F.J., et al., *Increased expression of TRPV1 in the cortex and hippocampus from patients with mesial temporal lobe epilepsy.* J Mol Neurosci, 2013. 49: p. 182-93.

[127] Bhaskaran, M.D. and B.N. Smith, *Effects of TRPV1 activation on synaptic excitation in the dentate gyrus of a mouse model of temporal lobe epilepsy.* Exp Neurol, 2010. 223: p. 529-36.

[128] Gonzalez-Reyes, L.E., et al., *TRPV1 antagonist capsazepine suppresses 4-AP-induced epileptiform activity in vitro and electrographic seizures in vivo.* Exp Neurol, 2013. 250: p. 321-32.

[129] Manna, S.S. and S.N. Umathe, *Involvement of transient receptor potential vanilloid type 1 channels in the pro-convulsant effect of anandamide in pentylenetetrazole-induced seizures.* Epilepsy Res, 2012. 100: p. 113-24.

[130] Ryu, H.J., et al., *Endothelial transient receptor potential conical channel (TRPC)-3 activation induces vasogenic edema formation in the rat piriform cortex following status epilepticus.* Cell Mol Neurobiol, 2013. 33: p. 575-85.

[131] Carreno, O., et al., *SNP variants within the vanilloid TRPV1 and TRPV3 receptor genes are associated with migraine in the Spanish population.* Am J Med Genet B Neuropsychiatr Genet, 2012. 159B: p. 94-103.

[132] You, I.J., et al., *Alterations in the emotional and memory behavioral phenotypes of transient receptor potential vanilloid type 1-deficient mice are mediated by changes in expression of $5\text{-}HT_{1A}$, $GABA_A$, and NMDA receptors.* Neuropharmacology, 2012. 62: p. 1034-43.

[133] Fogaca, M.V., et al., *The endocannabinoid and endovanilloid systems interact in the rat prelimbic medial prefrontal cortex to control anxiety-like behavior.* Neuropharmacology, 2012. 63: p. 202-10.

[134] John, C.S. and P.J. Currie, *N-arachidonoyl-serotonin in the basolateral amygdala increases anxiolytic behavior in the elevated plus maze.* Behav Brain Res, 2012. 233: p. 382-8.

[135] Micale, V., et al., *Anxiolytic effects in mice of a dual blocker of fatty acid amide hydrolase and transient receptor potential vanilloid type-1 channels.* Neuropsychopharmacology, 2009. 34: p. 593-606.

[136] Casarotto, P.C., et al., *Opposing roles for cannabinoid receptor type-1 (CB_1) and transient receptor potential vanilloid type-1 channel (TRPV1) on the modulation of panic-like responses in rats.* Neuropsychopharmacology, 2012. 37: p. 478-86.

[137] Heiser, J.H., et al., *TRPC6 channel-mediated neurite outgrowth in PC12 cells and hippocampal neurons involves activation of RAS/MEK/ERK, PI3K, and CAMKIV signaling.* J Neurochem, 2013. 127: p. 303-13.

[138] Leuner, K., et al., *Hyperforin--a key constituent of St. John's wort specifically activates TRPC6 channels.* FASEB J, 2007. 21: p. 4101-11.

[139] Leuner, K., et al., *Hyperforin modulates dendritic spine morphology in hippocampal pyramidal neurons by activating Ca^{2+}-permeable TRPC6 channels.* Hippocampus, 2013. 23: p. 40-52.

[140] Tu, P., et al., *Diacylglycerol analogues activate second messenger-operated calcium channels exhibiting TRPC-like properties in cortical neurons.* J Neurochem, 2009. 108: p. 126-38.

[141] Gibon, J., et al., *The antidepressant hyperforin increases the phosphorylation of CREB and the expression of TrkB in a tissue-specific manner.* Int J Neuropsychopharmacol, 2013. 16: p. 189-98.

[142] Gibon, J., P. Richaud, and A. Bouron, *Hyperforin changes the zinc-storage capacities of brain cells.* Neuropharmacology, 2011. 61: p. 1321-6.

[143] Gibon, J., et al., *The over-expression of TRPC6 channels in HEK-293 cells favours the intracellular accumulation of zinc.* Biochim Biophys Acta, 2011. 1808: p. 2807-18.

[144] Yoon, I.S., et al., *Altered TRPC7 gene expression in bipolar-I disorder.* Biol Psychiatry, 2001. 50: p. 620-6.

[145] McQuillin, A., et al., *Fine mapping of a susceptibility locus for bipolar and genetically related unipolar affective disorders, to a region containing the C21ORF29 and TRPM2 genes on chromosome 21q22.3.* Mol Psychiatry, 2006. 11: p. 134-42.

[146] Perova, T., et al., *Hyperactive intracellular calcium dynamics in B lymphoblasts from patients with bipolar I disorder.* Int J Neuropsychopharmacol, 2008. 11: p. 185-96.

[147] Xu, C., et al., *TRPM2 variants and bipolar disorder risk: confirmation in a family-based association study.* Bipolar Disord, 2009. 11: p. 1-10.

[148] Xu, C., et al., *Association of the putative susceptibility gene, transient receptor potential protein melastatin type 2, with bipolar disorder.* Am J Med Genet B Neuropsychiatr Genet, 2006. 141B: p. 36-43.

[149] Xu, C., et al., *Association of the iPLA$_2$beta gene with bipolar disorder and assessment of its interaction with TRPM2 gene polymorphisms.* Psychiatr Genet, 2013. 23: p. 86-9.

[150] Roedding, A.S., et al., *Effect of oxidative stress on TRPM2 and TRPC3 channels in B lymphoblast cells in bipolar disorder.* Bipolar Disord, 2012. 14: p. 151-61.

[151] Marinelli, S., et al., *Capsaicin activation of glutamatergic synaptic transmission in the rat locus coeruleus in vitro.* J Physiol, 2002. 543: p. 531-40.

[152] Brown, T.E., et al., *Loss of interneuron LTD and attenuated pyramidal cell LTP in Trpv1 and Trpv3 KO mice.* Hippocampus, 2013. 23: p. 662-71.

[153] Gibson, H.E., et al., *TRPV1 channels mediate long-term depression at synapses on hippocampal interneurons.* Neuron, 2008. 57: p. 746-59.

[154] Ciura, S., W. Liedtke, and C.W. Bourque, *Hypertonicity sensing in organum vasculosum lamina terminalis neurons: a mechanical process involving TRPV1 but not TRPV4.* J Neurosci, 2011. 31: p. 14669-76.

[155] Sinke, A.P. and P.M. Deen, *The physiological implication of novel proteins in systemic osmoregulation.* FASEB J, 2011. 25: p. 3279-89.

[156] Mori, F., et al., *TRPV1 channels regulate cortical excitability in humans.* J Neurosci, 2012. 32: p. 873-9.

[157] Musella, A., et al., *TRPV1 channels facilitate glutamate transmission in the striatum.* Mol Cell Neurosci, 2009. 40: p. 89-97.

[158] Marinelli, S., et al., *Activation of TRPV1 in the VTA excites dopaminergic neurons and increases chemical- and noxious-induced dopamine release in the nucleus accumbens.* Neuropsychopharmacology, 2005. 30: p. 864-70.

[159] Marinelli, S., et al., *Presynaptic facilitation of glutamatergic synapses to dopaminergic neurons of the rat substantia nigra by endogenous stimulation of vanilloid receptors.* J Neurosci, 2003. 23: p. 3136-44.

6

Peptide and Protein Neurotoxin Toolbox in Research on Nicotinic Acetylcholine Receptors

Victor Tsetlin and Igor Kasheverov

1. Introduction

The chapter briefly covers the history of protein and peptide neurotoxins in research on nicotinic acetylcholine receptors (nAChR). It all started with a great help of α-bungarotoxin and other similar α-neurotoxins from snake venoms in isolation from the *Torpedo* ray electric organ of the muscle-type nAChR as a first individual membrane receptor. The next contribution of α-neurotoxins was the discovery with their aid of the first neuronal nAChR in the brain now known as homooligomeric α7 nAChR. An overview of various α-neurotoxins (so-called three-finger toxins) is presented below showing the structural differences between them, as well as the benefits of their current application for identification and quantification of different nAChR subtypes at normal state and at various pathologies such as Alzheimer's and Parkinson's diseases, psychiatric diseases and nicotine addiction. A special emphasis is placed on the work at our institute, starting with the first detection of nAChRs as targets for the so-called weak or "non-conventional" neurotoxins. Recently, in proteomic studies of snake venoms, novel structural types have been discovered, such as covalently connected dimeric α-cobratoxin or, on the contrary - azemiopsin, the first peptide from venoms which does not contain disulfide bonds but still blocks selectively the muscle-type nAChR.

A generous source for sophisticated tools in research on nAChRs is combinatorial peptide libraries from the venoms of *Conus* marine snails. In particular, they contain α-conotoxins which not only distinguish muscle nAChRs from neuronal ones, but some of them block specifically distinct neuronal nAChR subtypes. At present, combinations of snake and snail toxins are widely used in fundamental research and in pharmacological studies.

The chapter briefly summarizes information on the spatial organization and subunit composition of different nAChR subtypes, but considers in more detail important contributions of peptide and protein neurotoxins into elucidation of the topography of the nAChR binding sites. The information mainly came from the X-ray structures of their complexes with the acetylcholine-binding protein (AChBP), an excellent structural model of the ligand-binding domain of nAChRs. These complexes are considered as initial blocks for design of novel drugs.

2. Muscle-type, neuronal and "non-neuronal" nAChRs — Brief overview

Before considering in detail protein and peptide neurotoxins on which the Chapter is mostly focused, it is reasonable to give very shortly the information about various types of nAChR which will make easier later discussions of the specificity of one or another toxin to a particular nAChR subtype.

As mentioned in the Introduction, α-bungarotoxin made possible identification and isolation in a pure form of the nAChR from the *Torpedo* ray electric organ. Later it was found that this receptor is composed of 5 subunits arranged around the central axis along which an ion channel should be arranged (Figure 1, A). The subunits in the order of their increasing molecular masses (estimated from the SDS-gel electrophoresis) have been named α, β, γ and δ. The molecular mass of the receptor complex is around 250 kD and it should contain two α subunits and by one of the "non- α" subunits. When nucleotide sequences of the *Torpedo* nAChR subunits and of those from mammalian muscles were established it became clear that those receptors are highly homologous. In fact, the mammalian embryonic nAChR has the same subunit stoichiometry (2α, β, γ and δ), but in the mature form it has an ε subunit instead of γ. Although the relevant information at present is available in numerous biochemistry books and reviews [1-4], it should be mentioned here that nAChRs are ligand-gated ion channels: binding of a ligand (acetylcholine, nicotine or other specific agonists) will result in the channel opening and passing sodium or calcium ions will activate a variety of signaling cascades. On the other hand, binding at the same sites of competitive antagonists such as α-bungarotoxin will prevent both binding of agonists and subsequent channel opening; some so-called non-competitive antagonists, like phencyclidine, bind directly to the channel moiety but they are not discussed here.

Earlier it was thought that the ligand-binding sites of nAChRs lie within the α-subunits, hence there should be two binding sites on the muscle-type nAChRs. To-day we know that, indeed, the main contributions to binding of agonists or competitive antagonists are donated by the α-subunits. Moreover, even isolated α-subunit and its fragment in the amino-acid region 170-200 can bind α-bungarotoxin, although with lower affinity than the whole-size receptors [5,6]. However, now it is well established that the binding sites are situated at the interfaces of the α-subunits with their neighbors, and it is the variability of functional groups brought to the binding sites by less conservative "non-alpha" subunits which underlies the differences in specificity between individual nAChR subtypes [4].

What are the types and subtypes of nicotinic acetylcholine receptors? As mentioned above, binding of radioactive α-bungarotoxin to brain membranes finally brought to life the nAChR presently known as homopentameric α7 nAChR that is composed of five identical α7-subunits. Thus, we have an example of homooligomeric receptor belonging to the family of neuronal nAChRs. Neuronal heteromeric nAChRs are composed of two types of subunits: α and β. At present there are 9 types of neuronal α-subunits (α2-α10) and three types of β subunits (β2-β4); α and β subunits in the muscle-type receptors presumed to be α1 and β1 ones. The characteristic feature of α-subunit is a vicinal disulfide between two neighboring Cys residues in the binding site (Cys192-Cys193 in the amino-acid sequence of the *Torpedo* α-subunit) which is not present in β or other "non-α" subunits. In recent years it became clear that diverse nAChRs are very much widespread and play different functional roles also outside the neuromuscular junctions or central nervous system. In fact, neuronal nAChR subunits were found on the immune system cells, skin, lung tissue and other. The respective receptors got the name of "non-neuronal" nAChRs thus making a third group of nicotinic acetylcholine receptors (see reviews [7,8]).

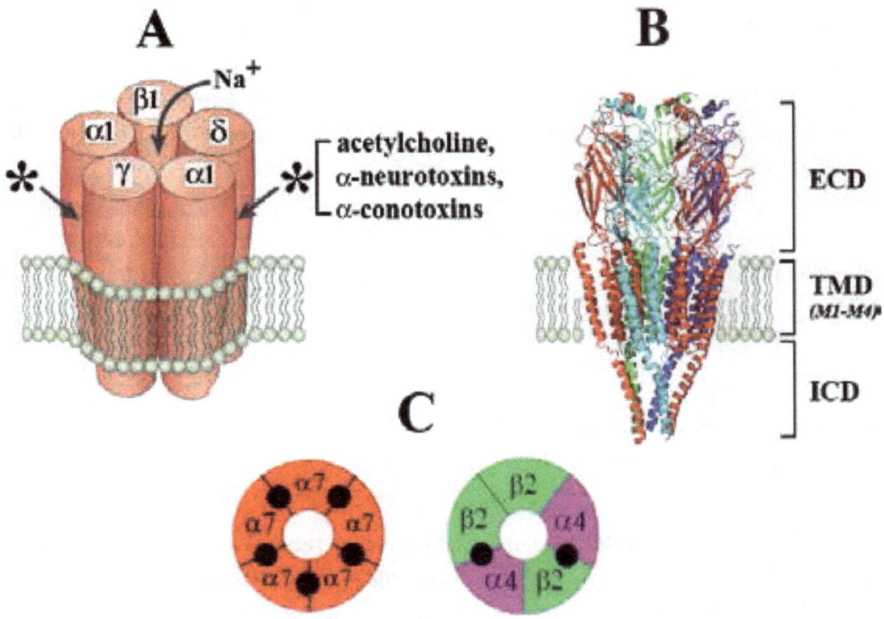

Figure 1. Spatial organization of nAChRs. A – Schematic presentation of *Torpedo* nAChR, consisting of 5 subunits with the ion channel along the central axis. Two binding sites of agonists (acetylcholine and others) and competitive antagonist (α-neurotoxins from snakes, α-conotoxins from *Conus* mollusks and others) are located at the interfaces of the α1/γ and α1/δ-subunits and marked with asterisks. B – Spatial organization of *Torpedo marmorata* nAChR derived from its cryo-electron microscopy structure. Subunits α1, β1, γ and δ are colored in red, green, cyanic and blue, respectively. Three main domains of the receptor – extracellular (ECD), transmembrane (TMD), consisting of 4 α-helical fragments (M1-M4), and intracellular (ICD) are shown. C – Schematic presentation of two representatives of neuronal nAChRs – homooligomeric and heterooligomeric ones. The probable binding sites of agonists and competitive antagonist are marked with black circles.

Structurally, the *Torpedo* nAChR is a prototype for all members of the nAChR family. First of all, it is a pentamer (composed of 5 subunits) as follows from the cryo-electron microscopy structure of the *Torpedo marmorata* receptor (see Figure 1, B). There are no structural data of this sort for any other nAChR, but their pentameric composition was presumed from computer modeling and from some indirect data like electrophysiology analysis. At present there are no doubts that all nAChRs are indeed either pentameric homooligomers (made exclusively of 5 α-type subunits, like α7 nAChR, α9 nAChR or α9/α10 nAChR) or pentameric heterooligomers (composed of α and other subunits) (Figure 1, C) – for example, one of the best presented in the brain is $\alpha4\beta2$ nAChR [9]. As already mentioned, all nAChRs should be built similarly to *Torpedo* nAChR: namely, four transmembrane fragments M1-M4 in each subunit, the most inner ones M2 fragments lining the channel, the N-terminal extracellular fragments of each subunit together forming the ligand-binding domain excellently imitated by the X-ray structure of the acetylcholine-binding protein (AChBP) (see below). The long intracellular loops between transmembrane fragments M3 and M4 of each subunit together form the cytoplasmic (intracellular) domain.

The first and the most direct structural evidence for a common three-dimensional organization of all nAChRs came from the crystal structure of AChBP [10]. Today even more convincing are the recently solved high-resolution X-ray structures of the whole-size prokaryotic membrane proteins belonging to the same superfamily of Cys-loop ligand-gated ion channels as nAChRs [11-13]. These proteins, each composed of 5 identical subunits, do not have large cytoplasmic domains (which apparently made their crystallization much more simple than of nAChRs or other mammalian Cys-loop receptors), but in the transmembrane and ligand-binding domains they are surprisingly similar to *Torpedo* nAChR. Moreover, the same type of structure was found for a Cys-loop receptor from *Caenorhabditis elegans* [14]. Now, after having these major facts about nicotinic acetylcholine receptors, we can open our toolbox and have a closer look on protein and peptide neurotoxins.

3. Snake venom neurotoxins utilized in research on nAChRs — Primary and three-dimensional structure

The word "toolbox" in the chapter title in the first place is related to the snake venom proteins, at least historically. It was the component of *Bungarus multicinctus* venom which was found to block very efficiently the muscle-type nAChRs and could be considered as a good marker of those receptors. The history of the discovery of such a tool, namely protein neurotoxin α-bungarotoxin, is presented in a recent review [15]. There Prof. Chang shares his memories about this discovery (exactly 50 years ago!) which played such a crucial role in understanding the structure and function of both snake neurotoxins and of one of their targets, namely nAChRs. Soon after the discovery of α-bungarotoxin, similar proteins were found in other snakes, in particular in cobra venoms and the whole family got the name of α-neurotoxins (see reviews [15-17]).

3.1. α-Neurotoxins

There are two structural types of α-neurotoxins: short-chain α-neurotoxins (60-62 amino acid residues, 4 disulfide bridges) and long-chain ones (66-75 amino acid residues, 5 disulfide bonds). The first X-ray structures have been determined for the short-chain α-neurotoxins, namely for erabutoxins a and b [18,19] (see Figure 2, A). The molecule has three loops, with a predominant β-structure, fixed in the space by 4 disulfide bridges forming a sort of a knot. This folding gave the name of "three-finger proteins" to α-neurotoxins. Later spatial structures have been determined both by NMR and X-ray crystallography for different short- and long-chain α-neurotoxins, including α-bungarotoxin [20,21]. Long-chain α-neurotoxins have the same three -finger folding as the short ones, but contain a longer C-terminal tail and an additional 5th disulfide in the central loop II (Figure 2, B). In the structures of some long-chain α-neurotoxins (α-bungarotoxin, α-cobratoxin [22] or neurotoxin I from *Naja oxiana* [23]) a short α-helical fragment was found at the tip of the loop II (see Figure 2, B).

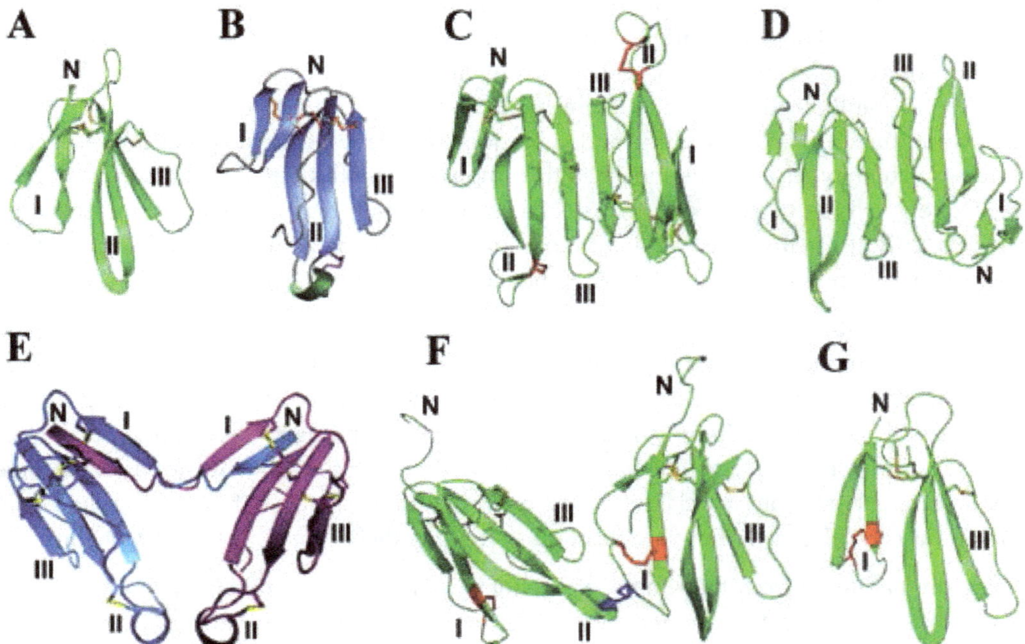

Figure 2. Spatial structures of snake 'three-finger' toxins interacting with nAChRs. The 'fingers' are marked with Roman numbers; N-termini are labeled as well. A - erabutoxin a (PDB ID: 5EBX). B – α-bungarotoxin (1KFH); the 5th disulfide bridge in loop II is colored in magenta (contrary to all other disulfides in orange) and α-helix at tip of this loop is colored intentionally in contrast green. C – κ-bungarotoxin (1KBA); 5th disulfide bridges in loops II are colored in red. D – haditoxin (3HH7). E – dimeric α-cobratoxin (4AEA), where disulfide bridges between Cys3 from one monomer and Cys20 from the second monomer stabilize the dimeric molecule; two monomers are shown in blue and magenta, respectively. F - irditoxin (2H7Z); 'non-conventional' disulfides in loops I are colored in red and disulfide bond between the monomers is shown in blue. G - candoxin (1JGK); disulfide in loop I is shown in red.

One of the characteristic features of α-neurotoxins is the stability of their three-dimensional structure fixed by 4 or 5 disulfide bridges. This conclusion is supported by high similarity of spatial structures determined by NMR at different conditions (varying pH and temperatures) and by X-ray crystallography. This may be one of the crucial factors explaining high efficiency of α-neurotoxin interactions with their targets, nicotinic acetylcholine receptors. As will be shown later, α-neurotoxins essentially preserve their conformation in complexes with the AChBP [24], with the ligand-binding domain of individual α1 subunit of nAChR [25] and with the chimera of AChBP and α7 nAChR extracellular domain [26].

3.2. Dimeric three-finger neurotoxins

First of all, we should mention here κ-bungarotoxins and several homologous neurotoxins which are dimers, but do not have covalent intermolecular bonds between monomers [27]. Each monomer is very similar to a typical long-chain α-neurotoxin: the same additional 5th disulfide at the tip of the central loop II, but a slightly shorter C-terminal tail (total number of amino acid residues 66 but not 75 as in α-bungarotoxin) (see Figure 2, C). The molecular targets of κ-bungarotoxins are neuronal nAChRs, but contrary to α-neurotoxins they have high affinity to neuronal α3β2 nAChR [28]. Interestingly, it was established about 20 years ago that there is one common property of α-neurotoxins and κ-neurotoxins, namely the additional disulfide in the loop II is essential for recognition of neuronal nAChRs. It was found that selective reduction of that disulfide and subsequent alkylation or removal of the respective cysteines in both types of toxins abolished their high affinity binding to α7 and α3β2 nAChRs, respectively (without decreasing the affinity of long-chain α-neurotoxins to muscle-type nAChRs [29,30]). On the other hand, introduction of additional disulfide into the central loop of short-chain α-neurotoxins considerably increased their affinity for α7 nAChR [31,32].

It is not yet absolutely clear why κ-bungarotoxins have preference for heteromeric nAChRs. There was a hypothesis that an important role in selectivity of κ-bungarotoxins towards α3β2 nAChRs belongs to the residue Lys26 [24]. However, its introduction to α-neurotoxin having a high affinity for α7 nAChRs only decreased considerably binding to this receptor but did not bring any affinity for α3β2 nAChRs [32]. Apparently, dimerization as such is important to force a protein, composed of two classical α-neurotoxins, to recognize a heteromeric neuronal nAChRs as can be seen on the example of other recently discovered dimeric neurotoxins.

One toxin, haditoxin from the King cobra venom [33] looks very similar to κ-bungarotoxin. Haditoxin is a non-covalent dimer composed of two short-chain α-neurotoxins, rather than of long-chain ones, and the monomers adopt a topological arrangement (Figure 2, D) reminiscent of that observed earlier for monomers in κ-bungarotoxin. Haditoxin can block not only muscle-type nAChRs, as typically observed for short-chain α-neurotoxins, but surprisingly it also blocks homooligomeric α7 and heterooligomeric α3β2 nAChRs. This finding appears to be in contradiction with the earlier found necessity of the additional disulfide in the central loop for recognition of neuronal nAChRs. However, it should be kept in mind that blocking of neuronal nAChRs by haditoxin was observed only at very high toxin concentrations [33]. It should be also mentioned that, strictly speaking, haditoxin cannot be assigned to classical short-chain α-neurotoxins because its homology to erabutoxin is only 50%, whereas it is 75-80% with the muscarinic toxin-like proteins (MTLP) having different targets [34].

Novel types of dimeric α-neurotoxins were recently discovered: contrary to κ-bungarotoxin or haditoxin, these are covalently bound where two molecules of α-cobratoxin are connected by two intermolecular disulfide bonds [35]. Before describing a biological activity of this new tool, it should be mentioned that such intermolecular disulfide is the first case of this post-translational modification found for the whole huge family of three-finger toxins. Dimeric α-cobratoxin retained, although at a lower level, the capacity to block α7 and muscle-type nAChRs and in addition acquired the ability to block α3β2 nAChR - again, with lower potency than did κ-bungarotoxin [35]. Interestingly, selective reduction of the disulfides in the loop II of dimeric α-cobratoxin abolished its activity against α7 nAChR. It could be expected in view of earlier described similar modification of α-cobratoxin itself, but this chemical modification even increased the affinity for α3β2 nAChR [36]. Since dimeric α-cobratoxin is present in the *Naja kaouthia* cobra venom only in minute amounts (0.01% in crude venom, as compared to 10% for α-cobratoxin itself or to 0.1% for κ-bungarotoxin), unequivocal localization of intermolecular disulfides by chemical means could not be done. Fortunately, dimeric α-cobratoxin has been recently crystallized (Figure 2, E) and the high-resolution X-ray structure revealed the disposition of the intermolecular disulfide bridges: the disulfide Cys3-Cys20 or Cys3′-Cys20′ in each monomer is not formed, but Cys3 of one monomer finds Cys20′ of another monomer, while Cys3′ of the latter makes a disulfide with Cys20 of the former [36].

As will be shown later, the main contribution to binding of α-neurotoxins both to nAChRs and to their models comes from the tip of the central loop II of α-neurotoxins. In dimeric α-cobratoxin the two tips are in close proximity and computer modeling showed impossibility of docking such a structure to AChBP, suggesting that some conformational changes should occur in the dimeric α-cobratoxin to ensure its binding observed in radioligand and electrophysiology experiments [36].

The discovery of dimeric α-cobratoxin was followed by finding another three-fingered toxin where monomers are connected by a disulfide bridge [37]. It was irditoxin isolated from Colubrid snake *Boiga irregularis*. In contrast to dimeric α-cobratoxin present in venom in minor amounts, irditoxin is a main component of boiga venom. Again, strictly speaking, irditoxin is neither a short- nor a long-chain α-neurotoxin: the monomers forming this toxin belong to non-conventional toxin type (see below) and each monomer contains an extra cysteine residue forming one disulfide bridge between two monomers (or protomers). None of these cysteines is present in classical α-neurotoxins. In the first protomer, the additional cysteine is located in loop I whereas in the second protomer it is in loop II. The three-dimensional structure of irditoxin [37] (see Figure 2, F) shows that the central loops II of the two protomers are oriented in a similar way as the central loops of dimeric α-cobratoxin (Figure 2, E).

3.3. Weak (non-conventional) three-fingered neurotoxins

A characteristic feature of this group of three-fingered toxins is the presence of additional disulfide bridge not in the central loop II, as in long-chain α-neurotoxins or in κ-bungarotoxins, but in the N- terminal loop I. Some representatives of this group were known long ago, but many of them did not have a strong toxicity (that is why their name was "weak toxins") and their targets were unknown. At present this group of toxins, consisting of 62-68 amino acid residues, is quite well investigated and has a more general name "non-conventional neurotoxins" [38]. The toxicities for the most of group members are very low (5-80 mg/kg) in contrast to classical α-neurotoxin with toxicities in the range from 0.04 to 0.3 mg/kg. However, some very potent toxins (like γ-bungarotoxin with LD50 of 0.15 mg/kg) are also included in the group of non-conventional toxins. Since, as mentioned above, molecular targets of weak (non-conventional) toxins for a long time were unknown, an important step in this field was the work [39] where was discovered that weak toxin (WTX) from *Naja kaouthia* cobra venom interacted with micromolar affinity with the $\alpha7$ and muscle-type nAChRs, the binding being practically irreversible. Later it was found [40] that candoxin (Figure 2, G), another non-conventional toxin, interacted both with $\alpha7$ and muscle-type nAChR with high affinity. An interesting feature of candoxin is that its attachment to the muscle-type receptor was easily reversible. Even more impressing species specificity was reported for denmotoxin, a non-conventional toxin isolated from Colubrid snake *Boiga dendrophila*: it was able to interact irreversibly and with high affinity with chick muscle nAChR, but only with low affinity with mouse receptors [41].

3.4. Three-finger snake neurotoxins having other targets than nicotinic acetylcholine receptors

Before considering in detail the mechanisms of interactions between α-neurotoxins and nAChRs and describing their earlier and current roles of tools, it is appropriate to say a few words about the whole family of three-finger proteins from snake venoms (see reviews [16,17]). They all have the same "three-finger" fold but are decorated with quite different functionally active amino-acid residue and, as a result, attack distinct targets. For example, in the preceding paragraph we considered WTX from *Naja kaouthia* venom which blocked nicotinic acetylcholine receptors. Its very low toxicity allowed testing of its behavioural activity on rats which suggested action on muscarinic acetylcholine receptors [42]. Indeed, subsequent radioligand analyses revealed the WTX interaction with the different subtypes of muscarinic acetylcholine receptors [43]. It should be noted here that we have a dualism of action for this group of the three-finger proteins from snake venom: namely, blocking of one acetylcholine receptor (the nicotinic one) belonging to the family of ligand-gated ion channels and another acetylcholine receptor, the muscarinic one which is a member of the superfamily of G-protein-coupled receptors (GPCR).

Much more strong effects on muscarinic acetylcholine receptors exert so-called muscarinic neurotoxins isolated from the green mamba *Dendroaspis angusticeps* [44-46]. Structurally these proteins are of the same type as short-chain α-neurotoxins. Interestingly, they can distinguish different subtypes (M1-M7) of muscarinic acetylcholine receptors and on some of them exert not the inhibitory, but the potentiating effects. There is not yet much information about how muscarinic toxins recognize their targets. A large series of mutations was performed both on the muscarinic toxin MT7 and on the M1 muscarinic receptor and the results of this pair-wise mutagenesis, analyzed by computer modelling, indicated that all three loops I-III should be involved in the interaction and the main binding site for this allosteric modulator is located in the extracellular loops of the receptor [46].

There are also several three-finger proteins from snake venoms (calciceptin, FS2) blocking Ca^{2+} channels [47,48]. We should also mention here fasciculin, a three-finger protein with 4 disulfides, targeting the acetylcholinesterase. Interestingly, the X-ray structures of fasciculin in complex with acetylcholinesterases were the first examples presenting a three-finger toxin bound to its biological target [49,50].

One of the most well-represented groups in the snake venoms are so-called cytotoxins (some of them were earlier called cardiotoxins) which apparently do not have a single well-defined target but disrupt the cell membranes thus inducing a multitude of effects (see reviews [51,52]). As a result of proteomic studies new three-finger proteins are being found in the snake venoms, and one of the minor components in the *Naja kaouthia* cobra venom was identified as a glycosylated cytotoxin I [53]. This post-translational modification, for the first time discovered for the family of three-finger toxins, considerably decreased the cytotoxicity of this protein, whereas enzymatic deglycosylation restored it to the level of cytotoxin I activity [53]. Another really a minor component of that venom (less than 0.01% in the crude venom) was a dimer of cytotoxin and α-cobratoxin connected by two intermolecular disulfide bridges which revealed a weak activity against neuronal nicotinic acetylcholine receptors [35].

We also would like to mention here the recent discovery of three-finger neurotoxins which interact with another group of GPCR, namely with the adrenoreceptors [54,55]. These toxins are most similar to muscarinic toxins and were also isolated from the eastern green mamba *Dendroaspis angusticeps*. One such toxin (ϱ-Da1a) has a very high affinity (0.35 nM) for the α1 adrenoreceptor, while another one (ϱ-Da1b) has a lower affinity but is more selective towards α2 types [55]. Interestingly, these toxins are considered as possible drugs against prostate hypertrophy.

Although it is not the topic of the present review, it is appropriate to mention here that there are three-finger proteins in nervous and immune system of mammals and insects belonging to the Ly6 family and some of them bind to nicotinic acetylcholine receptors and regulate their functioning *in vivo* (see [56-59] and recent publications from our institute [60-63]).

3.5. Peptides from snake venoms acting on nicotinic acetylcholine receptors

Such peptides are not as numerous as α-neurotoxins or non-conventional toxins targeting different subtypes of nAChR. Until recently the only group was that of waglerins isolated from the venom of South Asian snake *Tropidolaemus wagleri* which consist of 22-24 amino acids and contain one disulfide bridge [64,65]. These toxins bind with high affinity to muscle-type nAChR [66]. Interestingly, waglerins can distinguish embryonic ($\alpha1_2\beta1\ \gamma\delta$) and "mature" ($\alpha1_2\beta1\varepsilon\delta$) muscle-type nAChR: waglerin-1 efficiently blocks the ε-containing form, but not the γ-form of this receptor [67]. While snake venom α-neurotoxins bind with practically equal efficiency to the two binding sites (formed by two α-subunits with their non-α neighbors) in the muscle-type nAChRs, waglerin-1 binds 2100-fold more tightly to the α-ε than to the α-δ binding site of the mouse nAChR [68]. Several amino acid residues in the nAChR subunits participating in waglerin binding were identified by site directed mutagenesis [69], namely Asp59 and Asp173 were shown to be important for waglerin binding at both sites. On the other hand, the disulfide in waglerin was found to be essential for its activity, as well as several residues in its N-terminal part of the amino acid sequence [70].

A new peptide was recently found in the snake venom possessing a capacity to block muscle-type nAChR [71]. It is azemiopsin, isolated from the *Azemiops feae* viper venom, which consists of 21 amino acid residues. By the chain length azemiopsin is similar to waglerins and, moreover, shares with them a homologous C-terminal fragment. However, it possesses a unique structural feature: contrary to all earlier known proteins and peptides from the venoms of snakes or poisonous *Conus* mollusks (see below), whose structure is fixed by one or several S–S-bonds, azemiopsin contains no disulfides. It dose-dependently blocked acetylcholine-induced currents in *Xenopus* oocytes heterologously expressing human muscle nAChR, and was more potent against the adult ($\alpha 1_2\beta 1\varepsilon\delta$) than the fetal ($\alpha 1_2\beta 1\gamma\delta$) form. Ala-scanning and analysis of competition with α-bungarotoxin for binding to *Torpedo* nAChR resulted in identification of the azemiopsin residues essential for its activity which in general were found to be different from those responsible for the waglerin activity [71].

4. α-Conotoxins, peptides from poisonous marine snails *Conus*, acting on nicotinic acetylcholine receptors

Historically, snake venom α-neurotoxins were the first extremely important tools which made possible "digging out" in a purified form the first representative of the nAChR family, namely the muscle-type receptor from the *Torpedo* ray electric organ. Then, in the early 80[s], the peptide toxins were discovered in the marine mollusk *Conus geographus* venom which caused postsynaptic inhibition at the neuromuscular junction in frog and got the name of conotoxins [72]. The following studies brought to life a tremendous number of so-called conotoxins or conopeptides from different species of *Conus* snails. The number of *Conus* species living in different seas and oceans is about 1000 and the available data show that the venom of each species should contain in excess of 1000 conopeptides. Thus, *Conus* mollusks provide researchers with huge combinatorial libraries of peptides. The main task of slowly moving *Conus* mollusks is to immobilize their preys (small fishes, worms etc.), that is why their venoms contain a variety of peptides paralyzing the nervous systems of their targets. Evolutionary each *Conus* species is adjusted to a particular area and a distinct food source, hence the individuality of each venom. There are several types of conotoxins differing in their targets: α-conotoxins block nAChRs, μ-conotoxins are acting on Na^+-channels, κ-conotoxins interact with K^+-channels, ω-conotoxins block specifically certain Ca^{2+}-channels and one of such ω-conotoxins became a very potent analgesic (trade name Ziconotide or Prialt; see more about these and many other conotoxins and conopeptides in recent reviews [73-75]). The number of discovered conotoxins is rapidly increasing because nowadays they appear not so much due to isolation from *Conus* venoms (usually available only in minute amounts) but due to deciphering mRNAs obtained from the venom glands.

Since this chapter is devoted to neurotoxic proteins and peptides interacting with nicotinic acetylcholine receptors, below we will consider only those conotoxins which target these receptors. The major group is α-conotoxins, competitive antagonists of nAChRs. They have 12-19 amino-acid residues, as a rule amidated C-terminus and two disulfide bonds between Cys residues C^1–C^3 and C^2–C^4 (see Table). There are also several other groups of conotoxins acting on nAChRs (ψ-, αA-, αA_S-, αC-, αS- and αD), but they are not numerous, are not as widely used as α-conotoxins and will not be considered here.

Toxin	*Conus species*	Amino acid sequence [1]	Selectivity
3/5 α-conotoxins			
GI	*C. geographus*	ECCNPACGRHYSC*	α1β1γ/εδ
MI	*C. magus*	GRCCHPACGKNYSC*	α1β1γ/εδ
SIA	*C. striatus*	YCCHPACGKNFDC*	α1β1γ/εδ
4/3 α- conotoxins			
ImI	*C. imperialis*	GCCSDPRCAWRC*	α7, α9α10; α3β2; α3β4
RgIA	*C. regius*	GCCSDPRCRYRCR	α9α10
4/4 α- conotoxins			
BuIA	*C. bullatus*	GCCSTPPCAVLYC*	α3(α6)β2, α3(α6)β4
4/6 α- conotoxins			
AuIB	*C. aulicus*	GCCSYPPCFATNPDC*	α3β4
4/7 α- conotoxins			
PnIA	*C. pennaceus*	GCCSLPPCAANNPDYC*	α3β2
PnIB	*C. pennaceus*	GCCSLPPCALSNPDYC*	α7; α3β4
MII	*C. magus*	GCCSNPVCHLEHSNLC*	α3β2(β3); α6-containing
Vc1.1	*C. victoriae*	GCCSDPRCNYDHPEIC*	α9α10; α3β4, α3(α5)β2
TxIA	*C. textile*	GCCSRPPCIANNPDLC*	α3β2
ArIB	*C. arenatus*	DECCSNPACRVNNPHVCRRR	α7, α6α3β2β3, α3β2

[1] Scheme of disulfide closing for naturally-occurring α-conotoxins –

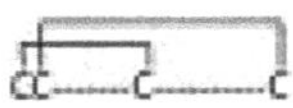

* indicates an amidated C-terminus; the names of α-conotoxins typed in italics mean that their structures were identified in cDNA libraries.

Table 1. Most studied members of naturally-occurring α-conotoxins.

α-Conotoxins are structurally subdivided into subgroups depending on the number of amino acid residues between the C^2–C^3 and C^3–C^4 cysteines (see Table) forming the first and second loops, respectively. This structural feature affects the α-conotoxin specificity to particular nAChR subtypes. All at present known 3/5 α-conotoxins are potent blockers of muscle type nAChRs (and conventionally can be called 'muscle' α-conotoxins). The members of other subgroups (4/3, 4/4, 4/6, 4/7) act on various neuronal nAChR subtypes (and can be called 'neuronal' α-conotoxins). It is very rare when naturally occurring neuronal α-conotoxin blocks specifically only one neuronal nAChR subtype, usually neuronal α-conotoxins interact with two or more nAChR subtypes (see Table).

Most of muscle 3/5 α-conotoxins can discriminate species-specifically two binding sites on muscle or *Torpedo* nAChRs. For example, α-conotoxins MI, GI or SIA have up to10000 times higher affinity for α1/δ- over α1/γ site in muscle nAChR [76,77]; in contrast to more effective binding of these peptides, although not with such a great difference, to α1/γ site in *Torpedo* receptor [78,79].

"Mutagenesis" studies of α-conotoxins (in fact not the mutagenesis as such, but substitutions of amino acid residues by solid-phase peptide synthesis) gave information about those residues which are the basis of the high affinity and selectivity to a particular receptor or receptor subgroup. For example, the crucial role of Arg9 in α-conotoxin GI, as well as of Pro6 and Tyr12 in α-conotoxin MI for discriminating the α1/γ- and α1/δ-sites was revealed [80-82]. Interestingly, Arg9 proved important for a neuronal 4/3 α-conotoxin RgIA for its α9α10 nAChR specificity [83]. Similar "mutagenesis" studies resulting in revelation of residues crucial for activity were done also for many other α-conotoxins (ImI, PnIA, MII, GID, Vc1.1, AuIB) [84-89].

Like in the analysis of interactions between different nAChR types and snake venom neurotoxins, when much efforts has been spent by many laboratories to establish the topography of their binding, similar studies have been undertaken to elucidate the mechanism of nAChR recognition by α-conotoxins. Among them were above-mentioned multiple substitutions in the amino acid sequences of naturally occurring α-conotoxins, making their structures more rigid, syntheses of radioactive, fluorescent and photoactivatable derivatives. Combination with mutagenesis of the receptor subunits (pair-wise mutagenesis) gave information about possible contact points between α-neurotoxins and nAChRs, as well as between α-conotoxins and nAChRs. The relevant information can be found in numerous reviews (see, for example, [90-92]), but will not be considered in detail here, because this chapter contains a special section where crystal structures of α-neurotoxins and α-conotoxins in complexes with the relevant biological targets will be discussed.

5. Three-dimensional structures of peptide and protein neurotoxins in complexes with the nicotinic receptor models and fragments

It was already mentioned that the crystal structure of the acetylcholine-binding protein (AChBP) provided an impressing jump in the structural analysis of not only nicotinic acetylcholine receptors but of all other members of the Cys-loop receptor family. This water-soluble protein was found to modulated synaptic transmission in glia of *Lymnaea stagnalis* fresh-water mollusk and was purified using affinity chromatography on a column with the attached α-bungarotoxin [93]. Sufficient amounts of AChBP were obtained by heterologous expression and the crystal structure was determined at 2.7 Å resolution [10]. This structure clearly showed that AChBP is an excellent structural model of N-terminal ligand-binding domains of all nAChRs: crystal AChBP was in a pentameric state, similarly to the whole-size nAChRs. In spite of low homology with the amino-acid sequences of extracellular domains of nAChR subunits (not more than 25%), AChBP contains all those amino acid residues which earlier in receptor studies were found essential for interacting with the cholinergic agonists and antagonist. The

AChBP crystal structure revealed that such residues are all clustered in the middle of AChBP, at the interfaces between its subunits (or protomers). At present, the X-ray structures of several molluscan AChBPs are known (from *Lymnaea stagnalis, Aplysia californica, Bulinus truncatus*), as well of their complexes with a wide variety of agonists and antagonists which gave quite a detailed picture of the respective binding sites in these AChBPs and of their contacts with ligands. Biochemical data and computer modeling show convincingly that these structures shed light on the receptor binding sites *per se* and on the ligand disposition in the binding sites of muscle and neuronal nAChRs. The relevant information can be found in recent original papers [94-97] and reviews [98,99], and below we will consider in detail only the crystal structures of complexes with protein and peptide neurotoxins.

Interestingly, the first AChBP crystal structure in complex with a competitive antagonist was that of *Lymanaea stagnalis* AChBP with bound α-cobratoxin [24]. (In parentheses it may be mentioned that later more structures were solved for the *Aplysia californica* AChBP complexes, but *L. stagnalis* AChBP has a much higher affinity for α-neurotoxins than AChBPs from other species). First of all, X-ray analysis revealed 5 α-cobratoxin molecules attached at the interfaces between 5 identical subunits (or protomers) of AChBP (Figure 3, A). The major role in the organization of the binding site is played by aromatic residues (so-called "aromatic box") of AChBP. Long before crystallographic studies, protein chemistry and mutagenesis revealed that these aromatic residues were important for binding different agonists and antagonists to diverse muscle-type and neuronal nAChRs. It was proposed that the binding sites are formed by three fragments (A, B, C) of polypeptide chain of one subunit and by three fragments (D, E, F) of the polypeptide chain of the other one on which these aromatic residues are located (see review [100]). The first three fragments in real receptors are on the α-subunits and form the main (principal) binding surface, while the last three are on non-α-subunits and compose the complementary binding surface. In the case of homopentameric receptors like α7 ones, the A-C loops are on the "front surface" of one α7-subunit and D-F on the "back surface" of the neighboring identical subunit. In general, the X-ray structure of the AChBP complex with α-cobratoxin is in accord with the earlier ideas on the α-neurotoxin binding to nAChRs formulated on the basis of chemical modification of α-neurotoxins, their mutagenesis, photoaffinity labeling and mutagenesis of receptors (see reviews [101,102]). Indeed, there is a multipoint binding of α-cobratoxin and the major role, as earlier shown by "wet biochemistry" methods, is played by the toxin central loop II.

The comparison with the NMR and X-ray structures for α-neurotoxins revealed that α-cobratoxin did not need to change its conformation dramatically to be accommodated in the binding region of AChBP. On the contrary, the AChBP loop C containing the disulfide between the neighboring cysteines (which is also a characteristic feature of all nAChR α-subunits) had to move to periphery up to 10 Å from the position which it occupied in the AChBP containing no bound ligand. (This movement should be supplemented with essential changes in conformation of loop F from complementary AChBP protomer.) Moreover, the earlier solved structure of AChBP with such agonist as nicotine revealed that, when agonist comes to the binding site, loop C embraces it and moves closer to the central axis of the molecule [94]. At present there are many crystal structures of various AChBPs in complexes with versatile specific or nonselective agonists and antagonists of the muscle-type and neuronal nAChRs and it appears to be a general rule: antagonists versus agonists induce movements of the loop C in the opposite directions.

5.1. X-ray structure of the extracellular domain of muscle nAChR α1 subunit in complex with α-bungarotoxin

Until now we were considering the X-ray and Electron microscopy structures of closely related but independent objects of studies: acetylcholine binding proteins and *Torpedo* nAChR. It should be emphasized that the structures of bound cholinergic agonists and antagonists until recently were available only for their complexes with AChBPs. That is why when researchers wished to analyze in three-dimensions the interactions of agonists or antagonists with the muscle-type or neuronal nAChRs, they had to rely on computer modeling. Fortunately, one of the bridges between the AChBPs and nAChRs spatial structures has been recently open: the X-ray structure has been determined for the α-bungarotoxin complex with heterologously expressed ligand-binding domain of mouse muscle nAChR α1 subunit [25]. Many laboratories have earlier tried, with the aid of heterologous expression, to obtain ligand-binding domains of α1 or α7 subunits as individual proteins and to determine their three-dimensional structure. Although in certain cases those proteins could bind α-bungarotoxin with relatively high affinity (but not with the nanomolar constants as intact receptors) [103-106], in no case the proteins could be crystallized. In view of the above-said, the work [25] is clearly a break-through. Using random mutagenesis, the authors have chosen a protein with a low tendency to aggregation. In spite of its having the mutation of Trp149 (localized in loop B and known to be important for binding agonists and antagonists), the protein could bind α-bungarotoxin. It was namely the complex of α-bungarotoxin rather than the free domain which was success-fully crystallized. (Thus, in addition to helping isolate the *Torpedo* nAChR and *L.stagnalis* AChBP, α-neurotoxins played again an important role, this time in crystallization of the nAChR subunit ligand-binding domain.) The structure of the complex has been solved at a very high resolution (1.94 Å) (see Figure 3, B).

Although this domain is a monomer, its spatial structure is very similar to an AChBP protomer in a pentameric complex. A molecule of bound α-bungarotoxin occupies the position similar to that of α-cobratoxin in complex with *L. stagnalis* AChBP (compare Figure 3, A and B). It should be emphasized that in the complex with α1 domain, α-bungarotoxin utilized for interaction only the principal side, while α-cobratoxin in complex with pentameric AChBP has contacts with both principal and complementary sides at the subunit interface. However, instead of this, α-bungarotoxin forms contacts with the sugar moiety present in the nAChR domain but absent in AChBPs.

5.2. X-ray structure of α-bungarotoxin with a chimera of L. stagnalis AChBP/ligand-binding domain of the human α7 subunit

This work can be considered as a further development of the recent breakthrough in the analysis of ligand binding domains of nAChRs when an important step was done in ascending from models to true receptors. The authors of [107] managed to substitute about

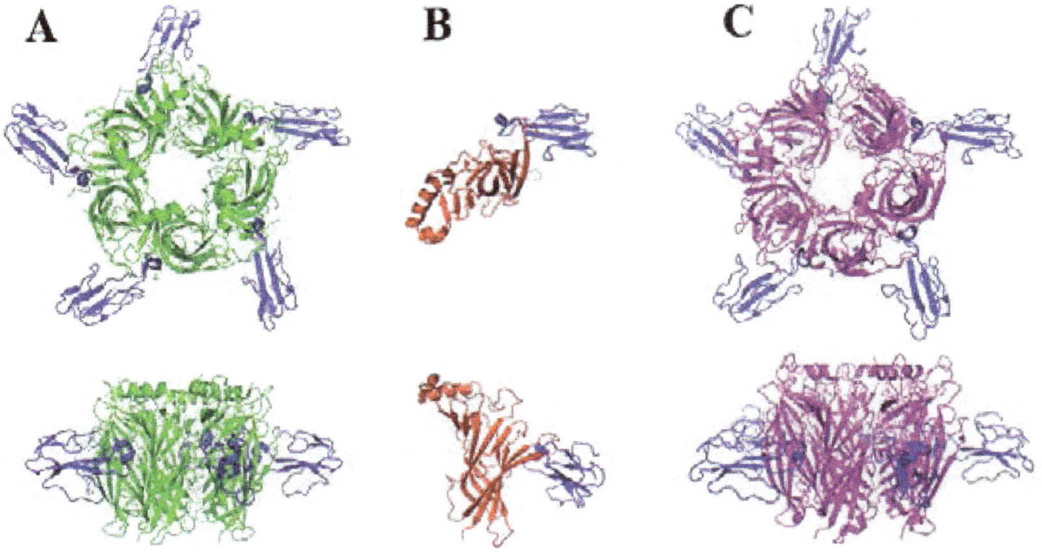

Figure 3. Crystal structures of the AChBP/nAChR domain-toxin complexes. Top and side views are in upper and lower lines, respectively. A - α-Cobratoxin bound to *L. stagnalis* AChBP (PDB ID: 1YI5); toxins and proteins are shown in blue and green. B – α-Bungarotoxin bound to the N-terminal domain of nAChR α1 subunit (2QC1); toxin and subunit are shown in blue and red; the sugar moiety presented in this complex were excluded for clarity. C - α-Bungarotoxin bound to the chimeric protein composed of N-terminal domain of nAChR α7 subunit and *L. stagnalis* AChBP (4HQP); toxins and chimeras are shown in blue and magenta.

70% of the amino-acid residues in *L. stagnalis*AChBP (not touching the less hydrophobic Cys-loop) for residues of the α7 subunit and crystallized this protein in free form and in complex with epibatidine, an potent but nonselective nAChR agonist[108]. The observed pentaoligomeric structure can be considered as the closest proximation to the 3D structure of the ligand-binding domain of the true α7 nAChR. Practically the same α7/AChBP chimera has been used to crystallize a complex with α-bungarotoxin [26]. Again, it was a pentaoligomer with 5 attached α-bungarotoxin molecules (see Figure 3, C). In general, disposition of α-bungarotoxin is very close to what was observed for α-bungarotoxin in complex with the α1 domain or for α-cobratoxin complex with the *L. stagnalis* AChBP (compare with Figure 3, B and A). Basing on the high-resolution structure of the α7/AChBP-α-bungarotoxin chimera, the authors designed a series of α7 nAChR mutants and from the analysis of their activities and efficiency of α-bungarotoxin binding collected a very detailed information about the intermolecular interactions which ensure the high affinity for α-bungarotoxin binding [26]. In particular, they not only confirmed the role of the "aromatic box", but also revealed the importance of amino-acid residues which in the amino acid sequence are direct neighbors of those aromatic residues.

5.3. X-ray structure structures of AChBP complexes with α-conotoxins

The first X-ray structure of the AChBP complex with α-conotoxin [109] has been solved soon after elucidation of the X-ray structure of the *L. stagnalis* AChBP complex with α-cobratoxin.

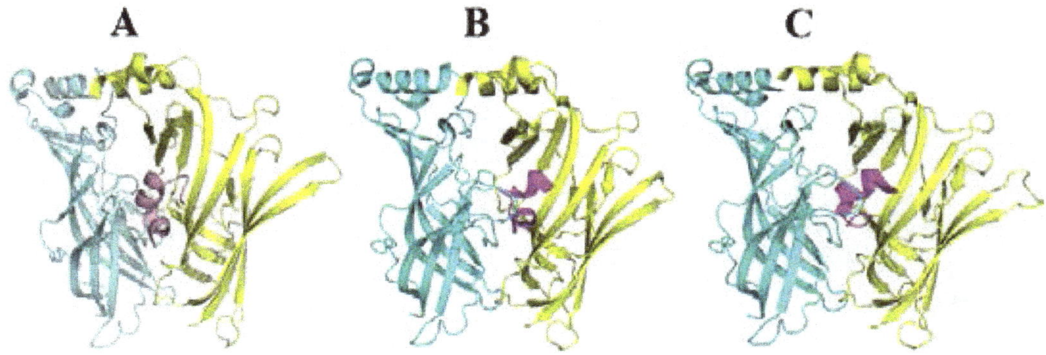

Figure 4. Spatial organization of complexes of α-conotoxins from different groups and *A. californica* AChBP derived from their crystal structures. Only two adjacent monomers of AChBP colored in cyan and yellow for clarity in side views are presented. All α-conotoxins are shown in magenta. A – complex with α-conotoxin PnIA[A10L, D14K] variant from 4/7 α-conotoxin group (PDB ID: 2BR8). B – complex with α-conotoxin ImI from 4/3 α-conotoxin group (2C9T). C - complex with α-conotoxin BuIA from 4/4 α-conotoxin group (4EZ1).

In this case it was another AChBP, namely the protein from the marine mollusk *Aplysia californica* [110]. First of all, contrary to the α-cobratoxin complex, it was a high-resolution (2.4 Å) structure and, secondly, it was the first X-ray structure for a representative of the huge conotoxin library in complex with a biological target. The crystals were raised for the complex of α-conotoxin PnIA analog having two substitutions ([A10L] and [D14K]) which had high affinity both for *L. stagnalis* and *A. californica* AChBPs and potently inhibited acetylcholine-induced currents in α7 nAChRs expressed in oocytes [109].

Hydrophobic contacts were found to play the major role in the interaction of α-conotoxin PnIA[A10L, D14K] with *A. californica* AChBP (Figure 4, A). As in other AChBP complexes with agonists or antagonists, at the principal side the contacts are formed mainly by highly conserved aromatic amino acid residues - Trp145, Tyr186, Tyr193. At the complementary side the contributions are from aliphatic residues (Val106, Met114, Ile116). It should be stressed again that loop C in the complex with α-conotoxin moves to the periphery of the AChBP molecule by more than 10 Å, as compared with its disposition in the "apo" form of *A. californica* AChBP. A similar shift was also observed, as mentioned above, for the α-cobratoxin complex [24], as well as for the majority of AChBP complexes with other antagonists (see reviews [98,111,112]). Thus, the conclusion that the most obvious distinction between the first steps in the binding modes of agonists versus antagonists is the induced movement of the loop C (to the central axis for the former and outwards for the latter) appears to be correct. However, there are some deviations from this trend: for example, strychnine is an antagonist both of the nAChRs and glycine receptors, but in the case of its complex with the *A. californica* AChBP, the loop C shift to the periphery was only very slight [113]. The changes in the disposition of the loop C were not pronounced also for AChBP complexes with partial agonists [96].

Another interesting feature of AChBP complexes was for the first time observed with partial agonists: in distinct binding sites within a pentameric AChBP molecule these compounds had different orientations [96]. Such multiplicity was first thought to be inherent only in partial agonists, but later altering dispositions in the 5 AChBP binding sites were observed for the complexes of such alkaloid antagonists as strychnine and d-tubocurarine [113]. Moreover, in several binding sites two alkaloid molecules managed to be accommodated simultaneously [113].

Variations of the ligand orientation in the binding sites of AChBPs and nAChRs are of undoubted interest. In the *A. californica* AChBP complex, all 5 bound α-conotoxin PnIA[A10L, D14K] molecules had the same conformation and orientation. This was also true for the later solved structures of α-conotoxin ImI complexes [114,115] (see Figure 4, B). These structures (very similar to those of α-conotoxin PnIA[A10L, D14K]) confirmed that, although bound α-conotoxin PnIA analog had two substitutions and was in this respect "unnatural α-conotoxin", the X-ray structure of its complex correctly revealed the structural principles of the α-conotoxin-AChBP recognition. Fine adjustments of such a recognition were brought to light by the structure of *A. californica* AChBP complex with the α-conotoxin TxIA[A10L] [116]. In general, the structure of this complex was very similar to those of α-conotoxin PnIA[A10L, D14K] or α-conotoxin ImI, but with a noticeable difference: this α-conotoxin derivative occupied exactly the same region as the two above-mentioned α-conotoxins, but it was turned around the central axis by about 20 degrees. The authors proposed that such rotation reflects certain differences in the selectivity of this particular α-conotoxin [116]. The latest published structure of the AChBP complex with α-conotoxin (November 2013) is announced by the Protein Data Bank (PDB) the structure with ID - 4EZ1. This is a complex of *A. californica* AChBP with α-conotoxin BuIA [117]. Despite the fact that α-conotoxin BuIA is a member of other subgroup of α-conotoxins (4/4) its position and orientation in the complex with AChBP (Figure 4, C) very close to that of both α-conotoxin PnIA analog (4/7 subgroup) and α-conotoxin ImI (4/3 subgroup) (compare Figure 4, A, B and C). In any case, from the four solved X-ray structures for AChBP complexes with α-conotoxins it followed that some variations in their attachment are possible. It might be expected that variations may be even more pronounced when α-conotoxins interact with true nAChRs, especially with heteroligomeric ones having different subunit interfaces.

Indeed, interpretation of the cross-linking of photoactivatable derivative of α-conotoxin GI to *Torpedo californica* nAChR in terms of the model built on the basis of the X-ray structure of the AChBP complex with α-conotoxin PnIA[A10L, D14K], suggested that for bound α-conotoxin two orientations are possible where the disposition of photoactivatable group differs by about 90 degrees [118]. Later a similar situation was demonstrated for an agonist, namely for the photoactivatable derivative of epibatidine [119]. This compound was shown to bind to only one site in the *T. californica* nAChR, but to 2 sites in the neuronal α4β2 nAChR which presumes two different dispositions of the bound ligand [119]. Naturally, cross-linking is not such a direct evidence as the X-ray structure, but the latter are available only for the AChBP complexes and the multiplicity of alkaloid antagonist orientations in the frames of one AChBP molecule [113] has been already mentioned.

6. Summary

In this chapter we tried to briefly present almost a 50-year history of using protein and peptide neurotoxins in fundamental and practical studies of nicotinic acetylcholine receptors (nAChRs). It was shown that the discovery of α-neurotoxins in the snake venoms was an extremely important step which made possible identification and isolation in individual form of the first nAChR from the *Torpedo* ray electric organ. Many laboratories comprehensively analyzed this receptor and it soon became clear that it is an appropriate model for nAChRs of all classes, namely muscle, neuronal and the so-called "non-neuronal" ones. Later, in addition to the three-finger α-neurotoxins, new shorter and smaller but not less efficient tools were found: namely, among a huge family of various peptides in the venoms of marine *Conus* mollusks, one particular group happened to be invaluable for research on nAChRs. Here we speak about α-conotoxins which not only discriminate the muscle-type from neuronal nAChRs, but some of them even are selective towards a particular neuronal nAChR subtype. One should not think that the discovery of α-conotoxins put the α-neurotoxins into archives. First of all, even to-day α-bungarotoxin and its radioactive and fluorescent derivatives are the most reliable tools for identification and measuring the levels of the functional $\alpha7$ nAChRs. Secondly, α-neurotoxins played another leading role a decade ago helping to purify the acetylcholine-binding protein (AChBP). The discovery and the X-ray structure of this protein, an ideal model for the ligand-binding domains of all nAChRs, was the major breakthrough in elucidating the three-dimensional structure of nAChRs and especially of their ligand-binding site topography. Our chapter also presented the data on the crystal structures of AChBP complexes both with α-neurotoxins and α-conotoxins that gave information about the topography of their interactions with the key residues in the binding site, thus providing a basis for new drug design. The next step was the establishment of the crystal structures of α-neurotoxins with chimera of AChBP and $\alpha7$ nAChR ligand-binding domain, which can be considered as a good mimic of the true $\alpha7$ receptor, as well as the X-ray structure of the α-bungarotoxin complex with a mutated nAChR $\alpha1$ subunit extracellular domain. In this chapter we were not discussing the bacterial pentameric ligand-gated ion channels (belonging to the same family as nAChRs), but at present not only high-resolution X-ray structures are available for them, but also for their complexes with different ligands. In particular, one of such receptors (ELIC) happened to be a close analog of the mammalian GABA-A receptors. We might hope that one day high resolution structures become available for nAChRs or their homologs in complexes with α-neurotoxins and/or α-conotoxins, to which the chapter is devoted. It will give new life to these still invaluable tools in fundamental research on nAChRs and in numerous practical applications.

Acknowledgements

The research was supported by RFBR grants and the grants of Presidium of RAS "Molecular and cellular biology" and "Fundamental principles of medicine".

Author details

Victor Tsetlin* and Igor Kasheverov

*Address all correspondence to: vits@mx.ibch.ru

Shemyakin-Ovchinnikov Institute of Bioorganic Chemistry, Russian Academy of Sciences, Moscow, Russian Federation

References

[1] Changeux JP. The nicotinic acetylcholine receptor: the founding father of the pentameric ligand-gated ion channel superfamily. Journal of Biological Chemistry 2012;287(48) 40207-40215.

[2] Kalamida D, Poulas K, Avramopoulou V, Fostieri E, Lagoumintzis G, Lazaridis K, Sideri A, Zouridakis M, Tzartos SJ. Muscle and neuronal nicotinic acetylcholine receptors. Structure, function and pathogenicity. FEBS Journal 2007;274(15) 3799-3845.

[3] Tsetlin V, Hucho F. Nicotinic acetylcholine receptors at atomic resolution. Current Opinion in Pharmacology 2009;9(3) 306-310.

[4] Sine SM, Engel AG. Recent advances in Cys-loop receptor structure and function. Nature 2006;440(7083) 448-455.

[5] Gershoni JM. Expression of the alpha-bungarotoxin binding site of the nicotinic acetylcholine receptor by Escherichia coli transformants. Proceedings of the National Academy of Sciences of the USA 1987;84(12) 4318-4321.

[6] Wilson PT, Hawrot E, Lentz TL. Distribution of alpha-bungarotoxin binding sites over residues 173-204 of the alpha subunit of the acetylcholine receptor. Molecular Pharmacology 1988;34(5) 643-650.

[7] Wessler I, Kirkpatrick CJ. Acetylcholine beyond neurons: the non-neuronal cholinergic system in humans. British Journal of Pharmacology 2008;154(8) 1558-1571.

[8] Fujii T, Takada-Takatori Y, Kawashima K. Basic and clinical aspects of non-neuronal acetylcholine: expression of an independent, non-neuronal cholinergic system in lymphocytes and its clinical significance in immunotherapy. Journal of Pharmacological Sciences 2008;106(2) 186-192.

[9] Picciotto MR, Kenny PJ. Molecular mechanisms underlying behaviors related to nicotine addiction. Cold Spring Harbor Perspectives in Medicine 2013;3(1) a012112. doi: 10.1101/cshperspect.a012112.

[10] Brejc K, van Dijk WJ, Klaassen RV, Schuurmans M, van Der Oost J, Smit AB, Sixma TK. Crystal structure of an ACh-binding protein reveals the ligand-binding domain of nicotinic receptors. Nature 2001;411(6835) 269-276.

[11] Hilf RJ, Dutzler R. X-ray structure of a prokaryotic pentameric ligand-gated ion channel. Nature 2008;452(7185) 375-379.

[12] Hilf RJ, Dutzler R. Structure of a potentially open state of a proton-activated pentameric ligand-gated ion channel. Nature 2009;457(7225) 115-118.

[13] Bocquet N, Nury H, Baaden M, Le Poupon C, Changeux JP, Delarue M, Corringer PJ. X-ray structure of a pentameric ligand-gated ion channel in an apparently open conformation. Nature 2009;457(7225) 111-114.

[14] Hibbs RE, Gouaux E. Principles of activation and permeation in an anion-selective Cys-loop receptor. Nature 2011;474(7349) 54-60.

[15] Chang CC. Looking back on the discovery of α-bungarotoxin. Journal of Biomedical Sciences 1999;6(6) 368-375.

[16] Tsetlin V. Snake venom α-neurotoxins and other 'three-finger' proteins. European Journal of Biochemistry 1999;264(2) 281-286.

[17] Kini RM, Doley R. Structure, function and evolution of three-finger toxins: mini proteins with multiple targets. Toxicon 2010;56(6) 855-867.

[18] Low BW, Preston HS, Sato A, Rosen LS, Searl JE, Rudko AD, Richardson JS. Three dimensional structure of erabutoxin b neurotoxic protein: inhibitor of acetylcholine receptor. Proceedings of the National Academy of Sciences of the USA 1976;73(9) 2991-2994.

[19] Tsernoglou D, Petsko GA. Three-dimensional structure of neurotoxin a from venom of the Philippines sea snake. Proceedings of the National Academy of Sciences of the USA 1977;74(3) 971-974.

[20] Love R, Stroud R. The crystal structure of α-bungarotoxin at 2.5 Å resolution: relation to solution structure and binding to acetylcholine receptor. Protein Engineering 1986;1(1) 37-46.

[21] Moise L, Piserchio A, Basus VJ, Hawrot E. NMR structural analysis of α-bungarotoxin and its complex with the principal α-neurotoxin-binding sequence on the $\alpha7$ subunit of a neuronal nicotinic acetylcholine receptor. Journal of Biological Chemistry 2002;277(14) 12406-12417.

[22] Betzel C, Lange G, Pal GP, Wilson KS, Maelicke A, Saenger W. The refined crystal structure of alpha-cobratoxin from Naja naja siamensis at 2.4-Å resolution. Journal of Biological Chemistry 1991;266(32) 21530-21536.

[23] Nickitenko AV, Michailov AM, Betzel C, Wilson KS. Three-dimensional structure of neurotoxin-1 from Naja naja oxiana venom at 1.9 Å resolution. FEBS Letters 1993;320(2) 111-117.

[24] Bourne Y, Talley TT, Hansen SB, Taylor P, Marchot P.Crystal structure of a Cbtx-AChBP complex reveals essential interactions between snake alpha-neurotoxins and nicotinic receptors. EMBO Journal 2005;24(8) 1512-1522.

[25] Dellisanti CD, Yao Y, Stroud JC, Wang ZZ, Chen L. Crystal structure of the extracellular domain of nAChR alpha1 bound to alpha-bungarotoxin at 1.94 Å resolution. Nature Neuroscience 2007;10(8) 953-962.

[26] Huang S, Li SX, Bren N, Cheng K, Gomoto R, Chen L, Sine SM. Complex between α-bungarotoxin and an α7 nicotinic receptor ligand-binding domain chimaera. Biochemical Journal 2013;454(2) 303-310.

[27] Dewan JC, Grant GA, Sacchettini JC. Crystal structure of κ-bungarotoxin at 2.3-A resolution. Biochemistry 1994;33(44) 13147-13154.

[28] Chiappinelli VA, Weaver WR, McLane KE, Conti-Fine BM, Fiordalisi JJ, Grant GA. Binding of native κ-neurotoxins and site-directed mutants to nicotinic acetylcholine receptors. Toxicon 1996;34(11-12) 1243-1256.

[29] Servent D, Winckler-Dietrich V, Hu HY, Kessler P, Drevet P, Bertrand D, Ménez A. Only snake curaremimetic toxins with a fifth disulfide bond have high affinity for the neuronal α7 nicotinic receptor. Journal of Biological Chemistry 1997;272(39) 24279-24286.

[30] Grant GA, Luetje CW, Summers R, Xu XL. Differential roles for disulfide bonds in the structural integrity and biological activity of κ-bungarotoxin, a neuronal nicotinic acetylcholine receptor antagonist. Biochemistry 1998;37(35) 12166-12171.

[31] Mourier G, Servent D, Zinn-Justin S, Ménez A. Chemical engineering of a three-fingered toxin with anti-α7 neuronal acetylcholine receptor activity. Protein Engineering 2000;13(3) 217-225.

[32] Lyukmanova EN, Shenkarev ZO, Schulga AA, Ermolyuk YS, Mordvintsev DY, Utkin YN, Shoulepko MA, Hogg RC, Bertrand D, Dolgikh DA, Tsetlin VI, Kirpichnikov MP. Bacterial expression, NMR, and electrophysiology analysis of chimeric short/long-chain α-neurotoxins acting on neuronal nicotinic receptors. Journal of Biological Chemistry 2007;282(34) 24784-24791.

[33] Roy A, Zhou X, Chong MZ, D'hoedt D, Foo CS, Rajagopalan N, Nirthanan S, Bertrand D, Sivaraman J, Kini RM. Structural and functional characterization of a novel homodimeric three-finger neurotoxin from the venom of Ophiophagus hannah (king cobra). Journal of Biological Chemistry 2010;285(11) 8302-8315.

[34] Kukhtina VV, Weise C, Muranova TA, Starkov VG, Franke P, Hucho F, Wnendt S, Gillen C, Tsetlin VI, Utkin YN. Muscarinic toxin-like proteins from cobra venom. European Journal of Biochemistry 2000;267(23) 6784-6789.

[35] Osipov AV, Kasheverov IE, Makarova YV, Starkov VG, Vorontsova OV, Ziganshin RK, Andreeva TV, Serebryakova MV, Benoit A, Hogg RC, Bertrand D, Tsetlin VI, Utkin YN. Naturally occurring disulfide-bound dimers of three-fingered toxins: a paradigm for biological activity diversification. Journal of Biological Chemistry 2008;283(21) 14571-14580.

[36] Osipov AV, Rucktooa P, Kasheverov IE, Filkin SY, Starkov VG, Andreeva TV, Sixma TK, Bertrand D, Utkin YN, Tsetlin VI. Dimeric α-cobratoxin X-ray structure: localization of intermolecular disulfides and possible mode of binding to nicotinic acetylcholine receptors. Journal of Biological Chemistry 2012;287(9) 6725-6734.

[37] Pawlak J, Mackessy SP, Sixberry NM, Stura EA, Le Du MH, Ménez R, Foo CS, Ménez A, Nirthanan S, Kini RM. Irditoxin, a novel covalently linked heterodimeric three-finger toxin with high taxon-specific neurotoxicity. FASEB Journal 2009;23(2) 534-545.

[38] Nirthanan S, Gopalakrishnakone P, Gwee MC, Khoo HE, Kini RM. Non-conventional toxins from Elapid venoms. British Journal of Pharmacology 2003;139(4) 832-844.

[39] Utkin YN, Kukhtina VV, Kryukova EV, Chiodini F, Bertrand D, Methfessel C, Tsetlin VI. "Weak toxin" from Naja kaouthia is a nontoxic antagonist of $\alpha 7$ and muscle-type nicotinic acetylcholine receptors. Journal of Biological Chemistry 2001;276(19) 15810-15815.

[40] Nirthanan S, Charpantier E, Gopalakrishnakone P, Gwee MC, Khoo HE, Cheah LS, Bertrand D, Kini RM. Candoxin, a novel toxin from Bungarus candidus, is a reversible antagonist of muscle ($\alpha\beta\gamma\delta$) but a poorly reversible antagonist of neuronal $\alpha 7$ nicotinic acetylcholine receptors. Journal of Biological Chemistry 2002;277(20) 17811-17820.

[41] Pawlak J, Mackessy SP, Fry BG, Bhatia M, Mourier G, Fruchart-Gaillard C, Servent D, Ménez R, Stura E, Ménez A, Kini RM. Denmotoxin, a three-finger toxin from the colubrid snake Boiga dendrophila (Mangrove Catsnake) with bird-specific activity. Journal of Biological Chemistry 2006;281(39) 29030-29041.

[42] Mordvintsev DY, Rodionov DI, Makarova MV, Kamensky AA, Levitskaya NG, Ogay AY, Rzhevsky DI, Murashev AN, Tsetlin VI, Utkin YN. Behavioural effects in mice and intoxication symptomatology of weak neurotoxin from cobra Naja kaouthia. Basic and Clinical Pharmacology and Toxicology 2007;100(4) 273-278.

[43] Mordvintsev DY, Polyak YL, Rodionov DI, Jakubik J, Dolezal V, Karlsson E, Tsetlin VI, Utkin YN. Weak toxin WTX from Naja kaouthia cobra venom interacts with both nicotinic and muscarinic acetylcholine receptors. FEBS Journal 2009;276(18) 5065-5075.

[44] Ménez A. Functional architectures of animal toxins: a clue to drug design? Toxicon 1998;36(11) 1557-1572.

[45] Olianas MC, Adem A, Karlsson E, Onali P. Action of the muscarinic toxin MT7 on agonist-bound muscarinic M1 receptors. European Journal of Pharmacology 2004;487(1-3) 65-72.

[46] Marquer C, Fruchart-Gaillard C, Letellier G, Marcon E, Mourier G, Zinn-Justin S, Ménez A, Servent D, Gilquin B. Structural model of ligand-G protein-coupled receptor (GPCR) complex based on experimental double mutant cycle data: MT7 snake toxin bound to dimeric hM1 muscarinic receptor. Journal of Biological Chemistry 2011;286(36) 31661-31675.

[47] de Weille JR, Schweitz H, Maes P, Tartar A, Lazdunski M. Calciseptine, a peptide isolated from black mamba venom, is a specific blocker of the L-type calcium channel. Proceedings of the National Academy of Sciences of the USA 1991;88(6) 2437-2440.

[48] Albrand JP, Blackledge MJ, Pascaud F, Hollecker M, Marion D. NMR and restrained molecular dynamics study of the three-dimensional solution structure of toxin FS2, a specific blocker of the L-type calcium channel, isolated from black mamba venom. Biochemistry 1995;34(17) 5923-5937.

[49] Bourne Y, Taylor P, Marchot P. Acetylcholinesterase inhibition by fasciculin: crystal structure of the complex. Cell 1995;83(3) 503-512.

[50] Harel M, Kleywegt GJ, Ravelli RB, Silman I, Sussman JL. Crystal structure of an acetylcholinesterase-fasciculin complex: interaction of a three-fingered toxin from snake venom with its target. Structure 1995;3(12) 1355-1366.

[51] Kumar TK, Jayaraman G, Lee CS, Arunkumar AI, Sivaraman T, Samuel D, Yu C. Snake venom cardiotoxins-structure, dynamics, function and folding. Journal of Biomolecular Structure and Dynamics 1997;15(3) 431-463.

[52] Konshina AG, Dubovskii PV, Efremov RG. Structure and dynamics of cardiotoxins. Current Protein and Peptide Science 2012;13(6) 570-584.

[53] Osipov AV, Astapova MV, Tsetlin VI, Utkin YN. The first representative of glycosylated three-fingered toxins. Cytotoxin from the Naja kaouthia cobra venom. European Journal of Biochemistry 2004;271(10) 2018-2027.

[54] Quinton L, Girard E, Maiga A, Rekik M, Lluel P, Masuyer G, Larregola M, Marquer C, Ciolek J, Magnin T, Wagner R, Molgó J, Thai R, Fruchart-Gaillard C, Mourier G, Chamot-Rooke J, Ménez A, Palea S, Servent D, Gilles N. Isolation and pharmacological characterization of AdTx1, a natural peptide displaying specific insurmountable antagonism of the alpha1A-adrenoceptor. British Journal of Pharmacology 2010;159(2) 316-325.

[55] Maïga A, Mourier G, Quinton L, Rouget C, Gales C, Denis C, Lluel P, Sénard JM, Palea S, Servent D, Gilles N. G protein-coupled receptors, an unexploited animal toxin

targets: Exploration of green mamba venom for novel drug candidates active against adrenoceptors. Toxicon 2012;59(4) 487-496.

[56] Miwa JM, Ibanez-Tallon I, Crabtree GW, Sánchez R, Sali A, Role LW, Heintz N. Lynx1, an endogenous toxin-like modulator of nicotinic acetylcholine receptors in the mammalian CNS. Neuron 1999;23(1) 105-114.

[57] Adermann K, Wattler F, Wattler S, Heine G, Meyer M, Forssmann WG, Nehls M. Structural and phylogenetic characterization of human SLURP-1, the first secreted mammalian member of the Ly-6/uPAR protein superfamily. Protein Science 1999;8(4) 810-819.

[58] Miwa JM, Stevens TR, King SL, Caldarone BJ, Ibanez-Tallon I, Xiao C, Fitzsimonds RM, Pavlides C, Lester HA, Picciotto MR, Heintz N. The prototoxin lynx1 acts on nicotinic acetylcholine receptors to balance neuronal activity and survival in vivo. Neuron 2006;51(5) 587-600.

[59] Tekinay AB, Nong Y, Miwa JM, Lieberam I, Ibanez-Tallon I, Greengard P, Heintz N. A role for LYNX2 in anxiety-related behavior. Proc Natl Acad Sci U S A. 2009 Mar 17;106(11):4477-82.

[60] Lyukmanova EN, Shenkarev ZO, Shulepko MA, Mineev KS, D'Hoedt D, Kasheverov IE, Filkin SY, Krivolapova AP, Janickova H, Dolezal V, Dolgikh DA, Arseniev AS, Bertrand D, Tsetlin VI, Kirpichnikov MP. NMR structure and action on nicotinic acetylcholine receptors of water-soluble domain of human LYNX1. Journal of Biological Chemistry 2011;286(12) 10618-10627.

[61] Shulepko MA, Lyukmanova EN, Paramonov AS, Lobas AA, Shenkarev ZO, Kasheverov IE, Dolgikh DA, Tsetlin VI, Arseniev AS, Kirpichnikov MP. Human neuromodulator SLURP-1: bacterial expression, binding to muscle-type nicotinic acetylcholine receptor, secondary structure, and conformational heterogeneity in solution. Biochemistry (Moscow) 2013;78(2) 204-211.

[62] Lyukmanova EN, Shulepko MA, Buldakova SL, Kasheverov IE, Shenkarev ZO, Reshetnikov RV, Filkin SY, Kudryavtsev DS, Ojomoko LO, Kryukova EV, Dolgikh DA, Kirpichnikov MP, Bregestovski PD, Tsetlin VI. Water-soluble LYNX1 residues important for interaction with muscle-type and/or neuronal nicotinic receptors. Journal of Biological Chemistry 2013;288(22) 15888-15899.

[63] Thomsen MS, Cinar B, Jensen MM, Lyukmanova EN, Shulepko MA, Tsetlin V, Klein AB, Mikkelsen JD. Expression of the Ly-6 family proteins Lynx1 and Ly6H in the rat brain is compartmentalized, cell-type specific, and developmentally regulated. Brain Structure and Function 2013. doi 10.1007/s00429-013-0611-x.

[64] Weinstein SA, Schmidt JJ, Bernheimer AW, Smith LA. Characterization and amino acid sequences of two lethal peptides isolated from venom of Wagler's pit viper, Trimeresurus wagleri. Toxicon 1991;29(2) 227-236.

[65] Schmidt JJ, Weinstein SA, Smith LA. Molecular properties and structure-function relationships of lethal peptides from venom of Wagler's pit viper, Trimeresurus wagleri. Toxicon 1992;30(9) 1027-1036.

[66] Tsai MC, Hsieh WH, Smith LA, Lee CY. Effects of waglerin-I on neuromuscular transmission of mouse nerve-muscle preparations. Toxicon 1995;33(3) 363-371.

[67] McArdle JJ, Lentz TL, Witzemann V, Schwarz H, Weinstein SA, Schmidt JJ. Waglerin-1 selectively blocks the epsilon form of the muscle nicotinic acetylcholine receptor. Journal of Pharmacology and Experimental Therapeutics 1999;289(1) 543-550.

[68] Molles BE, Rezai P, Kline EF, McArdle JJ, Sine SM, Taylor P. Identification of residues at the α and ε subunit interfaces mediating species selectivity of Waglerin-1 for nicotinic acetylcholine receptors. Journal of Biological Chemistry 2002;277(7) 5433-5440.

[69] Molles BE, Tsigelny I, Nguyen PD, Gao SX, Sine SM, Taylor P. Residues in the ε subunit of the nicotinic acetylcholine receptor interact to confer selectivity of waglerin-1 for the α-ε subunit interface site. Biochemistry 2002;41(25) 7895-7906.

[70] Schmidt JJ, Weinstein SA. Structure-function studies of waglerin I, a lethal peptide from the venom of Wagler's pit viper, Trimeresurus wagleri. Toxicon 1995;33(8) 1043-1049.

[71] Utkin YN, Weise C, Kasheverov IE, Andreeva TV, Kryukova EV, Zhmak MN, Starkov VG, Hoang NA, Bertrand D, Ramerstorfer J, Sieghart W, Thompson AJ, Lummis SC, Tsetlin VI. Azemiopsin from Azemiops feae viper venom, a novel polypeptide ligand of nicotinic acetylcholine receptor. Journal of Biological Chemistry 2012;287(32) 27079-27086.

[72] Gray WR, Luque A, Olivera BM, Barrett J, Cruz LJ. Peptide toxins from Conus geographus venom. Journal of Biological Chemistry 1981;256(10) 4734-4740.

[73] Halai R, Craik DJ. Conotoxins: natural product drug leads. Natural Product Reports 2009;26(4) 526-536.

[74] Teichert RW, Olivera BM. Natural products and ion channel pharmacology. Future Medicinal Chemistry 2010;2(5) 731-444.

[75] Lewis RJ, Dutertre S, Vetter I, Christie MJ. Conus venom peptide pharmacology. Pharmacological Reviews 2012;64(2) 259-298.

[76] Kreienkamp HJ, Sine SM, Maeda RK, Taylor P. Glycosylation sites selectively interfere with α-toxin binding to the nicotinic acetylcholine receptor. Journal of Biological Chemistry 1994;269(11) 8108-8114.

[77] Groebe DR, Dumm JM, Levitan ES, Abramson SN. α-Conotoxins selectively inhibit one of the two acetylcholine binding sites of nicotinic receptors. Molecular Pharmacology 1995;48(1) 105-111.

[78] Utkin YN, Kobayashi Y, Hucho F, Tsetlin VI. Relationship between the binding sites for an α-conotoxin and snake venom neurotoxins in the nicotinic acetylcholine receptor from Torpedo californica. Toxicon 1994;32(9) 1153-1157.

[79] Hann RM, Pagán OR, Eterović VA. The α-conotoxins GI and MI distinguish between the nicotinic acetylcholine receptor agonist sites while SI does not. Biochemistry 1994;33(47) 14058-14063.

[80] Groebe DR, Gray WR, Abramson SN. Determinants involved in the affinity of α-conotoxins GI and SI for the muscle subtype of nicotinic acetylcholine receptors. Biochemistry 1997;36(21) 6469-6474.

[81] Hann RM, Pagan OR, Gregory LM, Jacome T, Eterovic VA. The 9-arginine residue of α-conotoxin GI is responsible for its selective high affinity for the $\alpha\gamma$ agonist site on the electric organ acetylcholine receptor. Biochemistry 1997;36(29) 9051-9056.

[82] Jacobsen RB, DelaCruz RG, Grose JH, McIntosh JM, Yoshikami D, Olivera BM. Critical residues influence the affinity and selectivity of α-conotoxin MI for nicotinic acetylcholine receptors. Biochemistry 1999;38(40) 13310-13315.

[83] Ellison M, Feng ZP, Park AJ, Zhang X, Olivera BM, McIntosh JM, Norton RS. α-RgIA, a novel conotoxin that blocks the $\alpha9\alpha10$ nAChR: structure and identification of key receptor-binding residues. Journal of Molecular Biology 2008;377(4) 1216-1227.

[84] Servent D, Thanh HL, Antil S, Bertrand D, Corringer PJ, Changeux JP, Ménez A. Functional determinants by which snake and cone snail toxins block the $\alpha7$ neuronal nicotinic acetylcholine receptors. Journal of Physiology-Paris 1998;92(2) 107-111.

[85] Hogg RC, Hopping G, Alewood PF, Adams DJ, Bertrand D. α-Conotoxins PnIA and [A10L]PnIA stabilize different states of the $\alpha7$-L247T nicotinic acetylcholine receptor. Journal of Biological Chemistry 2003;278(29) 26908-26914.

[86] Everhart D, Cartier GE, Malhotra A, Gomes AV, McIntosh JM, Luetje CW. Determinants of potency on α-conotoxin MII, a peptide antagonist of neuronal nicotinic receptors. Biochemistry 2004;43(10) 2732-2737.

[87] Millard EL, Nevin ST, Loughnan ML, Nicke A, Clark RJ, Alewood PF, Lewis RJ, Adams DJ, Craik DJ, Daly NL. Inhibition of neuronal nicotinic acetylcholine receptor subtypes by α-conotoxin GID and analogues. Journal of Biological Chemistry 2009;284(8) 4944-4951.

[88] Halai R, Clark RJ, Nevin ST, Jensen JE, Adams DJ, Craik DJ. Scanning mutagenesis of α-conotoxin Vc1.1 reveals residues crucial for activity at the $\alpha9\alpha10$ nicotinic acetylcholine receptor. Journal of Biological Chemistry 2009;284(30) 20275-20284.

[89] Grishin AA, Cuny H, Hung A, Clark RJ, Brust A, Akondi K, Alewood PF, Craik DJ, Adams DJ. Identifying key amino acid residues that affect α-conotoxin AuIB inhibition of $\alpha3\beta4$ nicotinic acetylcholine receptors. Journal of Biological Chemistry 2013. doi: 10.1074/jbc.M113.512582.

[90] Kasheverov IE, Utkin YN, Tsetlin VI. Naturally occurring and synthetic peptides acting on nicotinic acetylcholine receptors. Current Pharmaceutical Design 2009;15(21) 2430-2452.

[91] Armishaw CJ. Synthetic α-conotoxin mutants as probes for studying nicotinic acetylcholine receptors and in the development of novel drug leads. Toxins (Basel) 2010;2(6) 1471-1499.

[92] Muttenthaler M, Akondi KB, Alewood PF. Structure-activity studies on α-conotoxins. Current Pharmaceutical Design 2011;17(38) 4226-4241.

[93] Smit AB, Syed NI, Schaap D, van Minnen J, Klumperman J, Kits KS, Lodder H, van der Schors RC, van Elk R, Sorgedrager B, Brejc K, Sixma TK, Geraerts WP. A glia-derived acetylcholine-binding protein that modulates synaptic transmission. Nature 2001;411(6835) 261-268.

[94] Celie PH, van Rossum-Fikkert SE, van Dijk WJ, Brejc K, Smit AB, Sixma TK. Nicotine and carbamylcholine binding to nicotinic acetylcholine receptors as studied in AChBP crystal structures. Neuron 2004;41(6) 907-914.

[95] Ulens C, Akdemir A, Jongejan A, van Elk R, Bertrand S, Perrakis A, Leurs R, Smit AB, Sixma TK, Bertrand D, de Esch IJ. Use of acetylcholine binding protein in the search for novel α7 nicotinic receptor ligands. In silico docking, pharmacological screening, and X-ray analysis. Journal of Medicinal Chemistry 2009;52(8) 2372-2383.

[96] Hibbs RE, Sulzenbacher G, Shi J, Talley TT, Conrod S, Kem WR, Taylor P, Marchot P, Bourne Y. Structural determinants for interaction of partial agonists with acetylcholine binding protein and neuronal α7 nicotinic acetylcholine receptor. EMBO Journal 2009;28(19) 3040-3051.

[97] Akdemir A, Rucktooa P, Jongejan A, Elk Rv, Bertrand S, Sixma TK, Bertrand D, Smit AB, Leurs R, de Graaf C, de Esch IJ. Acetylcholine binding protein (AChBP) as template for hierarchical in silico screening procedures to identify structurally novel ligands for the nicotinic receptors. Bioorganic and Medicinal Chemistry 2011;19(20) 6107-6119.

[98] Rucktooa P, Smit AB, Sixma TK. Insight in nAChR subtype selectivity from AChBP crystal structures. Biochemical Pharmacology 2009;78(7) 777-787.

[99] Yakel JL. Gating of nicotinic ACh receptors: latest insights into ligand binding and function. Journal of Physiology 2010;588(Pt 4) 597-602.

[100] [100] Hucho F, Tsetlin VI, Machold J. The emerging three-dimensional structure of a receptor. The nicotinic acetylcholine receptor. European Journal of Biochemistry 1996;239(3) 539-557.

[101] Fruchart-Gaillard C, Gilquin B, Antil-Delbeke S, Le Novere N, Tamiya T, Corringer PJ, Changeux JP, Menez A, Servent D. Experimentally based model of a complex be-

tween a snake toxin and the $\alpha 7$ nicotinic receptor. Proceedings of the National Academy of Sciences of the USA 2002;99(5) 3216-3221.

[102] Tsetlin VI, Hucho F. Snake and snail toxins acting on nicotinic acetylcholine receptors: fundamental aspects and medical applications. FEBS Letters 2004;557(1-3) 9-13.

[103] Gershoni JM, Hawrot E, Lentz TL. Binding of α-bungarotoxin to isolated α subunit of the acetylcholine receptor of Torpedo californica: quantitative analysis with protein blots. Proceedings of the National Academy of Sciences of the USA 1983;80(16) 4973-4977.

[104] Schrattenholz A, Pfeiffer S, Pejovic V, Rudolph R, Godovac-Zimmermann J, Maelicke A. Expression and renaturation of the N-terminal extracellular domain of Torpedo nicotinic acetylcholine receptor α-subunit. Journal of Biological Chemistry 1998;273(49) 32393-32399.

[105] Tsetlin VI, Dergousova NI, Azeeva EA, Kryukova EV, Kudelina IA, Shibanova ED, Kasheverov IE, Methfessel C. Refolding of the Escherichia coli expressed extracellular domain of $\alpha 7$ nicotinic acetylcholine receptor (Cys116 mutation diminishes aggregation and stabilizes the β structure). European Journal of Biochemistry 2002;269(11) 2801-2809.

[106] Zouridakis M, Zisimopoulou P, Eliopoulos E, Poulas K, Tzartos SJ. Design and expression of human $\alpha 7$ nicotinic acetylcholine receptor extracellular domain mutants with enhanced solubility and ligand-binding properties. Biochimica et Biophysica Acta 2009;1794(2) 355-366.

[107] Li SX, Huang S, Bren N, Noridomi K, Dellisanti CD, Sine SM, Chen L. Ligand-binding domain of an $\alpha 7$-nicotinic receptor chimera and its complex with agonist. Nature Neuroscience 2011;14(10) 1253-1259.

[108] Dukat M, Glennon RA. Epibatidine: impact on nicotinic receptor research. Cellular and Molecular Neurobiology 2003;23(3) 365-378.

[109] Celie PH, Kasheverov IE, Mordvintsev DY, Hogg RC, van Nierop P, van Elk R, van Rossum-Fikkert SE, Zhmak MN, Bertrand D, Tsetlin V, Sixma TK, Smit AB. Crystal structure of nicotinic acetylcholine receptor homolog AChBP in complex with an α-conotoxin PnIA variant. Nature Structural and Molecular Biology 2005;12(7) 582-588.

[110] Hansen SB, Talley TT, Radic Z, Taylor P. Structural and ligand recognition characteristics of an acetylcholine-binding protein from Aplysia californica. Journal of Biological Chemistry 2004;279(23) 24197-24202.

[111] Dutertre S, Lewis RJ. Toxin insights into nicotinic acetylcholine receptors. Biochemical Pharmacology 2006;72(6) 661-670.

[112] Tsetlin V, Utkin Y, Kasheverov I. Polypeptide and peptide toxins, magnifying lenses for binding sites in nicotinic acetylcholine receptors. Biochemical Pharmacology 2009;78(7) 720-731.

[113] Brams M, Pandya A, Kuzmin D, van Elk R, Krijnen L, Yakel JL, Tsetlin V, Smit AB, Ulens C. A structural and mutagenic blueprint for molecular recognition of strychnine and d-tubocurarine by different cys-loop receptors. PLoS Biology 2011;9(3) e1001034.

[114] Hansen SB, Sulzenbacher G, Huxford T, Marchot P, Taylor P, Bourne Y. Structures of Aplysia AChBP complexes with nicotinic agonists and antagonists reveal distinctive binding interfaces and conformations. EMBO Journal 2005;24(20) 3635-46.

[115] Ulens C, Hogg RC, Celie PH, Bertrand D, Tsetlin V, Smit AB, Sixma TK. Structural determinants of selective α-conotoxin binding to a nicotinic acetylcholine receptor homolog AChBP. Proceedings of the National Academy of Sciences of the USA 2006;103(10) 3615-3620.

[116] Dutertre S, Ulens C, Büttner R, Fish A, van Elk R, Kendel Y, Hopping G, Alewood PF, Schroeder C, Nicke A, Smit AB, Sixma TK, Lewis RJ. AChBP-targeted α-conotoxin correlates distinct binding orientations with nAChR subtype selectivity. EMBO Journal 2007;26(16) 3858-3867.

[117] Talley TT, Reger AS, Kim C, Sankaran B, Ho K, Taylor P, McIntosh J.M. Crystal structure of acetylcholine binding protein (AChBP) from Aplysia Californica in complex with α-conotoxin BuIA. 2013. doi: 10.2210/pdb4ez1/pdb.

[118] Kasheverov IE, Chiara DC, Zhmak MN, Maslennikov IV, Pashkov VS, Arseniev AS, Utkin YN, Cohen JB, Tsetlin VI. α-Conotoxin GI benzoylphenylalanine derivatives. ^{1}H-NMR structures and photoaffinity labeling of the Torpedo californica nicotinic acetylcholine receptor. FEBS Journal 2006;273(7) 1373-1388.

[119] Srivastava S, Hamouda AK, Pandhare A, Duddempudi PK, Sanghvi M, Cohen JB, Blanton MP. [(3)H]Epibatidine photolabels non-equivalent amino acids in the agonist binding site of Torpedo and $\alpha4\beta2$ nicotinic acetylcholine receptors. Journal of Biological Chemistry 2009;284(37) 24939-24947.

7

Neurochemical Communication: The Case of Endocannabinoids

Thomas Heinbockel

1. Introduction

The brain is equipped with a magnificent diversity of molecules that allow neurons to communicate with each other. Some of these molecules have been known to function as neurotransmitters for several decades such as GABA and glutamate while for others their involvement in brain signaling has been demonstrated more recently. Cannabinoids fall into the latter group. Even though the effects of cannabinoids as active ingredients in marijuana on human psyche and behavior have been experienced by humans for centuries or possibly millennia, their existence and production in the brain was described only some thirty years ago. Even more recently, their functional role in neural circuits of the brain has been discerned. This review focuses on these endogenously produced signaling molecules, endogenous cannabinoids or endocannabinoids (eCBs). Their functional role in the nervous system and interaction with other neurotransmitter systems will be described. One hallmark feature of endocannabinoid signaling is their ability to act as retrograde messengers in neural circuits. Two examples, one from the hippocampus and one from the main olfactory bulb, illustrate in detail this intercellular communication pathway.

Several features underscore the importance to understand the endocannabinoid system. Increasing evidence demonstrates the relevance of endocannabinoids in normal behaviors, including pain reception [1] and feeding [2, 3]. The therapeutic potential of cannabinoids has received increasing attention over the past few years [4]. endocannabinoids play a role in neuroprotection against acute excitotoxicity [5] and functional recovery after brain injury [6]. Endocannabinoids regulate human airway function and provide a means to treat respiratory pathologies [1]. Cannabinoids are in widespread use recreationally as psychoactive drugs and interact with other drugs of abuse. This fact emphasizes even more the need to understand the endocannabinoid system and the neurobiological substrate of their mood-altering capacity [7,

8]. Furthermore, the endocannabinoid system is crucially involved in processes of learning and memory, e.g., in the extinction of aversive memories [9].

2. The endocannabinoid system

Endocannabinoids are small lipids that regulate various aspects of brain function such as learning and memory including synaptic transmission and different forms of short-and long-term plasticity [10]. They also influence growth and development such as synapse formation and neurogenesis. Other biological functions modulated by endocannabinoids include eating and anxiety. Principally, two endocannabinoids, N-arachidonoylethanol-amide (anandamide, AEA) and 2-arachidonoylglycerol (2-AG) are the natural agonists/ligands of the most widely expressed cannabinoid receptor in the brain, CB1R [11] (Figure 1).

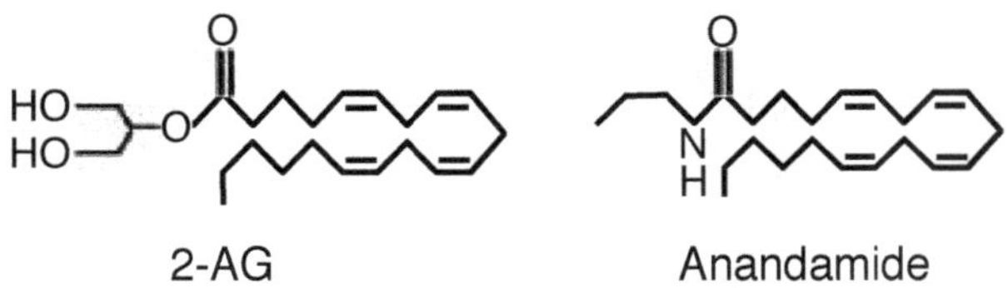

Figure 1. Two endocannabinoids, 2-arachidonoylglycerol (2-AG) and N-arachidonoylethanol-amide (anandamide, AEA), are the natural agonists/ligands of cannabinoid receptors, CB1Rs, in the brain.

Endocannabinoids, as fatty-acid derived endogenous ligands, together with their G-protein coupled cannabinoid receptors form the endocannabinoid system. This system also includes associated biochemical machinery with endocannabinoid precursors, synthetic and degradative enzymes for these lipidic neurotransmitters, and transporters [12-15]. Two different cannabinoid receptors have been cloned, CB1 and CB2 receptors. They share 44% amino acid sequence homology [16, 17]. The expression pattern of the two cannabinoid receptors in various body parts is distinctly different. In the brain, CB1R is the most abundant G-protein coupled receptor [18]. CB2R is primarily expressed in immune cells and peripheral tissues [17]. Some level of CB2R expression has also been detected in the brainstem, cortex and cerebellar neurons and microglia [19, 20].

Cannabinoid receptors are found at high levels in the brain [21, 22], specifically at presynaptic nerve terminals [23, 24]. They can be activated by cannabis-derived drugs. Δ9-Tetrahydrocannabinol, THC, is the bioactive ingredient of the drugs marijuana and hashish [25] and can artificially activate cannabinoid receptors as exogenous cannabinoids. Cannabinoid receptors exist in all normal brains [18, 21, 22] where they subserve many essential brain functions when activated by their natural ligands. Cannabinoid receptors in the nervous system are predominantly $G_{i/o}$-protein-coupled type 1 cannabinoid receptors (CB1 receptors, CB1Rs). Their ligands, endocannabinoids are synthesized from membrane lipids [26]. Endocannabinoids can diffuse through membranes and are thus able to activate receptors in the same manner as exogenously applied cannabinoids such as cannabis. Anandamide and 2-AG were discovered in the early 1990s [27-29, reviewed in 30] while their functional role in neuronal communication remained obscure for years. Since their discovery, the role of endocannabinoids as retrograde messengers that suppress both excitatory and inhibitory transmission has been well-established. Endocannabinoids mediate retrograde signals in the hippocampus [31-35], cerebellum [36-38], neocortex [39, 40], amygdala [41, 42], and olfactory bulb [43]. Termination of endocannabinoidsignalling is accomplished by reuptake into both neurons and glia. Subsequently, anandamide and 2-AG are hydrolyzed intracellularly by fatty acid amide hydrolase (FAAH) and monoacylglycerol lipase (MAGL), respectively [44].

3. Unusual and novel neurotransmitters

Endocannabinoids are different from conventional neurotransmitters because they are lipids that are not stored but rather are rapidly synthesized on demand at the site of need from components of the cell membrane. Upon cellular activation, they are released from places all over the cell. They are arachidonic acid-containing messengers generated by phospholipase action [45]. Stimuli that trigger release of endocannabinoids include rise of intracellular calcium levels inside the neuron or activation of certain G-protein-coupled receptors such as metabotropic glutamate receptors (mGluR5). Subsequent to their non-synaptic, non-vesicular release, endocannabinoids bind to cannabinoid receptors on nearby neurons such as presynaptic interneurons where they regulate presynaptic neurotransmitter release, e.g., through closure of specific ion channels.

Endocannabinoids are members of a loose family of unusual and novel neurotransmitters. Similar to endocannabinoids, other novel neurotransmitters such as nitric oxide (NO), carbon monoxide (CO), and hydrogen sulfide (H2S) do not adhere to the classic definition of neurotransmitters and challenge the notion of what constitutes a neurotransmitter [46, 47]. These synaptic molecules have changed markedly the definition of a neurotransmitter. They satisfy key neurotransmitter criteria but differ radically from classical transmitters. For example, endocannabinoids, nitric oxide and carbon monoxide are neither stored in synaptic vesicles nor released by exocytosis. Nitric oxide does not act via traditional receptors on postsynaptic membranes.

Like endocannabinoids, nitric oxide can serve as an intercellular messenger in the brain [48]. It acts as a retrograde factor at synapses and presynaptically regulates both glutamatergic and GABAergic synapses to alter release-probability in synaptic plasticity. Nitric oxide influences the synaptic machinery involved in transmitter release and, in a coordinated fashion, also the vesicular recycling mechanisms. Nitric oxide has a role in the coordination of local pre-and post-synaptic function during plasticity at individual synapses. It is involved in experience-dependent plasticity in the cerebral cortex. Likewise, cannabinoids mediate a variety of forms of short-and long-term synaptic plasticity that have been reviewed in detail elsewhere [49-51].

4. Depolarization-induced suppression of inhibition

The relevance of the endocannabinoid system for neural signaling and brain function in general has been explored only recently [13]. Endocannabinoids mediate a new type of neuronal communication, called DSI, **D**epolarization-induced **S**uppression of **I**nhibition (Fig. 2) (reviewed in [10, 12, 30]. A short rise in intracellular calcium concentration in a principal neuron, e.g., a pyramidal cell of the hippocampus, results in a transient decline of incoming inhibitory signals in the form of GABA arriving from other neurons. This observation led to the hypothesis that during DSI, some unknown messenger must travel from the postsynaptic cell to the presynaptic GABA-releasing one and somehow turns off neurotransmitter release. Conventional chemical synaptic signaling between two neurons involves activation of a presynaptic neuron resulting in transmitter release and subsequent activation of the postsynaptic neuron, e.g., a GABAergic inhibitory interneuron makes synaptic contacts with a glutamatergic pyramidal cell in the hippocampus. When the interneuron is activated it releases the inhibitory neurotransmitter GABA and inhibits the pyramidal cell. In contrast, during DSI, when a pyramidal cell is activated, e.g., through direct current injection, the inhibitory input onto that pyramidal cell is reduced. As a major breakthrough in our understanding of endocannabinoid signaling, endocannabinoids were found to act as retrograde signaling molecules that mediate communication between postsynaptic pyramidal cells and presynaptic inhibitory interneurons and evoke the reduction in GABA release. Since endocannabinoids are lipids, they do not diffuse over great distances in the watery extracellular environment of the brain. Rather, DSI acts as a short-lived local effect that enables individual neurons to disconnect briefly from their neighbors and encode information [12].

The announcement of this breakthrough has been given the Latin term 'Dies mirabilis' (wonderful day) by Alger [10]. In March of 2001 four independent labs described in three different journals their studies culminating in the conclusion that endocannabinoids function mainly as retrograde messengers. Elphick and Egertova [52] analyzed prior pharmacological and anatomical studies of the actions of cannabinoid receptor agonists and combined this with their knowledge of the localization of cannabinoid receptors and degradative enzymes for anandamide, fatty acid amide hydrolase (FAAH) to reason that endocannabinoids act as retrograde messengers. Pivotal work by Wilson and Nicoll [34] and Ohno-Shosaku et al. [32] established that DSI was mimicked by activating cannabinoid receptors whereas blockade of cannabinoid receptors prevented DSI. A corresponding phenomenon, DSE, **D**epolarization-induced **S**upression of **E**xcitation, mediated by retrograde action of endocannabinoids, was identified by Kreitzer and Regehr [36] at cerebellar excitatory synapses. DSI and DSE are based on a presynaptic effect as shown by an increase in calcium in the postsynaptic cells and corresponding changes in paired pulse ratio of neurotransmitter release.

G-protein coupled receptors (GPCRs) are involved in mediating the transduction of extracellular stimuli, such as neurotransmitters, into intracellular signaling cascades. Activation of specific G-protein coupled receptors triggers the release of endocananbinoids for many minutes, e.g., dopamine [53], metabotropic glutamate [33, 37, 54] or muscarinic M1/M3 acetylcholine receptors [55, 56]. Even though endocannabinoids are typically released in a

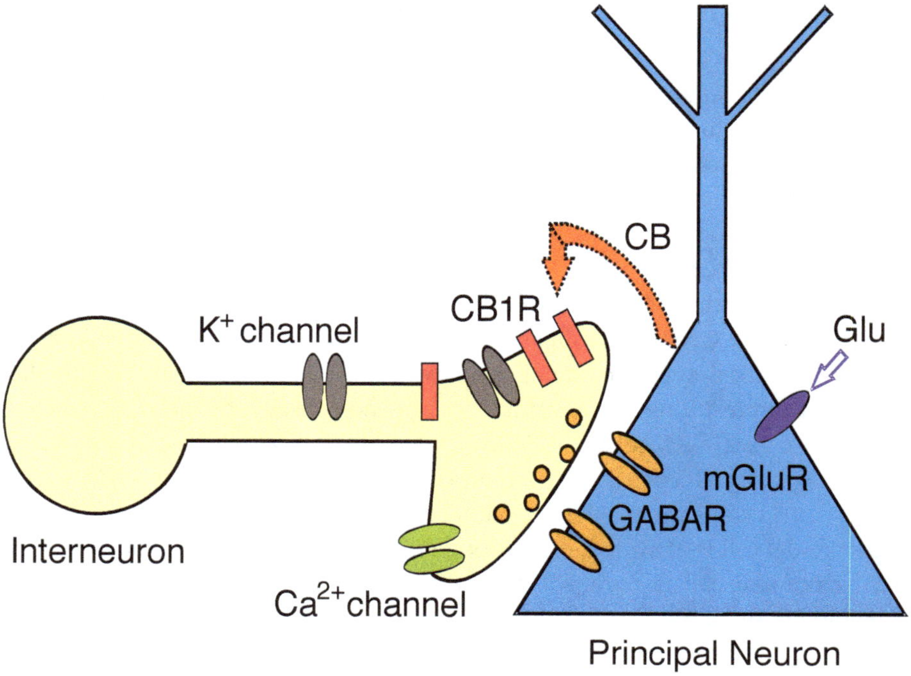

Figure 2. **D**epolarization-induced **S**uppression of **I**nhibition (DSI) is a model for retrograde signaling in the brain and allows assaying real time release of endocannabinoids from principal neurons as a brief cessation of GABA ouput. Activation of metabotropic glutamate receptors (mGluRs) on principal neurons or depolarization of postsynaptic principal cells evokes synthesis and release of cannabinoids (CBs). Cannabinoids bind to presynaptic cannabinoid receptors (CB1R) on GABAergic interneurons and transiently reduce GABA release from synaptic terminals. As a consequence, $GABA_A$ receptor-mediated synaptic currents and GABAergic inhibition are temporarily suppressed in postsynaptic principal neurons.

calcium-dependent manner [57, 58], in the mGluR-and mAChR-dependent pathways, no clear rise in intracellular calcium $[Ca^{2+}]_i$ [37, 55] is necessary. The release of endocananbinoids can be initiated even in the presence of high intracellular concentrations of calcium chelators, although endocannabinoids may nevertheless be sensitive to the ambient intracellular calcium concentration [59]. Studies by the Alger lab and others indicate that G-protein coupled receptor activation of postsynaptic cells leads to enhancement of DSI, e.g., glutamate acting on group I metabotropic glutamate receptors (mGluRs) directly generates endocannabinoids and enhances DSI ([37, 33]. It is now established that activation of many G-protein coupled receptors is linked to the use of endocannabinoids to deliver or fine-tune their messages to target cells [11].

The discovery of DSI has been a major advance in our understanding of the endocannabinoid system for brain function [60]. DSI is a type of short-term synaptic plasticity originally observed in the cerebellum and hippocampus [12, 14]. Endocannabinoids are retrograde signaling molecules that are released from depolarized principal neurons and travel to presynaptic inhibitory interneurons to reduce GABA release. DSI is a novel, regulatory process that manifests itself as a transient suppression of synaptic $GABA_A$ responses mediated by retrograde signaling of endocannabinoids from principal neurons (Fig. 3). Through the retrograde signaling process neurons alter the strength of synapses made onto them and thereby control their own synaptic excitability in an activity-dependent manner, which is functionally important in information processing by neuronal networks [14]. In the cerebellum, a retrograde signaling process that is similar to DSI reduces synaptic excitation by suppressing presynaptic glutamate release and is called DSE [61], see above.

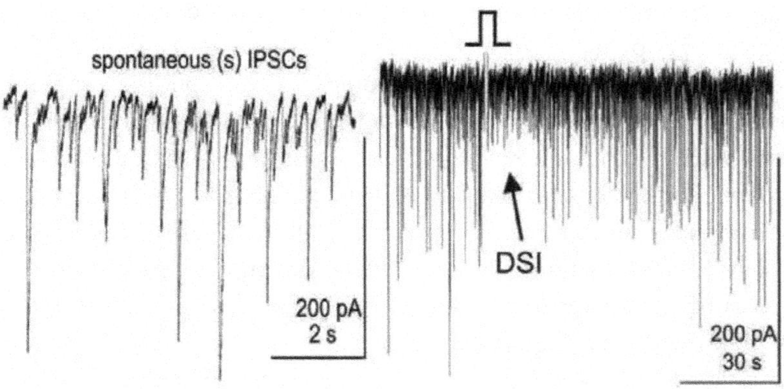

Figure 3. Right panel: Hippocampal pyramidal cells show spontaneous inhibitory postsynaptic currents (IPSCs). Left panel: In response to a 1-s voltage pulse the pyramidal cell reveals DSI, a transient reduction in IPSC activity as a result of endocannabinoids acting on CB1R on presynaptic GABAergic interneurons.

5. Hippocampal depolarization-induced suppression of inhibition

Endocannabinoids are lipids and, unlike classic neurotransmitters, are not stored but rather rapidly synthesized from components of the cell membrane. They are synthesized in, and released from, postsynaptic somatodendritic domains that are readily accessible to whole-cell patch electrodes. The effects of these lipid signals are detected electrophysiologically as CB1R-dependent alterations in conventional synaptic transmission, which, therefore, provide a sensitive means of bioassay in gendocannabinoid levels and actions. Endocannabinoid release can be triggered through Ca^{2+}-dependent or relatively Ca^{2+}-independent pathways, with different down-stream effects. As discussed above, endocannabinoids are released non-synaptically, non-vesicular from places all over cells when levels of calcium rise inside the neuron or when certain G-protein-coupled receptors are activated. After cellular release, endocannabinoids travel to cannabinoid receptors on nearby neurons and evoke a reversible, short-term depression of synaptic transmission, DSI. In activated hippocampal pyramidal cells, DSI leads to a transient reductionof GABA release from presynaptic terminals of inhibitory interneurons. Direct insights into the actions of endocannabinoids have been based primarily on pharmacological experiments. The hydrophobicity of endocannabinoids severely limits their penetration into brain tissue, and endocannabinoids are rapidly degraded by abundant endogenous lipases. These intrinsic properties of endocannabinoids make it difficult to directly study physiological effects of endocannabinoids. The development of a highly water-soluble caged anandamide that is inert to lipases circumvents these problems [62]. When perfused into hippocampal slice preparations, the caged anandamide serves as a latent endocannabinoid pool, and focal photolysis rapidly liberates highly hydrophobic anandamide *in situ* to activate CB1R. Photolysis is an alternative experimental approach to chemically stimulate synapses, cells, or circuits by directly applying neurotransmitter or neuromodulators. Often pharmacological approaches yield little control of the stimulation in terms of timing, space and specificity. However, photo-uncaging of caged neurotransmitters has made the pharmacological approach more sophisticated. Photo-uncaging uses localized, patterned light and yields higher spatial and temporal resolution. One application of photostimulation, the flash photolysis technique, can be used to determine signaling kinetics of the endocannabinoid system [60, 62]. The endocannabinoid system can be used as a tool for bioassaying the temporal dynamics or kinetics of lipid signaling. Combining whole-cell voltage patch-clamp recording, intracellular calcium measurements, and photorelease of caged glutamate and a novel, caged cannabinoid, anandamide (AEA) allows determining endocannabinoid signaling kinetics. Flash photolysis of caged compounds (photolysis using so-called molecular optical probes or photoprobes) is an important tool in this endeavor. Caged compounds are inert, biologically inactive (e.g., a caged cannabinoid or caged glutamate) until a flash of laser light breaks open the molecular cage, releases the caged molecule and generates a biologically active effector molecule in situ [63]. Chemically, the caged compound is a modified signal molecule. The modification of the molecule prevents its bioactivity until light absorption results in a photochemical change of the signal molecule such that its bioactivity is restored.

The lipid signaling pathway comprises several temporal components that can be determined to quantify the time that it takes from the DSI-inducing stimulus to the onset of DSI. These components contribute to the latency to onset of DSI (start of DSI-inducing stimulus to initial suppression of IPSCs). Among them is the rise of calcium to initiate endocannabinoid synthesis (t-Ca). The rise in intracellular calcium leads to endocannabinoid synthesis and release, followed by travel of these molecules to cannabinoid receptors on presynaptic interneurons, t-EC. The next step is the activation of CB1R and downstream effects, t-CB1R (t-DSI = t-Ca + t-EC + t-CB1R). Experiments carried out using the above-mentioned technological advances allowed determining the time for synthesis and release of eCB from the postsynaptic neuron, which was estimated to be around 150 ms at room temperature, comparable with the timescale of metabotropic signaling and at least an order of magnitude faster than previously thought. A major portion of the DSI onset time, t-DSI, reflects activation of presynaptic CB1Rs and downstream consequences. The data suggest that, far from simply serving long-term neuromodulatory functions, endocannabinoid signaling is sufficiently fast to exert moment-to-moment control of synaptic transmission. The DSI onset latency after a voltage step, t-DSI, is 350 to 400 ms. t-CB1R, the direct activation of CB1R by photoreleasing anandamide which results in suppression of sIPSCs, takes ~180ms (Fig. 4). A transient rise in intracellular calcium sufficient to obtain minimal DSI, t-Ca, is evoked by a 50-ms voltage step and takes ~60 ms. The time needed for endocannabinoid synthesis and release to occur, t-EC, is about 150 ms.

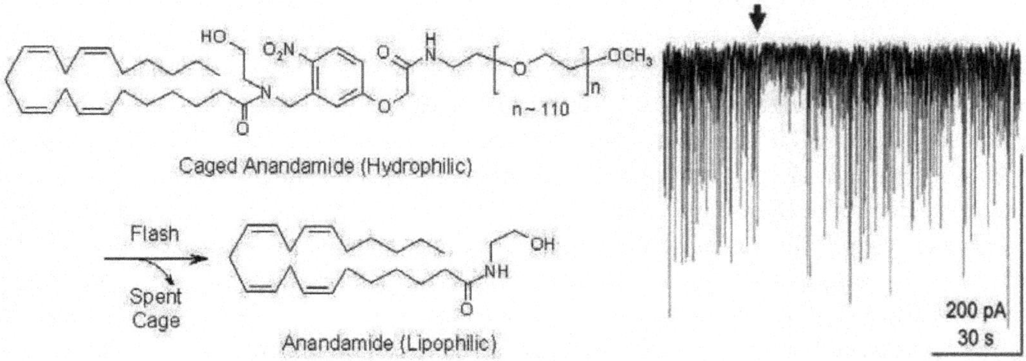

Figure 4. Left panel: Photolysis of caged anandamide yields bioactive anandamide. Right panel: Photorelease of anandamide suppresses sIPSCs after a delay of ~180 ms. Modified from [62] with permission of the Society for Neuroscience.

Voltage-activated DSI works through a rise in intracellular calcium concentration. However, release of endocannabinoids can be triggered even in the presence of high intracellular concentrations of calcium chelators, although they may nevertheless be sensitive to ambient intracellular calcium [59]. To test if these two pathways function on the same time scale, the dynamic components of the mGluR-induced endocannabionoid response on sIPSC frequency in pyramidal cells are compared (Fig. 5) [62]. The mean onset latency, duration and magnitude of the IPSC suppression evoked by uncaged glutamate are similar to that caused by uncaged AEA (Figs. 4, 5). No reduction in sIPSCs occurred for 221 ms (determined by extrapolation of the exponential fit to the control sIPSC level). The time-to-onset of IPSC suppression evoked by the mGluR-induced endocannabinoid process (time to mGluR-dependent suppression of inhibition, $t_{mGluRSI}$) is described by: t-mGluR-SI = 221 ms = t-eCB(mGluR) + t-CB1R, where t-eCB(mGluR) is the time for activation of the mGluR-dependent endocannabinoid synthesis and release, and t-CB1R is ~180 ms (see above). This leaves t-eCB(mGluR) to be < 50 ms, which is even faster than endocannabinoid synthesis and released evoked by a voltage step.

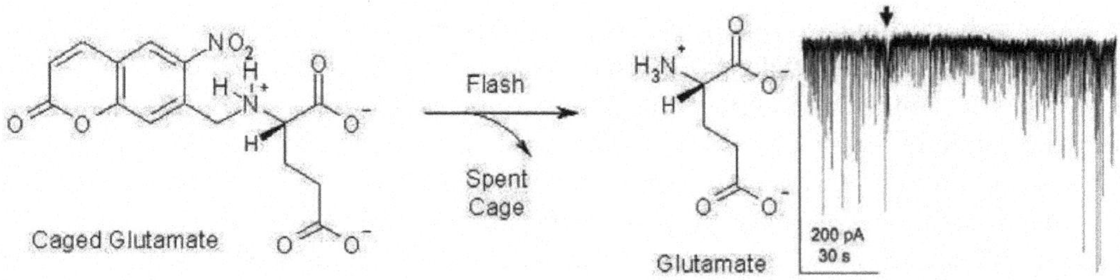

Figure 5. Dynamics of mGluR-dependent endocannabinoid suppression of sIPSCs in cultured hippocampal slices. Left panel: Photorelease of glutamate. Right panel: Recording from a pyramidal cell illustrates the transient reduction in spontaneous (s) IPSC frequency of CA1 pyramidal cells after flash photorelease of caged glutamate (photolysis induced suppression of inhibition, PSI). Arrow indicates laser flash. From [62] with permission of the Society for Neuroscience.

Anandamide can be released from its caged form by a UV-laser flash and rapidly activates presynaptic CB1Rs to suppress the release of GABA [62]. A specific CB1R antagonist, AM 251, blocks the suppression of spontaneous IPSCs. This establishes that uncagedanandamide can be used as a CB1R agonist to study activation of CB1R in the brain. Similarly, uncaged glutamate acts at mGluRs on hippocampal pyramidal cells to evoke cannabinoid release and subsequent suppression of presynaptic GABA release [62]. The data provide the first detailed attempt to determine the minimal time required for activation of an intercellular neuronal lipid messenger system. This signaling system requires a major portion of DSI onset time, t-DSI, for activation of presynaptic CB1R and downstream consequences. Endocannabinoids, and by extension similar lipid messengers, can be mobilized and evoke responses as quickly as conventional metabotropic, G-protein receptor-coupled neurotransmitters. The speed with which neuromodulators such as endocannabinoids act places critical constraints on the physiological roles they can play. Endocannabinoids and other lipids function in brain signaling not simply in homeostatic processes or slowly-activating forms of regulation, but rather lipids can affect neuronal excitability in moment-to-moment information processing.

6. Depolarization-induced suppression of inhibition in glomerular circuits of the olfactory bulb

The olfactory bulb is the first relay station in the CNS for processing of sensory information that comes from olfactory receptor cells in the nasal epithelium. Cannabinoid receptors are expressed at high levels in the olfactory bulb, specifically in the input region, the glomerular layer [21, 64-66]. Neurons in the glomerular layer are immunoreactive for enzymes that synthesize endocannabinoids [67-69]. Our understanding of the physiological role of endocannabinoids and cannabinoid receptors for neural signaling in the olfactory system is just emerging. Recent electrophysiological evidence has established that the endocannabinoid system plays a functional role in regulating neuronal activity and signaling in olfactory bulb glomeruli [43].

Neurons in the glomerular fall into three subpopulations: periglomerular (PG), external tufted (eTC), and short-axon (SA) cells. Periglomerular cells are neurochemically and functionally heterogeneous [70-72]. Periglomerular cells are GABAergic, short-axon cells express both GABA and dopamine, and external tufted cells are glutamatergic [72, 73]. Periglomerular cells receive input from the olfactory nerve or dendrodendritic glutamatergic input from external tufted or mitral cells, e.g., as spontaneous bursts of EPSCs [70, 73-74]. Periglomerular cells presynaptically inhibit olfactory receptor neurons through GABAergic transmission [76, 77]. External tufted cells receive spontaneous bursts of inhibitory postsynaptic currents (sIPSCs) from periglomerular cells at inhibitory GABAergic synapses as well as spontaneous glutamatergic EPSCs [74; 78]. In the glomerular layer, external tufted cells can be a potential source of endocannabinoids.

Cannabinoid receptors directly regulate membrane properties of periglomerular cells as shown by the effects of CB1R antagonist AM251 and agonist WIN in the presence of ionotropic glutamate and $GABA_A$ receptor blockers (synaptic blockers: CNQX, APV, gabazine) [43]. This indicates that the actions of cannabinoids on periglomerular cells are mediated through CB1R expressed by periglomerular cells. AM251 directly activates periglomerular cells and enhances their GABA release. Periglomerular cells are synaptically connected to external tufted cells. Therefore, any CB1R-mediated regulation of activity of periglomerular cells could affect GABA release and synaptic transmission to external tufted cells. CB1R is also expressed in external tufted cells and may participate in modulating external tufted cell activity.

In external tufted cells, neither AM251 nor WIN influences firing frequency or membrane potential [43]. However, in the presence of synaptic blockers cannabinoid drugs have a modest effect on external tufted cells. In this condition, AM251 slightly increases the firing rate of external tufted cells without membrane depolarization. In synaptic blockers, WIN slightly decreases firing of external tufted cells without a clear change in membrane potential. The effects of AM251 and WIN in the presence of synaptic blockers, i.e., during pharmacological isolation of external tufted cells, indicate that CB1R mediates a direct effect on external tufted cells. The direct excitatory effect of a CB1R antagonist on external tufted cells is opposed by increased GABAergic synaptic input from periglomerular cells onto external tufted cells, i.e., the enhanced GABA release from periglomerular cells triggered by a CB1R antagonist may dominate and mask the CB1R antagonist-evoked direct excitation of external tufted cells.

The CB1R effects on periglomerular and external tufted cell prompt the questions if DSI is present in the glomerular layer of the olfactory bulb. In external tufted cells, DSI can be induced with a 5-sec depolarizing voltage step from a holding potential of -60 mV to 0 mV (Fig. 5). In external tufted cells DSI is visible as a decrease in the amplitude and frequency of sIPSCs. The response to a single depolarizing step is a suppression of sIPSC area by ~40 % of control which then gradually recoveres. External tufted cells exhibit a distinct intrinsic bursting pattern [74]. In order to mimic spontaneous rhythmic bursting of an external tufted cell a train of depolarizing steps can be applied to the cell. This experimental paradigm allows determining a possible functional role of DSI in glomeruli. A train of depolarizing steps results in a transient 60% reduction in sIPSC area (20 steps, 0.75 Hz) (Fig. 4B, F). DSI can be completely eliminated in the presence of AM251, indicating that DSI is mediated by CB1R (Fig. 5C, F). The bursting frequency of external tufted cells ranges from 0.5 to 6.5 Hz with a mean frequency of 2.7 bursts/sec [74]. Depolarizing voltage pulses at 2 Hz (20 steps, pulse duration: 250 ms) evoke DSI as a reduction of sIPSCs in external tufted cells, similar to the results obtained with voltage steps at 0.75 Hz to 0 mV. In external tufted cells, single depolarizing voltage steps as well as a train of voltage steps evoke suppression of inhibition (DSI). This suggests that spontaneous rhythmic bursting of these cells triggers the release of endocannabinoids which function as retrograde messengers to reduce GABA release from periglomerular cells which in turn, regulates the activity of periglomerular cell synaptic targets such as external tufted cells.

Endocannabinoids regulate neuronal activity and signaling in olfactory bulb glomeruli. They function in the form of DSI through CB1R-mediated retrograde signaling among glomerular neurons. Endocannabinoids are released from external tufted cells and act as retrograde messengers to control the excitability of presynaptic neurons, i.e., periglomerular cells, and to regulate their transmitter release. Endocannabinoids are synthesized and

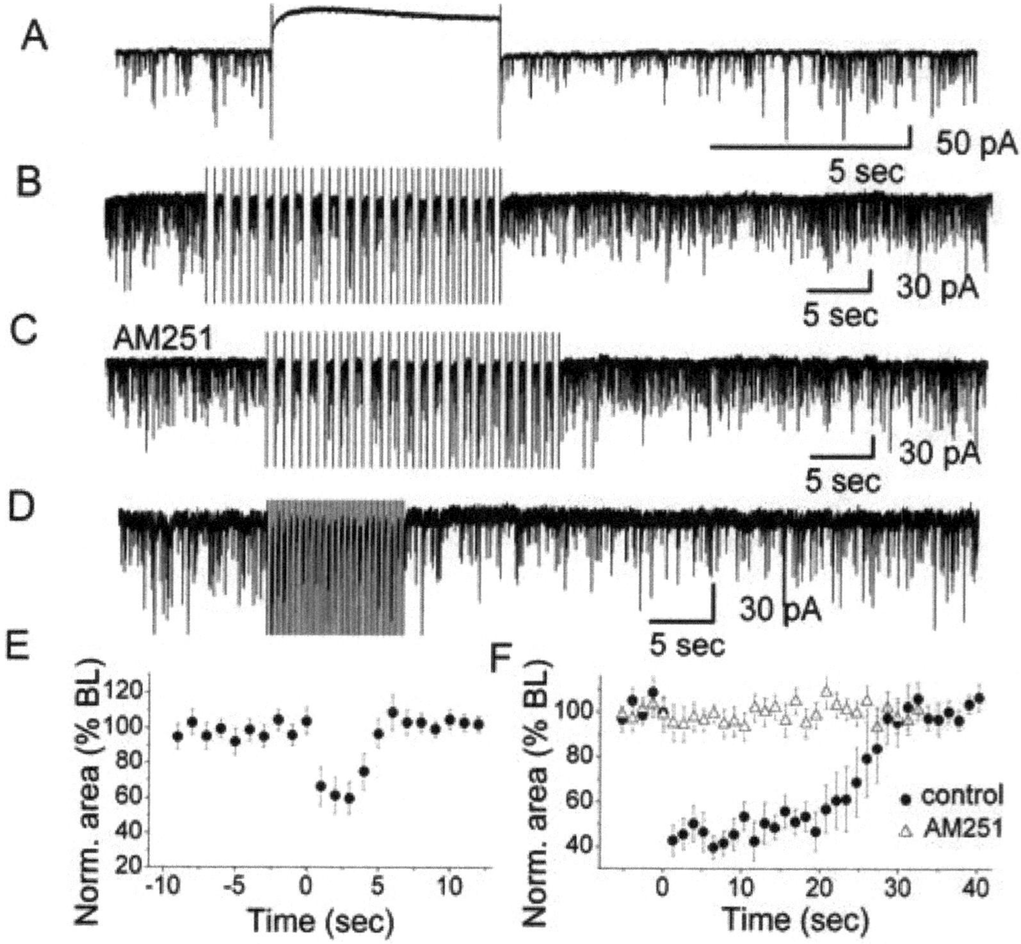

Figure 6. Depolarization-induced **S**uppression of **I**nhibition (DSI) in olfactory glomeruli. **A** A depolarizing voltage step evoked DSI in a representative external tufted cell. High Cl^--based pipette solution was used for recording sIPSCs. Depolarization was achieved by stepping from-60 mV holding potential to 0 mV for 5 sec. **B** In the presence of CNQX and 5-AP, a train of 20 voltage steps to 0 mV (0.75 Hz; step duration: 667 ms) transiently reduced sIPSCs in an external tufted cell. Holding potential was-60 mV. **C.** In the presence of AM251, no sIPSC suppression was observed. **D** A train of 20 voltage steps to-30 mV (2 Hz; step duration: 250 ms) transiently reduced sIPSCs in an external tufted cell (in CNQX and 5-AP). **E** Normalized sIPSCs area illustrating the magnitude and time course of DSI elicited by a 5-sec depolarizing pulse (n=7). The averaged values between 0 – 5 sec after the end of the voltage step were significantly different from the baseline (ANOVA and Bonferroni post-hoc analysis, $p< 0.05$). **F** Normalized sIPSC area illustrating the magnitude and time course of DSI elicited by a train of depolarizations to 0 mV (n=12) in control and in the presence of AM251 (n=10). In control conditions, the averaged values between zero to 2 5 seconds after the end of the train of voltage steps were significantly different from the baseline (ANOVA and Bonferroni post-hoc analysis, $p< 0.05$). From [43] with permission of the Society for Neuroscience.

released from neuronal cell bodies as a result of cellular excitation [11]. One potential source of endocannabinoids in the olfactory bulb is neurons that synapse onto presynaptic cells, i.e., periglomerular cells, and receive feedback synaptic inputs. This profile fits external tufted cells and they could be a potential endocannabinoid source in the olfactory bulb which is supported by the fact that DSI is found in external tufted cells. DSI in external tufted cells is subject to the level of cellular activation, i.e., voltage step duration and step number. DSI cannot be evoked with step durations of 1 sec or less while a step duration closer to 5 seconds evokes transient DSI. A train of depolarizing voltage steps (>3) generates particularly prominent DSI and strengthens the inhibition of sIPSCs. This suggests that excitation of external tufted cells in the form of rhythmic bursting triggers the release of endocannabinoids and regulates glomerular activity. Bursting is intrinsic to external tufted cells and mediated by several cell intrinsic conductances [79]. Bursting of neurons may modulate endocannabinoid release not only in the olfactory bulb but also in other brain systems and constitute a general phenomenon of endocannabinoidsignaling.

Olfactory sensory neurons form direct synaptic contacts with external tufted cells. Sensory or synaptic input to external tufted cells can trigger the release of endocannabinoids which have an inhibitory effect on CB1Rs in presynaptic periglomerular cells. Endocannabinoids thus reduce inhibitory input to external tufted cells and enhance external tufted cell sensitivity to weak sensory inputs by depolarizing the membrane potential closer to spike threshold. This CB1R-mediated inhibition of periglomerular cells reduces their GABA release and, in turn, modifies the firing pattern of external tufted cells and, potentially, also reduces inhibition of mitral cells and presynaptic olfactory nerve terminals. The functional relevance of this signaling pathway lies in a potential increase of the overall sensitivity of the glomerulus to sensory inputs resulting from activation of CB1R on periglomerular cells.

7. Endocannabinoid-evoked physiological responses and crosstalk with other neurotransmitters

Endocannabinoids can evoke physiological responses that are not mediated by presynaptic CB1Rs but rather by postsynaptic CB1Rs [14], e.g., via regulation of K^+ conductances present on the extrasynaptic dendritic surface of neurons or modulation of postsynaptic NMDA receptors or even non-CB1R, e.g., [80]. Several conventional CB1R ligands have been reported to have CB1R unspecific effects or activate non-CB1 receptors [14]. Electrophysiological evidence suggests that the CB1R agonist WIN55,212-2 produces non-CB1R mediated effects on the excitability of principal neurons in the basolateral amygdala [81], thus providing evidence for a non-CB1R site of action of WIN55,212-2 [82, 83]. Cannabinoid drugs can activate other 'non-CB' receptors, such as GPR55, peroxisome proliferator-activated receptors (PPARs), and vanilloid type TRP channels [84, 85].

The accepted view of endocannabinoid action is based on hippocampal studies demonstrating that endocannabinoids reduce synaptic inhibition of the principal cell (DSI), see above. Endocannabinoids were found to possess other properties, namely, to mediate self-modulation of neocortical pyramidal neurons [86] or long-lasting self-inhibition in neocortical GABA-containing interneurons [87]. This self-inhibition is mediated by autocrine release of endocannabinoids and does not depend on glutamatergic and/or GABAergic neurotransmission but rather on activity-dependent long-lasting hyperpolarization due to the activation of a K^+-conductance. Endocannabinoids released by these interneurons target the same cells and mediate a lasting hyperpolarization that is blocked by a CB1R antagonist. Self-inhibited cells can become hyperpolarized below spike threshold and are effectively removed from the neural circuit in which they reside.

The endocannabinoid system reciprocally modulates other neurotransmitter systems [88]. Examples include interactive cross-talk with the endogenous opioid system [89, 90]. Incidentally, like the endogenous opiate system, the endocannabinoid system was first discovered because it can be activated by a plant-derived compound – in the case of the endocannabinoids, this is Δ9-tetrahydrocannabinol, the bioactive ingredient of the drugs marijuana and hashish [25]. Other studies detected an interaction of the endocannabinoid system at the molecular and functional levels with other neurotransmitters such as the dopaminergic and adenosinergic systems [91-93]. Recent evidence has suggested cross-modulation between the endocannabinoid and hypocretinergic system [88]. This idea is based on the overlap observed in the neuroanatomical distribution of both systems as well as their putative functions. Functionally, both endocannabinoids and hypocretins can contribute to the regulation of appetite, reward and analgesia. Furthermore, biochemical and functional studies have demonstrated heterodimers between CB1 cannabinoid receptor and hypocretin receptor-1. Activation of hypocretin receptor-1 stimulates the synthesis of 2-arachidonoyl glycerol which through retrograde endocannabinoid signaling results in inhibition of neighboring cells. This interaction would allow endocannabinoids to contribute to hypocretin effects and provide potential therapeutic applications to currently existing drugs targeting these systems [88]. However, these two neuromodulatory systems exert antagonistic effects in the regulation of the sleep/wake cycle and anxiety-like responses which contributes even more to the excitement of performing research targeting the endocannabinoid system.

Acknowledgements

This work was supported in part by U.S.-PHS grants GM08016 and MD007597. I would like to gratefully acknowledge current and former collaborators Drs. Bradley E. Alger, Joseph P. Y. Kao, and Ze-Jun Wang.

Author details

Thomas Heinbockel*

Address all correspondence to: theinbockel@howard.edu

Department of Anatomy, Howard University College of Medicine, Washington, DC, USA

References

[1] Calignano A, Katona I, Desarnaud F, Giuffrida A, La Rana G, Mackie K, Freund TF, Piomelli D. Bidirectional control of airway responsiveness by endogenous cannabinoids. Nature 2000; 408:96-101.

[2] Cota D, Marsicano G, Lutz B, Vicennati V, Stalla GK, Pasquali R, Pagotto. Endogenous cannabinoid system as a modulator of food intake. Internat J Obesity 2003; 27:289-301.

[3] Soria-Gómez E, Bellocchio L, Reguero L, Lepousez G, Martin C, Bendahmane M, Ruehle S, Remmers F, Desprez T, Matias I, Wiesner T, Cannich A, Nissant A, Wadleigh A, Pape HC, Chiarlone AP, Quarta C, Verrier D, Vincent P, Massa F, Lutz B, Guzmán M, Gurden H, Ferreira G, Lledo PM, Grandes P, Marsicano G. The endocannabinoid system controls food intake via olfactory processes. Nat Neurosci 2014; 17:407-415.

[4] Iversen L, Chapman V. Cannabinoids: a real prospect for pain relief. Curr Opin Pharmacol 2002; 2:50-55.

[5] Marsicano G, Goodenough S, Monory K, Hermann H, Eder M, Cannich A, Azad SC, Cascio MG, Gutierrez SO, van der Stelt M, Lopez-Rodriguez ML, Casanova E, Schutz G, Zieglgansberger W, Di Marzo V, Behl C, Lutz B. CB1 cannabinoid receptors and on-demand defense against excitotoxicity. Science 2003; 302:84-88.

[6] Panikashvili D, Simeonidou C, Ben-Shabat S, Hanus L, Breuer A, Mechoulam R, Shohami E. An endogenous cannabinoid (2-AG) is neuroprotective after brain injury. Nature 2001; 413:527-531.

[7] Katona I, Rancz EA, Acsady L, Ledent C, Mackie K, Hajos N, Freund TF. Distribution of CB1 cannabinoid receptors in the amygdala and their role in the control of GABAergic transmission. J Neurosci 2001; 21:9506-9518.

[8] Valjent E, Mitchell JM, Besson MJ, Caboche J, Maldonado R. Behavioural and biochemical evidence for interactions between Delta9-tetrahydrocannabinol and nicotine. Br J Pharmacol 2002; 135:564-578.

[9] Marsicano G, Wotjak CT, Azad SC, Bisogno T, Rammes G, Cascio MG, Hermann H, Tang J, Hofmann C, Zieglgansberger W, Di Marzo V, Lutz B. The endogenous cannabinoid system controls extinction of aversive memories. Nature 2002; 418:530-534.

[10] Alger BE. Endocannabinoids at the synapse a decade after the dies mirabilis (29 March 2001): what we still do not know. J Physiol 2012; 590.10:2203–2212.

[11] Kano M, Ohno-Shosaku T, Hashimotodani Y, Uchigashima M, Watanabe M. Endocannabinoid-mediated control of synaptic transmission. Physiol Rev 2009; 89:309–380.

[12] Alger BE. Retrograde signaling in the regulation of synaptic transmission: focus on endocannabinoids. Prog Neurobiol 2002; 68:247-286.

[13] Alger BE, Kim J. Supply and demand for endocannabinoids. Trends Neurosci 2011; 34:304-315.

[14] Freund TF, Katona I, Piomelli D. Role of endogenous cannabinoids in synaptic signaling. Physiol Rev 2003; 83:1017-1066.

[15] Howlett AC, Breivogel CS, Childers SR, Deadwyler SA, Hampson RE, Porrino LJ. Cannabinoid physiology and pharmacology: 30 years of progress. Neuropharmacol 2004; 47:345-358.

[16] Matsuda LA, Lolait SJ, Brownstein MJ, Young AC, Bonner TI. Structure of a cannabinoid receptor and functional expression of the cloned cDNA. Nature 1990; 346, 561-564.

[17] Munro S, Thomas KL, Abu-Shaar M. Molecular characterization of a peripheral receptor for cannabinoids. Nature 1993; 365, 61–65.

[18] Herkenham M, Lynn AB, Little MD, Johnson MR, Melvin LS, de Costa BR, Rice KC. Cannabinoid receptor localization in brain. ProcNatlAcadSci USA 1990; 87:1932–1936.

[19] Van Sickle, M.D., Duncan, M., Kingsley, P.J., Mouihate, A., Urbani, P., Mackie, K., et al. Identification and functional characterization of brainstem cannabinoid CB2 receptors. Science 2005; 310:329-332.

[20] Núñez, E., Benito, C., Pazos, M.R., Barbachano, A., Fajardo, O., González, S., et al. Cannabinoid CB2 receptors are expressed by perivascular microglial cells in the human brain: an immunohistochemical study. Synapse 2004; 53:208-213.

[21] Herkenham M, Lynn AB, Johnson MR, Melvin LS, de Costa BR, Rice KC. Characterization and localization of cannabinoid receptors in rat brain: a quantitative in vitro autoradiographic study. J Neurosci 1991; 11:563-583.

[22] Matsuda LA, Bonner TI, Lolait SJ. Localization of cannabinoid receptor mRNA in rat brain. J Comp Neurol 1993; 327:535-550.

[23] Katona I, Sperlagh B, Sik A, Kafalvi A, Vizi ES, Mackie K, Freund TF. Presynaptically located CB1 cannabinoid receptors regulate GABA release from axon terminals of specific hippocampal interneurons. J Neurosci 1999; 19:4544-4558.

[24] Tsou K, Mackie K, Sanudo-Pena MC, Walker JM. Cannabinoid CB1 receptors are localized primarily on cholecystokinin-containing GABAergic interneurons in the rat hippocampal formation. Neurosci 1999; 93:969-975.

[25] Ameri A. The effects of cannabinoids on the brain. Prog Neurobiol 1999; 58:315-348.

[26] Di Marzo V, Melck D, Bisogno T & De Petrocellis L. Endocannabinoids: endogenous cannabinoid receptor ligands with neuromodulatory action. Trends Neurosci 1998; 21:521–528.

[27] Devane WA, Hanus L, Breuer A, Pertwee RG, Stevenson LA, Griffin G, et al. Isolation and structure of a brain constituent that binds to the cannabinoid receptor. Science 1992; 258:1946–1949.

[28] Mechoulam R, Ben-Shabat S, Hanus L, Ligumsky M, Kaminski NE, Schatz AR, Gopher A, Almog S, Martin BR, Compton DR, Pertwee RG, Griffin G, Bayewitch M, Barg J, Vogel Z. Identification of an endogenous 2-monoglyceride, present in canine gut, that binds to cannabinoid receptors. Biochem Pharmacol 1995; 50, 83–90.

[29] Sugiura T, Kondo S, Sukagawa A, Nakane S, Shinoda A, Itoh K, Yamashita A, Waku K. 2-Arachidonoylgylcerol – a possible endogenous cannabinoid receptor-ligand in brain. Biochem Biophys Res Commun 1995; 215:89–97.

[30] Nicoll R, Alger BE. The brain's own marijuana. Sci Amer 2004; 291:68-75

[31] Maejima T, Ohno-Shosaku T, Kano M. Endogenous cannabinoid as a retrograde messenger from depolarized postsynaptic neurons to presynaptic terminals. Neurosci Res 2001; 40:205-210.

[32] Ohno-Shosaku T, Maejima T, Kano M. Endogenous cannabinoids mediate retrograde signals from depolarized postsynaptic neurons to presynaptic terminals. Neuron 2001; 29:729-738.

[33] Varma N, Carlson GC, Ledent C, Alger BE. Metabotropic glutamate receptors drive the endocannabinoid system in hippocampus. J Neurosci 2001; 21:(RC188) 1-5.

[34] Wilson RI, Nicoll RA. Endogenous cannabinoids mediate retrograde signalling at hippocampal synapses. Nature 2001; 410:588-592.

[35] Wilson RI, Kunos G, Nicoll RA. Presynaptic specificity of endocannabinoid signaling in the hippocampus. Neuron 2001; 31:1-20.

[36] Kreitzer AC, Regehr WG. Cerebellar depolarization-induced suppression of inhibition is mediated by endogenous cannabinoids. J Neurosci 2001; 21:RC174.

[37] Maejima T, Hashimoto K, Yoshida T, Aiba A, Kano M. Presynaptic inhibition caused by retrograde signal from metabotropic glutamate to cannabinoid receptors. Neuron 2001; 31:463-475.

[38] Yoshida T, Hashimoto K, Zimmer A, Maejima T, Araishi K, Kano M. The cannabinoid CB1 receptor mediates retrograde signals for depolarization-induced suppression of inhibition in cerebellar Purkinje cells. J Neurosci 2002; 22:1690-1697.

[39] Trettel J, Levine ES. Endocannabinoids mediate rapid retrograde signaling at interneuron pyramidal neuron synapses of the neocortex. J Neurophys 2003; 89:2334-2338.

[40] Trettel J, Fortin DA, Levine ES. Endocannabinoidsignalling selectively targets perisomatic inhibitory inputs to pyramidal neurones in juvenile mouse neocortex. J Physiol (London) 2004; 556:95-107.

[41] Zhu PY, Lovinger DM. Retrograde endocannabinoid signaling in a postsynaptic neuron/synaptic bouton preparation from basolateral amygdala. J Neurosci 2005; 25:6199-6207.

[42] Kodirov SA, Jasiewicz J, Amirmahani P, Psyrakis D, Bonni K, Wehrmeister M, Lutz B. Endogenous cannabinoids trigger the depolarization-induced suppression of excitation in the lateral amygdala. Learning & Memory 2009; 17:43-49.

[43] Wang Z-J, Sun L, Heinbockel T. Cannabinoid receptor-mediated regulation of neuronal activity and signaling in glomeruli of the main olfactory bulb. J Neurosci 2012; 32:8475-8479

[44] Muccioli GG. Endocannabinoid biosynthesis and inactivation, from simple to complex. Drug Discov Today 2010; 15:474-483

[45] Di Marzo V. The endocannabinoid system: its general strategy of action, tools for its pharmacological manipulation and potential therapeutic exploitation. Pharmacol Res 2009; 60:77-84.

[46] Barañano DE, Ferris CD, Snyder SH. Atypical neural messengers. Trends Neurosci 2001; 24:99-106.

[47] Boehning D, Snyder SH. Novel neural modulators. Annu Rev Neurosci 2003; 26:105-31.

[48] Hardingham N, Dachtler J, Fox K. The role of nitric oxide in pre-synaptic plasticity and homeostasis. Front Cell Neurosci 2013; 31, 7:190.

[49] Cachope R. Functional diversity on synaptic plasticity mediated by endocannabinoids. Philos Trans R Soc Lond B BiolSci 2012; 367:3242-3253

[50] Castillo PE, Younts TJ, Chávez AE, Hashimotodani Y. Endocannabinoidsignaling and synaptic function. Neuron 2012; 76:70-81

[51] Katona I, Freund TF. Multiple functions of endocannabinoid signaling in the brain. Annu Rev Neurosci. 2012; 35:529-558.

[52] Elphick MR, Egertova M. The neurobiology and evolution of cannabinoid signalling. Philos Trans R SocLond B BiolSci 2001; 356:381–408.

[53] Giuffrida A, Parsons LH, Kerr TM, Rodriguez de Fonseca F, Navarro M, Piomelli D. Dopamine activation of endogenous cannabinoid signaling in dorsal striatum. Nat Neurosci 1999; 2:358-363.

[54] Ohno-Shosaku T, Shosaku J, Tsubokawa H, Kano M. Cooperative eCB production by neuronal depolarization and group I metabotropic glutamate receptor activation. Eur J Neurosci 2002; 15:953-961

[55] Kim J, Isokawa M, Ledent C, Alger BE. Activation of muscarinic acetylcholine receptors enhances the release of endogenous cannabinoids in the hippocampus. J Neurosci 2002; 22:10182-10191.

[56] Ohno-Shosaku T, Matsui M, Fukudome Y, Shosaku J, Tsubokawa H, Taketo MM, Manabe T, Kano M. Postsynaptic M1 and M3 receptors are responsible for the muscarinic enhancement of retrograde endocannabinoidsignalling in the hippocampus. Eur J Neurosci 2003; 18:109-116.

[57] Di Marzo V, Fontana A, Cadas H, Schinelli S, Cimino G, Schwartz JC, Piomelli D. Formation and inactivation of endogenous cannabinoid anandamide in central neurons. Nature 1994; 372:686-691.

[58] Stella N, Schweitzer P, Piomelli D. A second endogenous cannabinoid that modulates long-term potentiation. Nature 1997; 388:773-778.

[59] Hashimotodani Y, Ohno-Shosaku T, Tsubokawa H, Ogata H, Emoto K, Maejima T, Araishi K, Shin HS, Kano M. Phospholipase C_{β} serves as a coincidence detector through its Ca^{2+}dependency for triggering retrograde endocannabinoid signal. Neuron 2005; 45:257-268.

[60] Heinbockel T. Electrophysiological recording and imaging of neuronal signals in brain slices. In: Neuroscience. Heinbockel T (ed.), Rijeka, Croatia: Intech, 2012,ch 2, pp. 19-48.

[61] Kreitzer AC, Regehr WG. Retrograde inhibition of presynaptic calcium influx by endogenous cannabinoids at excitatory synapses onto Purkinje cells. Neuron 2001; 29:717-727.

[62] Heinbockel T, Brager DH, Reich C, Zhao J, Muralidharan S, Alger BE, Kao JPY. Endocannabinoid signaling dynamics probed with optical tools. J Neurosci 2005; 25: 9449-9459.

[63] Kao JPY. Controlling neurophysiology with light and caged molecules. In: Optical control of neural excitability. Keshishian H (ed), Washington, DC: Society for Neuroscience; 2008, pp. 1-12.

[64] Pettit DA, Harrison MP, Olson JM, Spencer RF, Cabral GA. Immunohistochemical localization of the neural cannabinoid receptor in rat brain. J Neurosci Res 1998; 51:391-402.

[65] Tsou K, Brown S, Sanudo-Pena MC, Mackie K, Walker JM. Immunohistochemical distribution of cannabinoid CB1 receptors in the rat central nervous system. Neurosci 1998; 83:393-411.

[66] Moldrich G, Wenger T. Localization of the CB1 cannabinoid receptor in the rat brain. An immunohistochemical study. Peptides 2000; 21:1735-1742.

[67] Allen Institute for Brain Science. Allen Mouse Brain Atlas [Online]. Seattle, WA. http://mouse.brain-map.org.; 2009

[68] Okamoto Y, Wang J, Morishita J, Ueda N. Biosynthetic pathways of the endocannabinoid anandamide. Chem Biodivers 2007; 4:1842-1857.

[69] Piomelli D. The molecular logic of endocannabinoid signaling. Nat Rev Neurosci 2003; 4:873-884.

[70] Ennis M, Hayar A, Hamilton KA. Neurochemistry of the main olfactory system. In: Handbook of Neurochemistry and Molecular Neurobiology (ed. Lajtha A), Sensory Neurochemistry, ed. Johnson DA. Springer: Heidelberg.; 2007, pp. 137-204.

[71] Shao Z, Puche AC, Kiyokage E, Szabo G, Shipley MT. Two GABAergic intraglomerular circuits differentially regulate tonic and phasic presynaptic inhibition of olfactory nerve terminals. J Neurophysiol 2009; 101:1988-2001.

[72] Kiyokage E, Pan YZ, Shao Z, Kobayashi K, Szabo G, Yanagawa Y, Obata K, Okano H, Toida K, Puche AC, Shipley MT. Molecular identity of periglomerular and short axon cells. J Neurosci 2010; 30:1185-1196.

[73] Hayar A, Karnup S, Ennis M, Shipley MT. External tufted cells: a major excitatory element that coordinates glomerular activity. J Neurosci 2004; 24:6676-6685.

[74] Hayar A, Karnup S, Shipley MT, Ennis M. Olfactory bulb glomeruli: external tufted cells intrinsically burst at theta frequency and are entrained by patterned olfactory input. J Neurosci 2004; 24:1190-1199.

[75] Hayar A, Shipley MT, Ennis M. Olfactory bulb external tufted cells are synchronized by multiple intraglomerular mechanisms. J Neurosci 2005; 25:8197-8208.

[76] Aroniadou-Anderjaska V, Zhou F-M, Priest CA, Ennis M, Shipley MT. GABA-B receptor-mediated presynaptic inhibition of sensory input to the olfactory bulb. J Neurophysiol 2000; 84:1194-1203.

[77] Murphy GJ, Darcy DP, Isaacson JS. Intraglomerular inhibition: Signaling mechanisms of an olfactory microcircuit. Nat Neurosci 2005; 8: 354-364.

[78] Hayar A, Ennis M. Endogenous GABA and glutamate finely tune the bursting of olfactory bulb external tufted cells. J Neurophysiol 2007; 98:1052-1056.

[79] Liu S, Shipley MT. Multiple conductances cooperatively regulate spontaneous bursting in mouse olfactory bulb external tufted cells. J Neurosci 2008; 28:1625-1639.

[80] Lozovaya N,Yatsenko N, Beketov A, Tsintsadze T, Burnashev N. Glycine receptors in CNS neurons as a target for nonretrograde action of cannabinoids. J Neurosci 2005; 25:7499-7506.

[81] Pistis M, Perra S, Pillolla G, Melis M, Gessa GL, Muntoni AL. Cannabinoids modulate neuronal firing in the rat basolateral amygdala: evidence for CB1-and non-CB1-mediated actions. Neuropharmacol 2004; 46:115-25.

[82] Breivogel CS, Griffin G, Di Marzo V, Martin BR. Evidence for a new G protein-coupled cannabinoid receptor in mouse brain. Mol Pharmacol 2001; 60:155-63.

[83] Hajos N, Ledent C, Freund TF. Novel cannabinoid-sensitive receptor mediates inhibition of glutamatergic synaptic transmission in the hippocampus. Neurosci 2001; 106:1-4.

[84] Kukkonen JP. A ménage à trois made in heaven: G-protein-coupled receptors, lipids and TRP channels. Cell Calcium 2011; 50:9-26.

[85] Pertwee RG, Howlett AC, Abood ME, Alexander SP, Di Marzo V, Elphick MR, et al. International Union of Basic and Clinical Pharmacology. LXXIX. Cannabinoid receptors and their ligands: beyond CB1 and CB2. Pharmacol Rev 2010; 62, 588-631.

[86] Marinelli S, Pacioni S, Cannich A, Marsicano G, Bacci A. Self-modulation of neocortical pyramidal neurons by endocannabinoids. Nat Neurosci 2009; 12, 1488–1490.

[87] Bacci A, Huguenard JR, Prince DA. Long-lasting self-inhibition of neocortical interneurons mediated by endocannabinoids. Nature 2004; 431:312-316.

[88] Flores A, Maldonado R, Berrendero F. Cannabinoid-hypocretin cross-talk in the central nervous system: what we know so far. Front Neurosci 2014; 7:256.

[89] Parolaro D, Rubino T, Viganò D, Massi P, Guidali C, Realini N. Cellular mechanisms underlying the interaction between cannabinoid and opioid system. Curr Drug Targets 2010; 11:393-405.

[90] Robledo P, Berrendero F, Ozaita A, Maldonado R. Advances in the field of cannabinoid-opioid cross-talk. Addict Biol 2008; 13:213-224.

[91] Carriba P, Ortiz O, Patkar K, Justinova Z, Stroik J, Themann A, et al. Striatal adenosine A2A and cannabinoid CB1 receptors form functional heteromeric complexes that mediate the motor effects of cannabinoids. Neuropsychopharmacol 2007; 32:2249-2259.

[92] Ferré S, Lluís C, Justinova Z, Quiroz C, Orru M, Navarro G, et al. Adenosine-cannabinoid receptor interactions. Implications for striatal function. Br J Pharmacol 2009; 160:443-453.

[93] Fernández-Ruiz J, Hernández M, Ramos JA. Cannabinoid-dopamine interaction in the pathophysiology and treatment of CNS disorders. CNS Neurosci Ther 2010; 16:e72-91.

Permissions

All chapters in this book were first published by InTech Open; hereby published with permission under the Creative Commons Attribution License or equivalent. Every chapter published in this book has been scrutinized by our experts. Their significance has been extensively debated. The topics covered herein carry significant findings which will fuel the growth of the discipline. They may even be implemented as practical applications or may be referred to as a beginning point for another development.

The contributors of this book come from diverse backgrounds, making this book a truly international effort. This book will bring forth new frontiers with its revolutionizing research information and detailed analysis of the nascent developments around the world.

We would like to thank all the contributing authors for lending their expertise to make the book truly unique. They have played a crucial role in the development of this book. Without their invaluable contributions this book wouldn't have been possible. They have made vital efforts to compile up to date information on the varied aspects of this subject to make this book a valuable addition to the collection of many professionals and students.

This book was conceptualized with the vision of imparting up-to-date information and advanced data in this field. To ensure the same, a matchless editorial board was set up. Every individual on the board went through rigorous rounds of assessment to prove their worth. After which they invested a large part of their time researching and compiling the most relevant data for our readers.

The editorial board has been involved in producing this book since its inception. They have spent rigorous hours researching and exploring the diverse topics which have resulted in the successful publishing of this book. They have passed on their knowledge of decades through this book. To expedite this challenging task, the publisher supported the team at every step. A small team of assistant editors was also appointed to further simplify the editing procedure and attain best results for the readers.

Apart from the editorial board, the designing team has also invested a significant amount of their time in understanding the subject and creating the most relevant covers. They scrutinized every image to scout for the most suitable representation of the subject and create an appropriate cover for the book.

The publishing team has been an ardent support to the editorial, designing and production team. Their endless efforts to recruit the best for this project, has resulted in the accomplishment of this book. They are a veteran in the field of academics and their pool of knowledge is as vast as their experience in printing. Their expertise and guidance has proved useful at every step. Their uncompromising quality standards have made this book an exceptional effort. Their encouragement from time to time has been an inspiration for everyone.

The publisher and the editorial board hope that this book will prove to be a valuable piece of knowledge for researchers, students, practitioners and scholars across the globe.

List of Contributors

Carlos Gutierrez-Merino, Dorinda Marques-da-Silva, Sofia Fortalezas and Alejandro K. Samhan-Arias
Dept. Biochemistry and Molecular Biology, School of Sciences, University of Extremadura, Badajoz, Spain

E.I. Zakharova and A.M. Dudchenko
Institute of General Pathology and Pathophysiology, Russian Academy of Medical Sciences, Moscow, Russia

Siddhartha Dalvi, Ngoc On, Hieu Nguyen, Michael Pogorzelec and Donald W. Miller
Departments of Pharmacology & Therapeutics, Center for Research and Treatment of Atherosclerosis, University of Manitoba, DREAM Manitoba Institute of Child Health, Canada

Grant M. Hatch
Departments of Pharmacology & Therapeutics, Center for Research and Treatment of Atherosclerosis, University of Manitoba, DREAM Manitoba Institute of Child Health, Canada
Biochemistry and Medical Genetics, Center for Research and Treatment of Atherosclerosis, University of Manitoba, DREAM Manitoba Institute of Child Health, Canada

Chloé Hegoburu
Center for Psychiatric Neuroscience, Prilly, University of Lausanne, Lausanne, Switzerland
CNRS, UMR 5292, Lyon Neuroscience Research Center, Olfaction: From Coding to Memory Team, Lyon, France
University Lyon, Lyon, France

Christian Harteneck
Institute of Pharmacology and Toxicology & Interfaculty Centre for Pharmacogenomics and Drug Research, Eberhard-Karls-University, Tübingen, Germany

Luc Denoroy
University Lyon, Lyon Neuroscience Research Center, BioRaN team, Lyon, France
University Lyon, Lyon, France

Anne-Marie Mouly
CNRS, UMR 5292, Lyon Neuroscience Research Center, Olfaction: From Coding to Memory Team, Lyon, France
University Lyon, Lyon, France

Sandrine Parrot
University Lyon, Lyon, France
INSERM, U1028, Lyon Neuroscience Research Center, NeuroDialyTics, Lyon, France

Kristina Leuner
Molecular und Clinical Pharmacy, Friedrich-Alexander-University Erlangen/Nürnberg, Germany

Victor Tsetlin and Igor Kasheverov
Shemyakin-Ovchinnikov Institute of Bioorganic Chemistry, Russian Academy of Sciences, Moscow, Russian Federation

Thomas Heinbockel
Department of Anatomy, Howard University College of Medicine, Washington, DC, USA

G. Ramírez-Rodríguez
Laboratory of Neurogenesis, Instituto Nacional de Psiquiatría, México City, México

Index

www.ingramcontent.com/pod-product-compliance
Lightning Source LLC
LaVergne TN
LVHW062237200926
848484LV00006B/1561